I0882068

The Psychology of Sports Injury

The Psychology of Sports Injury: From Risk to Retirement provides a critical overview of the psychology of sports injury, covering the 5Rs of sports injury: risk, response, rehabilitation, return to sport and retirement.

Drawing on a range of expert international perspectives from the fields of sport psychology and sport and exercise medicine, *The Psychology of Sports Injury* covers the psychological considerations associated with sports injuries, prior to the onset of injury through to supporting athletes with post-injury retirement. In addition to this injury lifespan perspective, the book features special interest topics including anterior cruciate ligament injury, sport-related concussion, spinal cord injury and the role of coaches in achieving athlete and team medical outcomes. Additionally, case studies provide the opportunity to apply learning from each chapter.

By covering the sports injury journey from risk factors to retirement and including athlete mental health during sports injury, *The Psychology of Sports Injury* is an essential text for students, instructors and practitioners in sports psychology, sport and exercise medicine and other related fields.

Dr Adam Gledhill is Course Director in Sport, Exercise and Health Sciences at Leeds Beckett University, UK. He is a Fellow of the British Association of Sport and Exercise Sciences (BASES) and a BASES Accredited Sport and Exercise Scientist. Dr Gledhill is the Chair of the BASES Division of Psychology and developed the psychology of sports injury and rehabilitation standards for the British Association of Sports Rehabilitators and Trainers Education Framework.

Dr Dale Forsdyke is Senior Lecturer in Sports Injury Management at York St John University, UK and a Society of Sports Therapists Accredited Sports Therapist. Dale is an experienced educator and practitioner, with 20 years' experience of teaching on sports injury related courses, research interests in psychological factors and return to sport outcomes, and over 10 years' experience as an injury practitioner across a range of sports.

The Psychology of Sports Injury

FROM RISK TO RETIREMENT

Edited by Adam Gledhill
and Dale Forsdyke

Routledge
Taylor & Francis Group
LONDON AND NEW YORK

First published 2021
by Routledge
2 Park Square, Milton Park, Abingdon, Oxon OX14 4RN

and by Routledge
52 Vanderbilt Avenue, New York, NY 10017

Routledge is an imprint of the Taylor & Francis Group, an Informa business

British Library Cataloguing-in-Publication Data
A catalogue record for this book is available from the British Library

Library of Congress Cataloging-in-Publication Data
Names: Gledhill, Adam, editor. | Forsdyke, Dale, editor.
Title: The psychology of sport injury: from risk to retirement / edited by Adam Gledhill, Dale Forsdyke.
Description: Milton Park, Abingdon, Oxon; New York, NY: Routledge, 2021. | Includes bibliographical references and index.
Identifiers: LCCN 2020034378 (print) | LCCN 2020034379 (ebook) | ISBN 9780367028664 (hardback) | ISBN 9780367028695 (paperback) | ISBN 9780429019227 (ebook)
Subjects: LCSH: Sports injuries—Psychological aspects.
Classification: LCC RD97 .P788 2021 (print) | LCC RD97 (ebook) | DDC 617.1/027—dc23
LC record available at https://lccn.loc.gov/2020034378
LC ebook record available at https://lccn.loc.gov/2020034379

ISBN: 978-0-367-02866-4 (hbk)
ISBN: 978-0-367-02869-5 (pbk)
ISBN: 978-0-429-01922-7 (ebk)

Typeset in Palatino
by KnowledgeWorks Global Ltd.

For Harry. This one's for you, little man. After all, you kept me company, you sat on my knee, you pressed some of the buttons and you kept me smiling. Thanks for keeping me company during this, although we both know that you really just wanted to write a book with 'Uncle Dale' ☺

Daddy will keep you safe, warm and loved, always.

Adam

Of most importance I would like to dedicate this book to my seminal influences, my family. To my wife Sophie and children Isla and Leo, you are beautiful, talented and funny in equal measure, and you are my driving force. Additionally, I would also like to thank the injured athletes that I have learnt from over the years, as I have become a better educator, practitioner and researcher as a result.

Dale

CONTENTS

Foreword *ix*
SUE SMITH

Preface *x*

Acknowledgements *xiii*

Contributors *xiv*

Part I
The role of psychology in sports injury risk and injury risk reduction 1

Chapter 1 **The injury-prone athlete: Psychosocial risk factors in sports injury 3**
PROFESSOR URBAN JOHNSON

Chapter 2 **Prevention is better than cure: The role of psychological interventions in sports injury risk reduction 16**
DR ANDREAS IVARSSON

Part II
Psychological responses to sports injury 31

Chapter 3 **Personal and situational factors affecting psychological response to sport injuries 33**
DIANE M. WIESE-BJORNSTAL

Chapter 4 **The downside of sports injury: Poor mental health in injured athletes 63**
DR ADAM GLEDHILL

Chapter 5 **The upside of sports injury and disability: Personal growth following adversity 76**
DR CHRIS HAMMER, DR LESLIE PODLOG AND DR ADAM GLEDHILL

Part III
Enhancing sports injury rehabilitation experiences for injured athletes 91

Chapter 6 **Believe in your ability to create change: Psychosocial factors influencing sports injury rehabilitation adherence 93**
DR ADAM GLEDHILL AND DR ANDREAS IVARSSON

Chapter 7 **Are you a buffer or an amplifier? The role of social support in the effective return to sport following injury 107**
DR DALE FORSDYKE

Chapter 8 **Seeing is believing: The role of imagery in sports injury rehabilitation 117**
DR ADAM GLEDHILL AND DR DALE FORSDYKE

Chapter 9 **Does it pay to pay attention? Making a case for mindfulness-based approaches in injury rehabilitation 126**
DR ADAM GLEDHILL

Part IV
The psychology of return to sport decisions 137

Chapter 10 **Is my athlete really ready to return to sport? Psychological factors and returning to sport following injury 139**
DR DALE FORSDYKE AND DR ADAM GLEDHILL

Chapter 11 **They think it's all over: Injury-related retirement from sport 152**
DR ADAM GLEDHILL AND DR DALE FORSDYKE

Part V
Special interests in sports injury 161

Chapter 12 **The psychological aspect of anterior cruciate ligament injuries 163**
DR KATE E. WEBSTER

Chapter 13 **'It's my concussion story, and I want it to be heard': Understanding the psychology of concussion experience 181**
DR OSMAN HASSAN AHMED, DR ERIC E. HALL AND DR CAROLINE J. KETCHAM

Chapter 14 **Spinal cord injury and sport 193**
DR TONI LOUISE WILLIAMS

Chapter 15 **'But I need you to play': Coach influences on athlete and team medical outcomes 202**
DR ADAM GLEDHILL

Chapter 16 **The coffee break to close the book … Where do we go from here? 211**
DR ADAM GLEDHILL AND DR DALE FORSDYKE

Index 216

FOREWORD

Having been an international footballer for over 15 years my career was certainly touched by sports injury. Throughout a long career you have to live with risk of becoming injured and hope that you are lucky enough to avoid significant injury. It was in 2012 when making a club debut that I wasn't lucky. The game started off fantastically for me as I scored a debut goal; however, it ended with me being stretchered off having ruptured my anterior cruciate ligament. Personally, and professionally sustaining this injury like this was a disaster as I was a 32 years old footballer in the twilight of her career and because of the injury I missed out on a once in a lifetime chance of representing my country at an Olympic games. During the recovery from the injury, while I could cope with the physical restrictions and pain, I found the psychological side a real challenge. Fear, anxiety, guilt, isolation, frustration and doubt are just some of the things I felt. No-one really prepares you for this either before injury or afterwards. While I was unlucky to get injured, I was lucky in the sense I had an understanding and supportive team around me and I was able to return to football and remain relatively injury free. This allowed me to keep motivated, picked me up when I was down, and managed my expectations. However, I know of many players that weren't so lucky. For me books such as this are really important in allowing people to manage injured players like me. From preventing injury to returning to sport and then retirement, I am sure this book will provide a comprehensive and valuable resource to everyone that works with athletes. Looking back, I wished I hadn't got injured because of the negative impact on my career and when I did return to football I never really felt psychologically ready so this book really resonates with my journey as an international footballer.

Sue Smith

England footballer 93 caps

International player of the year 1999, 2001

PREFACE

Even though we live in a scientifically advanced era, the burden of sports injury is high to the extent that it can be seen as an almost inevitable part of regular sports participation (Ardern et al., 2016). For every sports injury there is a significant and negative impact on the athlete regardless of performance level. At best an injury might be a minor nuisance that interrupts normal loading patterns; however, at worse injury can lead to once-in-a-lifetime missed opportunities, career termination and long-term health implications impacting quality of life. Additionally, we are also beginning to understand the broader impact as injury has negative consequences for sports teams and organizations in the form of reduced success and financial costs (Eliakim, Morgulev, Lidor & Meckel, 2020; Raysmith & Drew, 2016). As such, there should be collective focus on how the risk of injury can be reduced, and, for athletes that do get injured, enhancing the injury experience to augment return to sport outcomes. This is where theory and research indicate that psychological factors can play an important prognostic function.

While psychological factors are potentially important, in comparison to physical or biological factors they are underrepresented in research and applied practice (Forsdyke, Smith, Jones & Gledhill, 2016). Anecdotally, it is only when presented with complex injuries where progress is not as expected that psychological factors are finally considered. Why then is this the case? First, we contend that the dogma of the biomedical model encouraged a tradition of research and practice that is unidimensional in nature (i.e., concerned with physical and biological variables; Farre & Rapley, 2017). Even today, despite the emergence of biopsychosocial approaches, the legacy of the biomedical approach remains, as theory and research often view what happens to the body and the mind during sports injury as separate processes. A possible second reason might be that practitioners working with injured athletes may feel over challenge and ill-equipped to recognize, monitor and intervene with psychological factors (Alexanders, Anderson & Henderson, 2015). In comparison to physical and biological factors, psychological factors may be more dynamic, less predictable and 'recover' on different timescales to physical factors and as such this presents a significant challenge to manage (Podlog & Eklund, 2007). Of importance, practitioners that are exposed to more psychology of sport injury educational resources tend to feel more empowered to deal with this important aspect of athlete care (Heaney, Rostron, Walker & Green, 2017). This book has been put together with these points in mind by 'banging the drum' about the importance of psychological aspects of sport injury and providing rich evidence-informed content that may, in part, serve to empower and equip practitioners to work with injured athletes more holistically.

This book intends to provide a comprehensive overview of psychological factors and sports injury by including sections focusing on the five R's: risk, response, rehabilitation experience, return to sport and retirement (Gledhill & Forsdyke, 2015). A common theme across the chapters in this book is that a proactive approach (vs reactive) is advocated to firstly reduce the risk of injury in athletic populations and then secondly better manage the injury process in order to optimize return to sport outcomes for athletes. For example, whether this is providing interventions aimed at reducing psychological risk factors of injury or creating a pre-injury action plan of how injured athletes may be supported effectively. Rarely, when managing athletes is a 'fire-fighting' approach effective. The special interest chapters are centred on specific pathologies that frequently lead to significant negative consequences for athletes (i.e., ACL injury, sports concussion). As such, this book provides some contemporary injury-specific context. Each chapter concludes with a high-fidelity case study to give readers the opportunity to reinforce and apply the content they have engaged with. The single 'voice' from all the chapters in the book is that psychological factors are important consideration when trying to solve real-world sports injury problems. Therefore, we encourage readers to apply the knowledge gained through reading this book to their own research, practice and experience.

The book idea was born about 15 years ago when two blokes from Yorkshire were chatting and said: 'wouldn't it be cool if we wrote a psychology of sports injury book?' Of course, back then, we were nowhere near ready. Now, of course, this book is the product of countless hours of talking to and learning from fellow practitioners and injured athletes; years of research, teaching and applied practice experience; feeling like we're a bit closer to being ready, and as equally important, gallons of strong coffee!

We are delighted to have collaborated with some of our favourite authors and practitioners that are world-leading authorities in this field. One of the perks of editing a book is that you get to assemble your own 'dream team' of chapter authors and, particularly against the backdrop of COVID-19, being able to closely collaborate with national and international colleagues has been a pleasure. Additionally, how to prevent injury and enhance return to sport outcomes is an international problem, so assembling chapters written by authors from around the world was important to us. By including chapters written by researchers, practitioners and athletes we hope we have achieved the right blend and that this book resonates with all readers whatever their professional background. This book has content aimed at improved knowledge and understanding but also content directed at enhancing applied practice. We are keen for this book to stimulate reflection on practice, professional discussions, new exciting lines of research and support practitioner to work with injured athletes in a slightly different way. So, take some time, grab a brew and enjoy reading about the psychology of sport injury.

References

Alexanders, J., Anderson, A., & Henderson, S. (2015). Musculoskeletal physiotherapists' use of psychological interventions: A systematic review of therapists' perceptions and practice. *Physiotherapy*, 101(2), 95–102.

Ardern, C.L., Glasgow, P., Schneiders, A., Witvrouw, E., Clarsen, B., Cools, A., Gojanovic, B., Griffin, S., Khan K. M., Moksnes, H., Mutch, S. A., Phillips, N., Reurink, G., Sadler, R., Silbernagel, K. G., Thorborg, K., Wangensteen, A., Wilk, K. E., & Bizzini, M. (2016). 2016 Consensus statement on return to sport from the First World Congress in Sports Physical Therapy, Bern. *British Journal of Sports Medicine*, 50, 853–864.

Eliakim. E., Morgulev, E., Lidor, R., & Meckel, Y. (2020). Estimation of injury costs: Financial damage of English Premier League teams' underachievement due to injuries. *BMJ Open Sport & Exercise Medicine*, 6, e000675. doi: 10.1136/bmjsem-2019-000675

Farre, A., & Rapley, T. (2017). The new old (and old new) medical model: Four decades navigating the biomedical and psychosocial understandings of health and illness. *Healthcare (Basel, Switzerland)*, 5(4), 88.

Forsdyke, D., Smith, A., Jones, M., & Gledhill, A. (2016). Psychosocial factors associated with outcomes of sports injury rehabilitation in competitive athletes: A mixed studies systematic review. *British Journal of Sports Medicine*, 50, 537–544.

Gledhill, A., & Forsdyke, D. (2015, June). *Rehabilitating the athlete, not just the injury*. Invited International webinar for the British Association of Sport and Exercise Sciences and Human Kinetics. Available from: https://www.youtube.com/watch?v=p89x1_9s9fI

Heaney, C.A., Walker, N., Green, A.J., & Rostron, C.L. (2017). The impact of a sport psychology education intervention on physiotherapists. *European Journal of Physiotherapy*, 19(2), 97–103.

Podlog, L., & Eklund, R.C. (2007). The psychosocial aspects of a return to sport following serious injury: A review of the literature from a self-determination perspective. *Psychology of Sport and Exercise*, 8(4), 535–566.

Raysmith, B.P., & Drew, M.K. (2016). Performance success or failure is influenced by weeks lost to injury and illness in elite Australian track and field athletes: A 5-year prospective study. *Journal of Science and Medicine in Sport*, 19(10), 778–783.

ACKNOWLEDGEMENTS

As our first foray into editing a book of this nature, we naturally have a number of people that we would like to acknowledge for playing key roles in the book's development. First, our sincere gratitude goes to the authors of each of the chapters, for your excellent contributions to the book. Thank you for producing your chapters in a timely manner, providing us with feedback on the process and for engaging in the critical debate that one would expect of a project of this nature. We hope you are pleased with the end product.

Next, thanks to Routledge for initially approaching us about the project and then subsequently commissioning the book. Special thanks for your understanding during the different setbacks over the past 18 months, not least of which was that little matter of COVID-19! Christina and Danielle, you've both been a great help with your timely replies, clear guidance and always being willing to be on the other end of a video call when we needed you. It has been a rocky road at times.

Next, thank you to our respective employers, Leeds Beckett University and York St. John University, for supporting us in our endeavours with this project. Special thanks from Adam goes to Drs Andrew Manley and Emily Williams at Leeds Beckett University for your support with balancing the 'day job' alongside completing the latter stages of the book.

Finally, this book was an idea about 15 years in the making, but really this double act has been doing the rounds since 2001. During that time, we've been so fortunate to have careers in education, sport, research and publishing that have allowed us to engage with some amazing athletes, coaches, parents of athletes, academic and applied colleagues, all of whom have enriched our development as practitioners and academics. For every class, debate, conversation, argument, chat over a coffee, journal club, case consultation…we could go on…thank you for allowing us into your lives and for contributing to our development.

CONTRIBUTORS

Dr Osman Ahmed is a Senior Lecturer in Sports Therapy within the Department of Rehabilitation and Sports Sciences at Bournemouth University, England. He is a Chartered Physiotherapist with 18 years of experience working in a variety of clinical settings. He undertook his postgraduate education at the University of Otago in New Zealand, where he was awarded his Postgraduate Diploma in Sports Physiotherapy in 2006 and his PhD in 2013. He has worked at two Paralympic Games (Beijing 2008 and Rio de Janiero in 2016) and currently works as a Physiotherapist for the Football Association in England within their elite disability football programme. He has published and presented widely in the areas of concussion in sport, disability sport and the intersection of technology and healthcare. In addition to his employed roles, Osman holds a number of additional advisory and committee roles. He is an Associate Editor at the British Journal of Sports Medicine, Head of Medical at the International Federation of Cerebral Palsy Football and Medical Committee member at the International Blind Sports Association. He is also a committee member of the Institute of Sport and Exercise Medicine, and a member of the scientific advisory group of the British Association of Sports and Exercise Medicine.

Dr Dale Forsdyke is a Senior Lecturer in Sports Injury Management at York St John University in the UK with a background in sports therapy, strength and conditioning and sport and exercise science. He is an experienced educator and practitioner with a developing research portfolio in psychological factors and return to sport outcomes. He has had the opportunity to speak at several national and international conferences on his research area. Dale is an accredited member of The Society of Sports Therapists (MSST) and a Certified Strength and Conditioning Specialist (CSCS). Much of his applied work is in elite women's and girls' football where he has over 10 years of coordinating a multidisciplinary performance team to support and develop athletes. This has allowed him to implement his own research findings in order to better manage sports injury. Away from work Dale is a keen exerciser and enjoys taking part in long-distance running and triathlon events, spending time with his family, and is also a grassroots community football coach.

Dr Adam Gledhill is a Course Director: Sport, Exercise and Health Sciences at Leeds Beckett University, England. He is a British Association of Sport and Exercise Sciences (BASES) Accredited Sport and Exercise Scientist (Support, Research and Pedagogy; Psychology; Sport Performance) with over 15 years' experience working as an applied practitioner in a range of sporting environments, including Head of Sport Science and Head of Psychosocial Development roles within women's and girls' football. In recognition of his approaches to applied practice, Adam was the recipient of the 2020 BASES Applied Practitioner Award. Away from applied sport consultancy, Adam has also held a number of education consultancy, advisory and committee roles. He has fulfilled education consultancy roles in the UK, Europe, Africa and Asia; sits on the BASES Education Endorsement Committee; developed the psychology of sports injury and rehabilitation standards for the British Association of Sports Rehabilitators and Trainers Education Framework (8th Edition); is the sitting Chair of the BASES Division of Psychology; serves as an Associate Editor (Psychology of Sports Injury) for the British Journal of Sports Medicine; and, in 2019, was awarded Fellowship of BASES in recognition of his esteemed contributions to sport and exercise science.

Dr Eric Hall is a professor of exercise science and the faculty athletics representative at Elon University in North Carolina. He received his undergraduate degree from Miami University and did his graduate work at the University of Illinois at Urbana-Champaign in Kinesiology. His primary research interest is in the area of exercise neuroscience as it relates to physical activity and mental health, as well as the impact of concussions on student-athletes. Additionally, he is interested in the influence of high-impact practices on student development, as well as, the importance of high-quality mentorship in undergraduate research and other high-impact practices. He has authored over 80 research articles, 6 book chapters and is the co-editor of a recent book on concussion management. He currently serves as co-director for the Elon Brain-CARE Research Institute (www.elon.edu/braincare), which has concussion advocacy and positive mental wellness as the primary goals. He has served on the NCAA Committee on Competitive Safeguards and Medical Aspects of Sports and is currently on the NCAA Committee on Academics and the NCAA Concussion Protocol Committee. He has received numerous awards for mentoring and scholarship during his time at Elon.

Dr Chris Hammer earned a PhD in Exercise and Sport Science from the University of Utah (Salt Lake City, Utah). Following completion of his doctoral studies, Chris became the triathlon coach at Davis and Elkins College (Elkins, West Virginia), where he also teaches a course on the psychosocial aspects of sport. Chris' research interests include para sport and posttraumatic growth, which stem from his experiences as a Paralympian. Outside of training as a triathlete, Chris enjoys watching sports, playing board games and outdoor activities with his wife and two daughters.

Dr Andreas Ivarsson is an Associate Professor in Sport and Exercise Psychology at Halmstad University in Sweden. His research interests include psychological aspects related to sports injuries, motivational aspects related to sport and exercise participation, statistical and methodological issues within psychological research and mindfulness. He is currently Associate Editor for the Psychology of Sport and Exercise and section editor for the Scandinavian Journal of Medicine and Science in Sports and Measurement in Physical Education and Exercise Science. Andreas has experience as a sport psychology consultant with elite soccer teams; he is the current Head of Psychology and Personal Development Research at Arsenal FC.

Urban Johnson, Phd is Professor in Sport & Exercise Psychology at Halmstad University, Sweden. He has an elite-trainer certificate in handball, in which he has worked as a coach for many years. His main research focus is about psychological aspects of sports injury, prevention, rehabilitation and intervention. He also conducts research in areas such as health psychology and exercise science. Dr. Johnson has vast experience in working with applied sport psychology, especially for team sport athletes. He has been a member of the Medical Committee at the Swedish Football Federation since 2001, and he was a member of the managing council of FEPSAC 2003-2011. Currently Dr. Johnson is a member of the scientific committee at the Swedish National Centre for Research in Sports.

Dr Caroline J. Ketcham is Professor and Chair of Exercise Science at Elon University. Caroline's expertise is in the area of movement neuroscience and her current research focuses on understanding the control and coordination in the execution of movements foundational to development and functional participation for neurodiverse populations. In addition, she is co-director of Elon BrainCARE Research Institute, which has concussion advocacy and positive mental wellness as the primary goals for Elon students and student-athletes. Caroline has a co-edited book, more than 50 peer-reviewed publications, and over 100 scholarly presentations. Caroline is also engaged in high-impact practice research including co-mentoring undergraduate research for student and faculty development, student-athlete access and engagement and capstone experiences. She has been recognized for her high-quality teaching, scholarship and mentoring with college and university awards.

Dr Leslie Podlog's research focuses primarily on the psychological aspects of sport injury rehabilitation. His interest in the topic stems from his personal injury experiences as a former amateur wrestler at Simon Fraser University in Burnaby, British Columbia, Canada. Following completion of his doctoral studies (2006) at the University of Western Australia, Les held faculty positions at Charles Sturt University (Bathurst, Australia), the German Sport University (Cologne, Germany) and Texas Tech University (Lubbock, Texas). He has been a faculty member at the University of Utah since 2011 where he has taught classes in sport psychology, exercise psychology, motivation theory and the psychology of sport injury. He has over 100 peer reviewed publications and chapters in edited books. He enjoys travelling, hiking and spending time with his wonderful family.

Dr Kate Webster is Professor in the College of Science, Health and Engineering at La Trobe University, Melbourne, Australia. Her personal research interests cover a range of topics pertaining to knee orthopaedics, including surgical techniques and outcomes, biomechanical changes after knee surgery and return to sport issues, with a focus on the psychological impact of returning to sport participation. She was the lead developer of the Anterior Cruciate Ligament Return to Sport after Injury (ACL-RSI) scale. Kate has received several awards for her research including 3 best paper of the year awards from the American Journal of Sports Medicine, Orthopeadic Journal of Sports Medicine and Journal of Orthopaedic Research and has over 200 scientific publications. She is a current member of the ACL Study Group and past recipient of their Traveling Scientist Fellowship. She is a member of the Electronic Media Board for the American Journal of Sports Medicine and has appointments for many other advisory boards and international research working groups. Kate also teaches evidence-based practice to undergraduate Allied Health students. She is committed to providing high-quality research supervision and is one of the research mentors for the OrthoSport Victoria orthopaedic fellowship program.

Diane M. Wiese-Bjornstal is a Professor of Sport and Exercise Psychology and Associate Director of the School of Kinesiology at the University of Minnesota Twin Cities. She is a Fellow in the National Academy of Kinesiology and the Association for Applied Sport Psychology, and a Certified Mental Performance Consultant. As Director of the Sports Medicine Psychology Laboratory, her scholarship focuses on theory, research and practice in the psychological, behavioural and sociocultural aspects of sports injury prevention and care among physically active populations across the lifespan. Diane and her collaborator, Dr. Aynsley Smith, are recognized for their integrated model of psychological response to the sport injury and rehabilitation process. Her involvement with the Tucker Center for Research on Girls & Women in Sport resulted in collaborations focusing on female athletes and concussions, sport injuries among female children and youth and the psychosocial aspects of developing physically active girls. Diane trained as a physical education teacher, head coached volleyball and softball teams at youth and collegiate levels and studied biomechanics and sport psychology in her graduate work. These interdisciplinary experiences ground her research publications on psychological responses to sport injuries and her applied contributions to sport coach and athletic trainer education.

Dr Toni L. Williams is a Senior Lecturer in Sport and Exercise Psychology at Leeds Beckett University. Her research in physical activity and disability focuses on understanding the physical activity experiences of people with spinal cord injury and effective physical activity promotion. Toni's research also explores the use and development of qualitative research methods and methodologies to conceptually advance sport and exercise psychology research. This includes the use of qualitative meta-synthesis and novel methods of data collection such as timelining and story completion. Her work in these areas has been published in international journals such as *Health Psychology Review, Qualitative Research in Sport, Exercise and Health, Psychology of Sport and Exercise* and she has contributed to leading books including the *International Handbook of Qualitative Methods in Sport and Exercise* (2016) and the *International Encyclopedia of Sport Psychology* (2020). Toni is also involved in various professional and scholarly activities. For example, she was co-chair of the highly successful 4th International Conference on Qualitative Research in Sport and Exercise (QRSE2014) and continues to be a member of the scientific committee. She is also a founding member and treasurer of the new International Society for Qualitative Research in Sport and Exercise (@QRSEsoc, qrsesoc.com) launched in 2020.

Part I

THE ROLE OF PSYCHOLOGY IN SPORTS INJURY RISK AND INJURY RISK REDUCTION

As the old adage goes: 'An ounce of prevention is worth a pound of cure'. This really provides the essence of this first section of the book.

Sports injury, particularly severe or recurrent sports injury, can have serious and long-term health effects for athletes (Putukian, 2016) and are the leading cause of retirement for top level athletes (Ristolainen et al., 2012). Increased occurrence of injury is associated with less successful performance on the pitch, with fewer competitions won by team who have more injuries (Hägglund, et al., 2013). Injuries also have significant impact off the pitch, with injuries estimated to cost of £45 million per season in the English Premier League (Eliakim et al., 2020). Consequently, injury practitioners and sports organization more broadly have a duty of care to their athletes, their profession and their employers to be doing everything possible to reduce the burden of injury (Gledhill & Forsdyke, 2018).

Given the awareness of psychological risk factors for sports injury (e.g. Ivarsson et al., 2017), as well as the increasingly accepted role of psychologically informed interventions in reducing sports injury risk (e.g. Ivarsson et al., 2017), it would be remiss of us to have started this book with anything other than chapters devoted to the role of psychology within injury risk and risk reduction.

Throughout this section, Urban Johnson and Andreas Ivarsson will guide you through the established and emerging areas of research within this body of knowledge. Urban's chapter will provide a theoretical and applied overview of the major psychological risk factors within sports injury. It considers the most established model of sports injury risk, the model of stress and athletic injury (Williams & Andersen, 1998), as well as examining more contemporary approaches such as the biopsychosocial model of athletic injury and health (Appaneal & Perna, 2014). As an important contribution, Urban's chapter will consider various psychobiological, psychosocial and neurocognitive explanations behind sports injury risk.

Following Urban's introduction, Andreas Ivarsson will walk you through the body of research into the role of psychological intervention within sports injury prevention. Andreas argues throughout the chapter that injury prevention is indeed better than injury rehabilitation, wherever possible. Let's be frank here: even the leading authorities on sports injury prevention argue that preventing injury in sport is nigh impossible; however we do have a responsibility to reduce injury risk using clinically meaningful methods (Ivarsson et al., 2017). Given that sport psychology as an injury prevention tool is relatively under-utilized in professional sport and the reasons behind this often relate to sports medicine practitioners' uncertainty over the efficacy or effectiveness of the different approaches (Gledhill et al., 2018), Andreas' practical evidence-informed approach to the chapter will support an increased awareness in this area.

References

Appaneal, R. & Perna, F. (2014). Biopsychosocial model of injury. In R. Eklund & G. Tenenbaum (Eds.), *Encyclopedia of sport and exercise psychology* (pp. 74–76). Thousand Oaks: SAGE Publications.

Eliakim, E., Morgulev, E., Lidor, R., & Meckel, Y. (2020). Estimation of injury costs: Financial damage of English Premier League teams' underachievement due to injuries. *BMJ Open Sport & Exercise Medicine*. DOI: 10.1136/bmjsem-2019-000675.

Gledhill, A., & Forsdyke, D. (2018). An ounce of prevention is better than a pound of cure: Shouldn't we be doing EVERYTHING to reduce sports injury incidence and burden? *British Journal of Sports Medicine, 52*, 1292–1293.

Gledhill, A., Forsdyke, D., & Murray, E. (2018). Psychological interventions used to reduce sports injuries: A systematic review of real-world effectiveness. *British Journal of Sports Medicine, 52*, 967–971.

Hägglund, M., Waldén, M., Magnusson, H., Kristenson, K., Bengtsson, H., & Ekstrand, J. (2013). Injuries affect team performance negatively in professional football: An 11-year follow-up of the UEFA Champions League injury study *British Journal of Sports Medicine, 47*, 738–742.

Ivarsson, A., Johnson, U., Andersen, M. B., Tranaeus, U., Stenling, A., & Lindwall, M. (2017). Psychosocial factors and sports injuries: Meta-analyses for prediction and prevention. *Sports Medicine, 47*, 353–365.

Putukian, M. (2016). The psychological response to injury in student athletes: A narrative review with a focus on mental health. *British Journal of Sports Medicine, 50*, 145–148.

Ristolainen, L., Ketunen, J. K., Kujala, U. M., & Heinonen, A. (2012). Sports injuries as the main cause of sports career termination among Finnish top-level athletes. *European Journal of Sport Science, 12*, 274–282.

Williams, J., & Andersen, M. (1998) Psychosocial antecedents of sport injury: Review and critique of the stress and injury model. *Journal of Applied Sport Psychology, 10*(1), 5–25.

1 THE INJURY-PRONE ATHLETE

PSYCHOSOCIAL RISK FACTORS IN SPORTS INJURY

Professor Urban Johnson

INTRODUCTION

Participation in competitive sports is associated with high physiological, biomechanical and psychological demands. Difficulties in coping with these types of demand are related to increased risks of becoming injured (see e.g. Soligard et al., 2016). Sport injuries are ubiquitous and represent substantial economic, health, personal and community costs. In Europe approximately 4.5 million athletes are annually treated for sport injuries (Kisser & Bauer, 2010). Severe sport injuries are related to negative emotional responses, such as sadness, anger and depression (Wiese-Bjornstal, 2010), and decreased psychological and physiological well-being (Putukian, 2016). Moreover, recent research has conceptualized some sport injuries as career-changing events that can have substantial impact on athletes' careers and trajectories (e.g. Ivarsson et al., 2016). With the high rates of injury within sport, together with the negative consequences that may follow, it seems warranted as a first step, to identify psychosocial risk factors that might increase the risk of becoming injured, but also to suggest applied strategies to decrease injury risk in sport.

At the start of this chapter, I initially present some models focusing on psychological risk factors in sports injury, with a special attention on the model of stress and athletic injury (Williams & Andersen, 1998), but also more contemporary models. A literature review of some of the more characteristic psychosocial risk factors in sport follows after the presentation of the models, with a focus on traditional risk factors such as personality, history of stressors and coping resources. Attention will also be paid to less researched areas including psychological risk factors and overuse injuries, risk factors among younger athletes but also psychological perspectives of the injury-prone athlete. Suggestions for applied recommendations as well as future research directions are provided. In addition, a case study, built on the core of the literature review, will be presented followed by questions derived from the chapter.

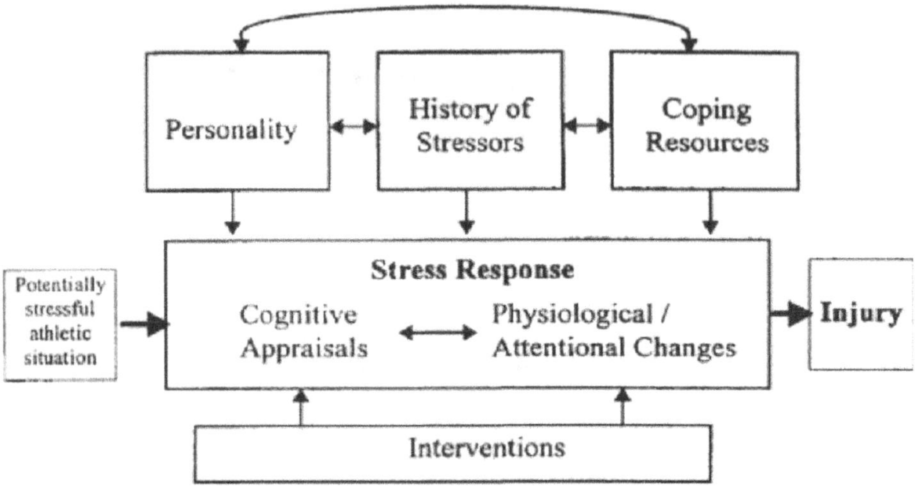

Figure 1.1 The model of stress and athletic injury (Williams & Andersen, 1998)

THE MODEL OF STRESS AND ATHLETIC INJURY

The model of stress and athletic injury is probably the most cited model in the area of psychology and injury prediction/injury prevention (Johnson & Ivarsson, 2017). According to the model, injury risk may be influenced by the athlete's stress responses that are suggested to have a bidirectional relationship with the athlete's appraisal of a potential stressful situation (e.g. game, competition) (see Figure 1.1). Both the magnitude of the stress reaction and the athlete's appraisal of the situation are suggested to be influenced by the interplay between various psychosocial factors, which are divided into three categories: personality factors, history of stressors and coping resources. In the early version of the model, Andersen and Williams (1988) suggested that only the history-of-stressors variable directly influenced the stress response, whereas both personality and coping variables had an indirect effect on stress responses through history of stressors. Ten years later, however, they argued that an athlete's history of stressors could influence the development of both an athlete's traits and coping mechanisms and, therefore, placed bidirectional arrows between the three psychosocial categories (Williams & Andersen, 1998). Also, in the model, intervention approaches are suggested to influence/buffer the stress response. This buffering effect could probably, in turn, decrease the injury risk an athlete is exposed to. When discussing the model, it is important to state that it is developed as a framework for traumatic injuries – that is where the injury has a sudden onset in association with a known trauma (Olsen et al., 2005).

THE BIOPSYCHOLOGICAL SPORT INJURY RISK PROFILE

Based on the biopsychosocial model of sport injury rehabilitation (Brewer et al., 2002), Wiese-Bjornstal (2010) developed the "biopsychological sport injury risk profile", specifically focusing risk factors for injury. Here, it is suggested that internal/personal variables, such as biological (e.g. allostatic load, body composition, nutrition and hydration, fatigue, recovery status and health status) as well as psychological (e.g. perfectionism, coping, attitudes, attentional focus, life event stress, mood state and risk behaviours), will influence the injury risk that an athlete is exposed to. In complement to the internal/personal risk variables also, external/environmental variables, such as physical (e.g. weather, medical care, sport type, opponent size and skill and intensity of play) as well as sociocultural (e.g. social resources, rules, organizational stress, sport norms and coaching quality), will also influence the likelihood for an athlete to become injured. The complex interaction of the internal/personal and external/environmental factors will, in turn, influence the athlete behaviour and risk vulnerability based on the resultant exposures, choices and hazards.

A WORKING MODEL OF PSYCHOLOGICAL RISK FACTORS FOR OVERUSE INJURIES

Complementing Williams and Andersen (1998) by exploring overuse injuries more specifically, Tranaeus et al. (2014) produced the model of psychological risk factors for overuse injuries. Tranaeus et al. (2014) noted that different psychosocial risk factors, such as stress load, exposure over time and limited communication within and between athletes and coaches/managers (see Tranaeus et al., 2014 for an overview), precede the overuse injury compared to the acute injury in sport. In their working model, it is suggested that the history of stressors, person factors, psycho-physiological factors, psychosocial factors and an athlete's coping resources influence injuries over time (see Figure 1.2). For instance, an athlete competing on a team and lacking the possibility of venting his/her concerns about stress or exhaustion (history of stressors) may be at risk of sustaining an overuse injury. This is probably particularly important for those athletes who have a limited social network outside of their sport (psychosocial factor), for instance those who have recently moved to a new team and/or a new town. In addition, if the athlete is showing signs of carelessness with body and lack of recovery (person and psycho-physiological factors), the risk of sustaining an overuse injury is plausible. It is proposed a division of coping resources into two broad categories: effective/adaptive coping and ineffective/maladaptive coping (Johnson, 2011), which

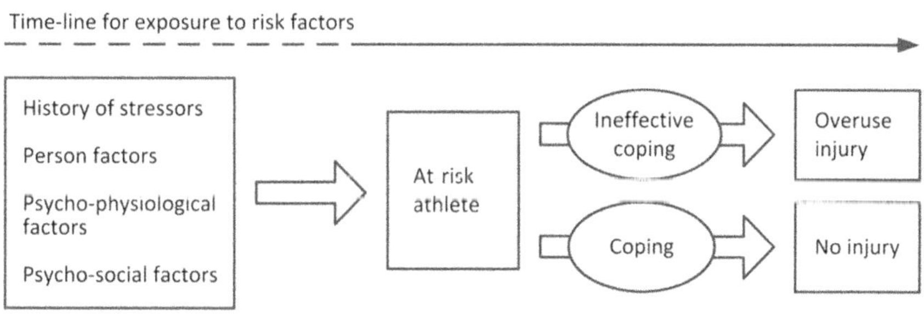

Figure 1.2 A working model of psychological risk factors for overuse injuries

are suggested to result in beneficial behavioural changes after an intervention is completed. It is tentatively hypothesized that effective coping leads to decreasing the proneness to overuse injuries, while ineffective coping makes the athlete more vulnerable to overuse injuries. The outcome of the working model is outlined as either an injury or no injury (characteristic of a sliding scale there between), with an assumption that effective coping results in less overuse injuries. Several combinations of factors are likely to contribute to the risk of sustaining overuse injuries, such as stress in life, high athletic identity, lack of recovery and limited communication with head coaches. Being exposed over time to a combination of these factors challenges the athlete's stress tolerance and coping recourses, which is proposed to influence whether an overuse injury occurs or not.

PSYCHOSOCIAL RISK FACTORS IN SPORTS INJURY

Researchers have examined many of the psychosocial risk factors specifically articulated in Williams and Andersen's (1998) model but also recognized in the biopsychological sport injury risk profile (Wiese-Bjornstal, 2010).

Personality

Several personality characteristics have been found to influence the strength of the stress–injury relationship. Personality characteristics may predispose individuals to perceive fewer situations and events as stressful, or they may dispose individuals to be more susceptible to the effects of stressors, such as major life events and daily hassles. Relationships have been found between injury outcome and risk factors, such as passion for sport (Steffen et al., 2009), trait anxiety (Li et al., 2017), state anxiety (Sibold et al., 2011), trait irritability (Ivarsson & Johnson, 2010), locus of control (Kerr & Minden, 1988) and stress susceptibility (Johnson & Ivarsson, 2011). Most of this research was conducted on male, elite or competitive athletes. In addition, based on biomechanical analyses, Swanik et al. (2007) found that neurocognitive differences were associated with the loss of neuromuscular control and coordination errors, predisposing athletes to noncontact anterior cruciate ligament injuries. Wilkerson (2012) also found that neurocognitive reaction time seemed to be an indicator of elevated risk for lower extremity sprains and strains among football players. Findings among high school and collegiate athletes similarly indicate that preinjury somatization symptoms may contribute to reported post-concussive symptom recovery via their influence on acute post-concussive symptoms (Nelson et al., 2016). Importantly, there are some inconsistent findings regarding the influence of personality factors on injury risk. For instance, researchers using nonspecific sport measures have found inconclusive results regarding trait anxiety and incidence of athletic injury (see Kleinert, 2002, for a review).

History of stressors

Since Holmes' seminal study in (Holmes, 1970), many others have examined the relationship of life stress to athletic injury. The vast majority of these studies have found a positive relationship between injury and high life stress (Steffen et al., 2009), daily hassles (Ivarsson et al., 2013) and life changes (Sibold et al., 2011). For example, Rogers and Landers (2005) found that negative life event stress increased the likelihood that athletes experienced a narrowing of their peripheral vision, which in turn increased the likelihood of injury. Similarly, Ivarsson et al. (2013) found that trait anxiety and negative life event stress influenced athletes' tendency to experience daily hassles. One recent review paper, targeting the categories of risk factors suggested in the model of stress and athletic injury (Williams & Andersen, 1998), concluded that psychosocial variables can influence the risk of incurring traumatic injuries among athletes (Ivarsson et al., 2017). More specifically, the numbers of perceived stressors in combination with the magnitude of individuals' stress responses were the factors that had the strongest relationships with injury risk. Singh and Conroy (2017) also found that approximately 75% of identified studies in both athletic and occupational contexts indicated a positive association between stress and injury occurrence, concluding that the consistency of findings suggests strong stress-related injury vulnerability for both exposures and responses. The cumulative influence of daily hassle subsequently increased athletes' susceptibility to injury. These findings suggest that preoccupation with life change and chronic daily hassles may negatively impact concentration on training and competition, increasing the likelihood of injury.

Coping resources

Coping resources includes a wide variety of behaviours and social networks that help the individual deal with the problems, joys, setbacks and stresses of life. Coping resources may come from the environment (e.g. friends, family) or from personal resources (e.g. social competence, healthy diet). The presence of good coping resources may directly protect the individual against injury or may attenuate the negative effects of stressors or the effects of personality. Some studies have supported the link between general coping resources and athletic injury. For instance, Devantier (2011) reported statistically significant lower level of coping with adversity between injured and non-injured athletes. Perna et al. (2003) also reported that athletes practicing cognitive behavioural stress management reported fewer injury days than athletes in the control group. However, several studies report inconclusive or non-significant results regarding coping between injured and non-injured sport populations (see Johnson et al., 2014 for a review).

PSYCHOLOGICAL RISK FACTORS IN OCCURRENCE OF OVERUSE INJURY

In addition to the three stated psychosocial risk factors of injury that primarily is about acute injuries, research related to psychological risk factors for sporting overuse injuries is slowly gaining traction (see also Figure 1.2). Even though the amount of studies has increased the last 5–10 years, still few researchers have systematically examined the potential influence of psychosocial risk factors in the development of overuse injuries. This research limitation is perhaps surprising because it is estimated that 30–40% of the sport injuries reported can be classified as overuse injuries (Yang et al., 2012). Studies targeting psychosocial risk factors' relationships with overuse injuries have stated that personality traits (e.g. perfectionism; Martin, 2018), sport sociocultural norm and rules (Tranaeus et al., 2014) and perceived negative life event stress connected to poor coach–athlete relationships (Pensgaard et al., 2018) might be important risk factors that could influence overuse injury risk through a variety of pathways (e.g. maladaptive behaviours stemming from trying to comply with cultural imperatives) (see also Richardson et al., 2008). Bittencourt et al. (2016) express it suitably saying that overuse injuries are not likely to result from "the linear interaction between isolated predictive factors, but from the complex interaction among a web of determinants" (p. 1). Cleary, this research area is in its early stages but will likely generate substantially more reports in the years to come, not least in light of the preventive conclusions that can be given for future and applied research in the area.

PSYCHOLOGICAL RISK FACTORS AND SPORTS INJURY – A YOUTH SPORT PERSPECTIVE

Compared to adult competitive athletes, it is not uncommon for younger and prosperous athletes, for example 12–15 years, to be exposed to high physical and psychological demands that they sometime may not be fully mature to manage. Findings from a systematic review of dropout from organized sport among children and youth (aged between 5 and 19 years) indicated that intrapersonal and interpersonal constraints are more frequently associated with dropping out of sport than structural constraints. Among five major areas that emerged in the review, physical factors, and not least injuries, were clearly outlined as reasons for dropout from sport (Crane & Temple, 2015). As sport is the leading cause of injury among children and adolescents (e.g. Keats et al., 2012), further exploration of the relationship between injuries and disengagement from sport seems warranted. According to Wiese-Bjornstal (2003), children and adolescents have seldom been studied in sport injury psychology research. This is a bit unexpected because tendencies seen in the literature (e.g. Patel & Nelson, 2000) show that about 50 per cent of youth sport athletes experience at least one injury during each athletic season. Of those injuries, about two-thirds are classified as minor (i.e. less than 1-week rehabilitation). For instance, recent research points to the problematic situation of early sport specialization and the risk of injury outcome that potentially follows (Meyer et al., 2015). Specifically, young athletes who exceeded volume recommendations have been found to be more likely to have a history of overuse injuries (Post et al., 2017). Two psychological factors seem to be especially related to injury occurrence among young athletes, that is, perceived stress-symptoms and communication with coaches (see e.g. Steffen et al., 2009). Research shows that particularly perceived high quality in the communication with soccer coaches was related to reduce injury risk (Johnson & Ivarsson, 2018). Other psychosocial factors such as emotional instability, insufficient and lack of mature coping strategies and a self-esteem and personal identification reliant on physical attractiveness seem to be potential risk factors making young athletes prone to injury. Undoubtedly, more research, ideally based on a biopsychological perspective, is needed here.

THE PERSPECTIVE OF THE INJURY-PRONE ATHLETE

A rather commonly discussed concept that has gained modest research space is about the injury-prone athlete. As a supplement to the psychosocial risk factors for injury presented earlier, some new theoretical perspectives are given that might attract attention to psychological perspectives of the injury-prone athlete. In the development of model such as the biopsychological sport injury risk profile, researchers more and more acknowledge the multifaceted pathogenesis of injuries. Historically, different lines of research have been proposed to explain the injury-prone athlete. One such a line of research, based on psychodynamic theory (e.g. Suchman, 1970), consider unconscious psychological motives such as self-destructiveness to cause repeated injuries. According to this view, dysfunctional behaviour is the result of the subjects attempt to handle unconscious conflicts. In psychodynamic terms, the subject's ambivalence towards aggressiveness is a determining factor in whether he or she experiences tension and anxiety. This ambivalence is nourished by the fact that physical aggressiveness is encouraged in competitive sport, especially team sports. For many individuals, this produces a classical conflict situation, one of approach-avoidance (Roth & Cohen, 1986). On the one hand, an athlete may wish to participate (approach) in the competition since it offers victory and prestige. On the other hand, an athlete may wish to avoid competition since it may result in an outflow of self-assertive aggression, through succumbing to injury. The tension and worry associated with an unconscious conflict can negatively influence performance, increasing the risk of injury (an actual injury or a faked one), this representing an unconscious defence. A different approach, in some respects previously touched upon in the chapter, is about possible relationships between injury-proneness and specifically stress. For instance, in a classical study by Bramwell et al. (1975), the relationship between injury-proneness and psychological well-being in a broad sense, focusing on different socially stressful events as identified through the Social and Athletic Readjustment Rating Scale (SARRS). The study included American football players, and at the end of the first season, the athletes were divided into an injured and a non-injured group, with the injured group subdivided into low-, medium- and high-risk group on the bases of SARRS scores. It was found that 30% of the players in the low-risk group, 50% in the medium group and 73% in the high-risk group had lost time from practice because of injury. Many other researchers, like Kerr and Minden (1988), Rogers and Landers (2005) and Yang et al. (2015), have used similar approaches and modified versions of SARRS or the Life Experience Survey. Within this line of research, it is hypothesized that athletes who are subject to acute injury, particularly serious and complex ones have experienced major life change in lifestyle to a greater extent than athletes with fewer injuries; thus, this could be labelled as a potentially injury-prone athlete.

APPLIED RECOMMENDATIONS FOR REDUCING INJURY RISK IN SPORT

As more and more scientific documentation emerges regarding the relationship between psychological risk factors and the occurrence of injury in sport, increased conditions are given for creating tailor-made and scientifically sustainable intervention programs. In this context, it is important to translate the findings so that coaches and sport organizations can integrate the findings into their practice and in this way hopefully minimize the injury occurrence among children, youth and senior athletes. One such strategy to prevent sport injuries, identified in the literature review above, is for coaches, to ensure that they establish good communication with their players (Johnson & Ivarsson, 2018). Encouraging positive communication between athletes and coaches is a step towards the development of a safe and secure sport environment that has low interpersonal stress and is relatively free of threat. For instance in a study by Ekstrand et al. (2019), it was found that the injury burden and incidence of severe injuries were significantly higher in teams with low quality of communication between the head coach/manager and the medical team compared with teams with moderate or high-quality scores. Thus, it seems as this sort of environment has the potential to buffer the other stressors that inevitably come with competitive sport and may lower injury risk by addressing some of the main predictors of injury (e.g. stress and social support). More specifically, it is important for coaches to think about how their behaviours fit with their thoughts, norms (personal as well as the club/context/culture) to create constructive and non-judgemental communication, thereby reducing the potential injury risk associated with physical activity and sport, not at least in youth sport. Clement et al. (2017) and Kolar et al. (2016) also emphasize the importance of improving the communication between athletes and coaches, taking the opinion of an athlete into account, and the athlete's active involvement in preparation of the sport injury prevention program. Another recommendation for sporting organizations is to develop interdisciplinary medical teams (e.g. physicians, physiotherapists, athletic trainers, sport psychology practitioners) who can work with injury prevention from a biopsychological perspective. It is also important that the medical teams have good relationships with the coaches, because this might also influence the risk of the athletes becoming injured through the pathways of good communication and solid social support from the professional parties who are involved in athlete health and welfare on a variety of levels (Ekstrand et al., 2019).

FUTURE RESEARCH DIRECTIONS

Previous researchers have suggested that the interplay between physiological and psychological factors might increase the injury risk (e.g. Bahr & Krosshaug, 2005). However, there is a scarcity of studies that have tested a prevention program based on a combination of physiological and psychological interventions. Thus, a recommendation for research could be to integrate neuromuscular (Hägglund et al., 2013) and neurocognitive exercises (Faltus, 2014) into the same prevention program. Such programs can, potentially, reduce injury rates due to increased strength, reduced motor control problems and improved perceptual capacity (Grooms & Onate, 2016). It seems warranted to investigate if a prevention program based on such a combination of approaches will be even more effective than past prevention programs in reducing sport injuries. Research studies focused on overuse injury for younger athletes are also a prioritized area to further explore, not least because young athletes are vulnerable group but because many of them have not yet acquired adaptive coping strategies to handle stressful event in life (Johnson & Ivarsson, 2018). Another suggested line of research is to use prospective designs and to investigate how sociocultural factors might influence injury risk through stress responses and risky behaviours that stem from subcultural imperatives (e.g. play with pain, keep silent about minor injuries). Researchers can, for example, investigate how the perceived environments within sport (e.g. sociocultural norms and expectations, quality of the interaction with coach and teammates) are related to injury risk through stress responsivity and culturally mandated harmful overtraining behaviours.

SUMMARY

As a start of this chapter, three different models were presented in relation to psychosocial risk factors in sport; the stress and athletic injury, the biopsychological sport injury risk profile and the working model of psychological risk factors for overuse injuries. Several psychosocial risk factors were identified related to three overall categories and well adapted to especially the stress and athletic model: personality, history of stressor and coping resources. In addition, special attention was given towards some psychological risk factors preceding sports-related injury that has not be well represented in research, such as overuse injury in sport, risk factors in youth sport as well as perspective of the injury-prone athlete. In the final part of the chapter, two different types of applied recommendation for reducing injury risk in sport were given: establishment of good communication players–coaches and development of interdisciplinary medical teams that work with injury prevention. In addition, future research directions such as integration of neuromuscular and neurocognitive exercise into the same intervention program, and the need of studies focusing overuse injuries for younger athletes is discussed.

Case study

Sally is 17 years old and a promising soccer player, practicing several times a week in the soccer academy where she moved last year to study and play. She is characterized as being an outgoing, caring, talented and happy girl who loves to practice and play matches. Sally has previously had quite a few serious injuries in connection with her sports, but at some point, she has earlier been on sick leave from school as a result of worried "stomach" and occasionally she has felt great homesickness for her family who live a few hours away. Sally also has a very close and caring relationship with her grandmother, with whom she has spent a lot of time in her earlier life. Recently, however, the usually positive and happy Sally has felt progressively more and more subdued and worried. The main reason for this condition is probably due to the occurrence of some events that happened at about the same time. First and probably most importantly is that Sally's grandmother ended up in the hospital after a serious car accident with uncertain future forecast some days ago. In addition, Sally and her team have increased their physical training considerably before the upcoming regional playoffs, where Sally's team is top ranked to win the desired trophy, which has the potential to open up for games at national level. As an addition, Sally's position is as a starting central defender; she is expected to organize the team's central backline, which is considered the key to success for the team. At the day of playoff, Sally is unable to fully focus on the game, and unlike usual, she feels worried and tense for the first game. In her mind, she repeatedly comes back to her severely injured grandmother. Moreover, the hard physical stress of recent weeks seems to remain in the body. In fact, Sally doesn't feel ready to play at all. She is aware that the girls in the team and not least the coaches see her as a core player, but this insight hardly helps her. In her thoughts, she repeats all the time "I am not ready for this; I am not ready for this…." In a moment of poor concentration, Sally badly twists her ankle, at a corner early in the match. The sports medicine specialist indicates that he has a third-degree ankle sprain and ruptured ligaments. After visiting the doctor, Sally is informed that she will be out of play for several months. She is devastated by the news and the problems this potentially causes for herself but also for her hard-working teammates. But somewhere deep inside her she also feels a relief; now she has a legitimate excuse to go and meet her sick grandmother.

Questions

1. Williams and Andersen's stress and athletic injury model suggests that there are three categories of psychological factors that will influence an athlete's appraisal of the situation, potentially leading to an injury. Give examples of different psychological risk factors mentioned within each category.
2. Recent literature suggests different psychosocial risk factors as possibly responsible for the occurrence of overuse injuries in competitive sport. Give example of such factors and discuss in what way these factors differentiate from risk factors traditionally associated with the acute injury.
3. Identify three distinct psychosocial risk factors in the case of Sally that potentially caused her third-degree ankle sprain to happen.
4. Sally's inability to focus on the upcoming match is likely due to a combination of different biopsychological risk factors. What factors do you ascribe as to have the greatest impact on Sally's concentration problems? Is there any single factor that you think is particularly important here? If so, which and why?

References

Andersen, M. B., & Williams, J. M. (1988). A model of stress and athletic injury: Prediction and prevention. *Journal of Sport and Exercise Psychology, 10*, 294–306.

Bahr, R., & Krosshaug, T. (2005). Understanding injury mechanisms: a key component of preventing injuries in sport. *British Journal of Sports Medicine, 39*, 324–32.

Bittencourt, N. F. N., Meeuwisse, W. H., Mendonça, L. D., Nettel-Aguirre, A., Ocarino, J. M., & Fonseca, S. T. (2016). Complex systems approach for sports injuries: Moving from risk factor identification to injury pattern recognition—Narrative review and new concept. *British Journal of Sports Medicine, 50*, 1309–1314.

Bramwell, S. T., Minoru, M., Wagner, N. N., & Holmes, T. H. (1975). Psychosocial factors in athletic injuries. Development and application of the social and athletic readjustment rating scale (SARRS). *Journal of Human Stress, 1*(2), 6–20.

Brewer, B. W., Andersen, M. B., & Van Raalte, J. L. (2002). Psychological aspects of sport injury rehabilitation: Toward a biopsychosocial approach. In D. L. Mostofsky & L. D. Zaichkowsky (Eds.), *Medical and psychological aspects of sport and exercise* (pp. 41–54).

Clement, D., Ivarsson, A., Tranaeus, U., Johnson, U., & Stenling, A. (2017). Investigating the influence of intra-individual changes in perceived stress symptoms on injury risk in soccer. *Scandinavian Journal of Medicine and Science in Sports, 28*, 1461–1466.

Crane, J., & Temple, V. (2015). A systematic review of dropout from organized sport among children and youth. *European Physical Education Review, 21*(1), 114–131.

Devantier, C. (2011). Psychological predictors of injury among professional soccer players. *Sport Science Review, 20*(5–6), 5–36.

Ekstrand, J., Lundqvist, D., Davison, M., D'Hooghe, M., & Pensgaard, A.-M. (2019) Communication quality between the medical team and the head coach/manager is associated with injury burden and player availability in elite football clubs. *British Journal of Sports Medicine, 53*, 304–308.

Faltus, J. (2014). Rehabilitation strategies addressing neurocognitive and balance deficits following a concussion in a female snowboard athlete: A case report. *International Journal of Sports Physical Therapy, 9*(2), 232–241.

Grooms, R. R., & Onate, J. A. (2016). Neuroscience Application to Noncontact Anterior Cruciate Ligament Injury Prevention. *Sport Health, 8*(2), 149–152.

Hägglund, M., Atroshi, I., Wagner, P., & Waldén, M. (2013). Superior compliance with a neuromuscular training programme is associated with fewer ACL injuries and fewer acute knee injuries in female adolescent football players: Secondary analysis of an RCT. *British Journal of Sports Medicine, 47*(15).

Holmes, T. H. (1970). Psychological screening. In *Football injuries* (pp. 211–214). Paper presented at a workshop sponsored by Subcommittee on Athletic Injuries, Committee on the Skeletal System, Division of Medical Science, National Research Council, February 1969. Washington, DC: National Academy of Science.

Ivarsson, A., & Johnson, U. (2010). Psychological factors as predictors of injuries among senior soccer players: A prospective study. *Journal of Sports Science and Medicine, 9*, 347–352.

Ivarsson, A., Johnson, U., Andersen, M. B., Tranaeus, U., Stenling, A., & Lindwall, M. (2017). Psychosocial factors and sport injuries: Meta-analyses for prediction and prevention. *Sports Medicine, 47*, 353–365.

Ivarsson, A., Johnson, U., & Podlog, L. (2013). Psychological predictors of injury occurrence: A prospective investigation of professional Swedish soccer players. *Journal of Sport Rehabilitation, 22*, 19–26.

Ivarsson, A., Stambulova, N., & Johnson, U. (2016). Injury as a career transition: Experiences of a Swedish elite handball player. *International Journal of Sport and Exercise Psychology, 16*(4), 365–381.

Johnson, U. (2011). Athletes' experience of psychosocial risk factors preceding injury. *Qualitative Research in Sport and Exercise, 3*(1), 99–115.

Johnson, U., & Ivarsson, I. (2011). Psychological predictors of sport injury among junior soccer players. *Scandinavian Journal of Medicine and Science in Sport, 21*, 129–136.

Johnson, U., & Ivarsson, A. (2018). Managing injuries among young athletes. In C. J. Knight, C. G. Harwood & D. Gould (Eds.), *Sport Psychology for Young Athletes* (pp. 174–184). Routledge Taylor and Francis Group.

Johnson, U., Tranaeus, U., & Ivarsson, A. (2014). Current status and future challenges in psychological research of sport injury prediction and prevention: A methodological perspective. *Revista de Psicología del Deporte*, *23*(2), 401–409.

Johnson, U., & Ivarsson, A. (2017). Psychosocial factors and sport injuries: Prediction, prevention and future research directions. *Current Opinion in Psychology*, *16*, 89–92.

Keats, M., Emery, C. A., & Finch, C. (2012). Are we having fun yet? Fostering adherence to injury preventive exercise recommendations in young athletes. *Sports Medicine*, *42*, 175–184.

Kerr, G., & Minden, H. (1988). Psychological factors related to the occurrence of athletic injuries. *Journal of Sport and Exercise Psychology*, *10*, 167–173.

Kisser, R., & Bauer, R. (2010). Sport injuries in the European Union. *Injury Prevention*, *16* (Suppl. 1):A1–A289.

Kleinert, J. (2002). Causative and protective effects of sport injury trait anxiety on injuries in German university sport. *European Journal of Sport Science*, *2*, 1–11.

Kolar, E., Pavletic, M. S., Smrdu, M., & Atikovic, A. (2016). Athletes' perception of the causes of injury in gymnastics. *The Journal of Sports Medicine and Physical Fitness*, *57*(5), 703–710.

Li, H., Moreland, J. J., Peek-Asa, C., & Yang, J. (2017). Preseason Anxiety and Depressive Symptoms and Prospective Injury Risk in Collegiate Athletes. *The American Journal of Sports Medicine*, *45*(9), 2148–2155.

Martin, S. (2018). Are perfectionistic and stressed athletes the main victims of the "silent epidemic"? A prospective study of personal and interpersonal risk factors of overuse injuries in sport (Unpublished master's thesis). School of Health and Welfare, Halmstad University, Sweden.

Myer, G. D., Jayanthi, N., Difiori, J. P., & Faigenbaum, A. D. (2015). Sport Specialization, Part I: Does Early Sports Specialization Increase Negative Outcomes and Reduce the Opportunity for Success in Young Athletes? *Sports Health*, *7*(5), 437–442.

Nelson, L. D., Tarima, A., LaRoche, A. A., Hammeke, T. A., Barr, W. B., Guskiewicz, K., Randolph, C., & McCrea, M. A. (2016). Preinjury somatization symptoms contribute to clinical recovery after sport-related concussion. *Neurology*, 86(20), 1856–1863.

Olsen, O. E., Myklebust, G., Engebretsen, L., Holme, I., & Bahr, R. (2005). Exercises to prevent lower limb injuries in youth sports: Cluster randomised controlled trail. *British Medical Journal*, *330*, 449.

Patel, D. R., & Nelson, T. L. (2000). Sport injuries in adolescents. *Medical Clinics of North America*, *84*(4), 983–1007.

Pensgaard, A.-M., Ivarsson, A., Nilstad, A., Solstad, B.-E., & Steffen, K. (2018). Psychosocial stress factors, including the relationship with the coach, and their influence on acute and overuse injury risk in elite female football players. *BMJ Open Sport Exercise Medicine*, *4*, e000317.

Perna, F. M., Antonio, H. M., Baum, A., Gordon, P., & Schneiderman, N. (2003). Cognitive behavioral stress management effects on injury and illness among competitive athletes: A randomized clinical trial. *Annals of Behavior Medicine*, *25*, 66–73.

Post, E. G., Trigsted, S. M., Riekena, J. W., Hetzel, B. S., McGuine, T. A., Brooks, M. A., & Bell, D. R. (2017). The association of sport specialization and training volume with injury history in youth athletes. *The American Journal of Sports Medicine*, *45*(6), 1405–1412.

Putukian, M. (2016). The psychological response to injury in student athletes: A narrative review with a focus on mental health. *British Journal of Sports Medicine, 50*, 145–148.

Richardson, S. O., Andersen, M. B., & Morris, M. (2008). *Overtraining athletes: Personal journeys in sport*. Human Kinetics.

Rogers, T. M., & Landers, D. M. (2005). Mediating effects of peripheral vision in the life event stress/athletic injury relationship. *Journal of Sport and Exercise Psychology, 27*, 271–288.

Roth, E., & Cohen, L. J. (1986). Approach, avoidance, and coping with stress. *American Psychologist, 4*(17), 813–819.

Sibold, J., Howard, A., & Zizzi, S. (2011). A comparison of psychosocial and orthopedic data in injured college athletes: Novel application of hurdle regression. *Athletic Insight, 13*, 1–12.

Singh, H., & Conroy, D. E. (2017). Systematic review of stress-related injury vulnerability in athletic and occupational contexts. *Psychology of Sport & Exercise, 33*, 37–44.

Soligard, T., Schwellnus, M., Alonso, J. M., Bahr, R., Clarsen, B., Dijkstra, H. P., Gabbett, T., Gleeson, M., Hägglund, M., Hutchinson, M. R., van Rensburg, C. J., Khan, K. M., Meeusen, R., Orchard, J. W., Pluim, B. M., Raftery, M., Budgett, R., & Engebretsen, L. (2016). How much is too much? (Part 1) International Olympic Committee consensus statement on load in sport and risk of injury. *British Journal of Sports Medicine, 50*(17), 1030–1041.

Suchman, E. A. (1970). Accident and social deviance. *Journal of Health and Social Behaviour, 11*, 4–15.

Swanik, C. B., Covassin, T., Stearne, D. J., & Schatz, P. (2007). The relationship between neurocognitive function and noncontact anterior cruciate ligament injuries. *The American Journal of Sports Medicine, 35*(6), 943–948.

Steffen, K., Pensgaard, A-M., & Bahr, R. (2009). Self-reported psychological characteristics as risk factors for injuries in female youth football. *Scandinavian Journal of Medicine and Science in Sport, 19*, 442–451.

Tranaeus, U., Johnson, U., Engström, B., Skillgate, E., & Werner, S. (2014). Psychological antecedents of overuse injuries among Swedish elite floorball players. *Athletic Insight, 6*(2), 155–172.

Wiese-Bjornstal, D. M. (2003). From skinned knees and Pee Wees to menisci and masters: Developmental sport injury psychology. In M.R. Weiss (Ed.), *Developmental sport and exercise psychology: A lifespan perspective* (pp. 525–568). Fitness Information Technology.

Wiese-Bjornstal, D. M. (2010). Psychology and socioculture affect injury risk, response, and recovery in high-intensity athletes: A consensus statement. *Scandinavian Journal of Medicine and Science in Sports, 20*(Suppl. 2), 103–111.

Wilkerson, G. B. (2012). Neurocognitive reaction time predicts lower extremity sprains and strains. *International Journal of Athletic Therapy and Training, 17*, 4–9.

Williams, J. M., & Andersen, M. B. (1998). Psychosocial antecedents of sport injury: Review and critique of the stress and injury model. *Journal of Applied Sport Psychology, 10*, 5–25.

Yang, J., Peek-Asa, C., Covassin, T., & Torner, J. C. (2015). Post-concussion symptoms of depression and anxiety in Division I collegiate athletes. *Developmental Neuropsychology, 40*(1), 18–23.

Yang, J., Tibbetts, A. S., Covassin, T., Cheng, G., Nayar, S., & Heiden, E. (2012) Epidemiology of overuse and acute injuries among competitive collegiate athletes. *Journal of Athletic Training, 47*, 198–204.

2 PREVENTION IS BETTER THAN CURE

THE ROLE OF PSYCHOLOGICAL INTERVENTIONS IN SPORTS INJURY RISK REDUCTION

Dr Andreas Ivarsson

Given the high injury rates associated with sport participation, combined with the negatively associated consequences both at individual and team/club, as well as community levels, preventive strategies for sport injuries are of great interest. To develop functional preventive strategies and programmes, it is important to, first, single out risk factors that are likely to increase the likelihood of sport injuries (Bahr, 2016). Risk factors and prevention research have, in most cases, focused on physiological and/or biomechanical factors (e.g. Almeida et al., 2014). Consequently, researchers have recently emphasized the importance of including different perspectives to extend the knowledge within the field. Wiese-Bjornstal (2010), for example, emphasized the importance of combining biological and behavioural, as well as social sciences, together into a biopsychosocial perspective, to advance the knowledge of sport injury prevention.

Based on identified risk factors, different injury prevention programmes have been developed. One of the most frequently implemented is the FIFA 11+ (Soligard et al., 2008). This program is based on a combination of strengthening, balancing and jumping/landing exercises. The FIFA 11+ program has been effective in reducing injuries in, for example, soccer (Thorborg et al., 2017). Other types of prevention programmes, effective in reducing injury rates, are balance board training and warm-up programmes (for more information, see, Leppänen et al., 2014). Unlike physical, physiological or biomechanical injury risk factors, even where prominent psychosocial factors (e.g. psychosocial stress) have been found to influence injury risk, few intervention programmes targeting these factors have been implemented. To extend the knowledge within the field of injury prevention, it is, however, important to include a biopsychosocial perspective into regular injury prevention work (Gledhill & Forsdyke, 2018; Gledhill et al., 2018).

The objectives of the chapter are to (1) review and summarize the psychological-based intervention studies conducted to decrease injury risk among athletes, (2) highlight and discuss some of the reasons for the lack of implementation of psychological strategies within injury prevention programmes, (3) discuss methodological considerations related to the developed interventions, (4) provide recommendations for the future work on psychological aspects related to sport injury prevention and (5) present a case where the reader can elaborate on how to justify, develop and implement an injury prevention programme.

PSYCHOLOGICAL INTERVENTION STUDIES AIMED AT REDUCING INJURY RISK

Concerning psychological risk factors for injury high levels of stress together with strong stress responses are found to, in a substantial number of studies, be related with increased risk of injuries (Ivarsson et al., 2017). In the model of stress and athletic injury, interventions based on psychological training programmes are suggested to decrease injury risk among athletes through decreasing the magnitude of stress responses (Williams & Andersen, 1998).

Targeting psychosocial risk factors several intervention studies have been successfully implemented (Ivarsson et al., 2017). More specifically, since the beginning of the 1990s, at least 12 intervention studies, based on psychological training programmes, have been conducted in the research field of sport injury prevention (see Table 2.1). During the last couple of years, at least, two systematic reviews on the topic have been published (Gledhill et al., 2018; Ivarsson et al., 2017). In a recent systematic review and meta-analysis on the role of psychological interventions in injury prevention, seven studies, all applying designs with one intervention and one (or several) control condition(s), were included (Ivarsson et al., 2017). The result from the meta-analysis showed an overall moderate effect size corresponding to fewer injuries in psychological intervention conditions compared to control conditions (Cohen's $d = -0.63$). In a more recent publication (Gledhill et al., 2018), 13 publications (containing 14 studies) were included. Of the included studies, 93% reported fewer injuries in the psychological intervention condition in comparison to the control condition (ES ranged between 0.2 and 1.21). There was, however, moderate overall risk of bias in reporting. Collectively, these two systematic reviews demonstrate that there is merit in considering psychological interventions if seeking to reduce the risk of sports injuries.

One of the first studies published within the area implemented stress management training (e.g. imagery, relaxation) in a sample of swimmers and football players (Davis, 1991). The result showed a 52% reduction in swimming injuries and a 33% reduction in football injuries, respectively. However, a control condition was not included, reducing the level of confidence in the findings.

Kerr and Goss (1996) study on elite gymnasts was one of the first prevention studies using a randomized controlled trail (RCT) approach. In the randomization process, the participants were matched on sex, age and performance level. The intervention programme was based on stress inoculating training. The

Table 2.1 Characteristics of the included studies

Study	*Design*	*Population (sample size)*	*Type of intervention*	*Length of the intervention/Number of sessions*	*Result*
Davis (1991)	Quasi-experimental	21 swimmers and football players	Relaxation training and imagery	1 swimming session, 2–5 football sessions a week	52% decrease in injuries for swimmers and 33 decrease in injuries for football players
Edvardsson et al. (2012)	Quasi-experimental	29 football players	Self-regulation techniques	9 weeks/7 sessions	Intervention group: 0.38 injury/player Control group: 1.0 injury/player
Ivarsson et al. (2015a)	RCT	42 football players	Experimental: mindfulness Control: sport psychology skills	7 weeks/7 sessions	Intervention group: 8 injuries Control group: 15 injuries
Johnson et al. (2005)	RCT	32 football players	Stress management	19 weeks/6 sessions	Intervention group: 0.22 injury/player Control group: 1.31 injury/player
Kerr & Goss (1996)	RCT	24 gymnasts	Stress management (stress inculcation training)	8 months/16 sessions	The participants in the intervention group experienced fewer injuries in comparison to the participants in the control group (Cohen's $d = 0.67$)
Kolt et al. (2004)	RCT	20 gymnasts	Stress management	24 weeks/12 sessions	Intervention group: 2.5 injuries/athlete Control group: 3.2 injuries/player
Maddison & Prapavessis (2005)	RCT	48 rugby players	CBT	4 weeks/6 sessions	Intervention group: 2.84 injuries/athlete Control group: 3.43 injuries/athlete

(*Continued*)

Table 2.1 Characteristics of the included studies (*Continued*)

Study	*Design*	*Population (sample size)*	*Type of intervention*	*Length of the intervention/Number of sessions*	*Result*
Noh et al. (2007)	Quasi-experimental	35 ballet dancers	Experimental group 1: Autogenic training Experimental group 2: Broad-based coping skills	12 weeks/36 sessions	Dancers in coping skills groups spent less time injured than the control group
Perna et al. (2003)	RCT	34 rowers	CBT	3 weeks/7 sessions	The intervention group experienced significantly fewer days out due to injuries in comparison to the control group
Olmedilla-Zafra (2017)	RCT	74 soccer players	Stress inoculation training	3 months/1 session/week	Intervention: 0.11 injuries/player Control: 0.24 injuries/player
Tranaeus et al. (2015a), Tranaeus et al. (2015b)	RCT	Study 1: 401 floorball players Study 2: 346 floorball players	Psychological skills training	6 weeks/6 sessions	Study 1: Intervention group: 0.49 injuries/player Control group: 0.53 injuries/player Study 2: Intervention group: 0.31 injuries/player Control group: 0.41 injuries/player
Zadeh et al. (2019)	RCT	45 soccer players	MAC	6 weeks/7 sessions	Intervention group: 0.45 injuries/player Control group: 2.82 injuries/player

results showed, in comparison to the control group, fewer injuries in the intervention group (the difference was, however, not statistically significant).

An additional study, applying stress inoculation training programme, was conducted in a sample of rowers (Perna et al., 2003). In this study, a large effect in the reduction of injury frequency between the two conditions was present (Cohen's $d = 0.99$), with fewer injuries reported in the intervention group compared to the control group.

Building on the previous presented studies, Johnson et al. (2005) argued that the next step was to, based on the categories of risk factors proposed in the stress-injury model (Williams & Andersen, 1998), test the potential intervention effect on at-risk athletes. After screening, 32 participants (soccer players) were considered to be at risk and were, therefore, randomized into an intervention and one control condition. The intervention programme was based on five themes (i.e., relaxation, stress management skills, goal setting, self-confidence training, reflections based on critical incident diary). The results showed that the participants in the intervention group experienced considerable fewer injuries ($n = 3$), in comparison to the control group ($n = 21$).

Following Johnson et al. study design, both Maddison and Prapavessis (2005) and Noh et al. (2007) screened for at-risk prior to the intervention. In the Maddison and Prapavessis (2005) study, conducted within a sample of elite rugby players, a cognitive behavioural stress management intervention was applied. The results showed fewer injuries in the intervention group, in comparison to the control group. Similar results were found in Noh et al. (2007). The difference between these two studies was that Noh et al. applied a quasi-experimental design on female ballet dancers where Maddison and Prapavessis (2005) used a RCT design. Also, in the Noh et al. study, two intervention groups (autogenic training group and broad-based coping skills) and one control group were present.

In two of the studies, resulting in three publications, a cluster randomization procedure (based on team belonging) was used to allocate participants into intervention and control conditions (Kolt et al., 2004; Tranaeus et al., 2015a, 2015b). In both studies, stress management interventions were tested in populations of gymnastics (Kolt et al., 2004) and floorball players (Tranaeus et al., 2015a, 2015b). In the Kolt et al. study, the participants in the control condition were offered a placebo programme containing anthropometric measurements and lectures on nutrition. In both studies, fewer injuries were reported in the intervention group compared to the control group. Whilst these differences were not statistically significant, they did demonstrate a potentially clinically meaningful reduction in injury frequency.

In comparison to most other studies conducted within the area, three slightly different intervention programmes have been tested in soccer samples. In one of the study, biofeedback training combined with relaxation and breathing exercises was implemented (Edvardsson et al., 2012). The participants in the intervention group reported fewer injuries compared to the control group (no statistically significant difference). In the other study, the intervention programme was based on the Mindfulness Acceptance Commitment (MAC) approach (Ivarsson et al., 2015b). The participants in the control condition received lectures on different sport psychological skills. The result showed fewer injuries in the intervention condition in comparison to the control condition (ES = 0.59). The MAC approach was also used in another study conducted on a sample of amateur soccer players (Zadeh et al., 2019). Also in this study, the intervention group experienced fewer injuries in comparison to the control group.

Another recent study published within the area was also conducted within a soccer population. The participants in the intervention condition, receiving a stress-management and muscle relaxation programme, reported fewer injuries compared to the participants in the control condition (Olmedilla-Zafra et al., 2017).

To sum up, the interventions have been conducted in a variety of different populations, such as soccer, gymnastics, rugby and floorball. Studies have also considered the spectrum of skill levels, from elite professional athletes through to high school students. Most of the studies have used an RCT design (n = 9), where three have applied a quasi-experimental (e.g. lack of control group, lack of randomization etc.). Concerning the structure of the interventions, they have had between 1 and 36 sessions, usually lasting between 30 and 60 min.

In all of the conducted interventions where control conditions have been used, the experimental group has, in comparison to the control groups, reported less number of injuries. Similar results have also been reported in the studies without control group where a reduction in injuries has been shown pre- to post-intervention.

POTENTIAL EXPLANATIONS FOR THE EFFECTS OF PSYCHOLOGICAL PROGRAMMES ON INJURY RISK

When discussing the potential explanations for the interventions, successful influence in reducing injury risk several can be listed. When discussing results in intervention studies, potential explanatory variables can be divided into two categories: specific factors and common factors (e.g. Mulder et al., 2017). The specific factors are related to the specific intervention content while the common factors are related to general and context related aspects.

Specific factors

One potential explanation for the results, even though there have been different conceptual approaches and designs, is that most of the studies have, however, applied programmes targeting stress management techniques (e.g. relaxation programmes, critical incident diaries, goal setting programmes). More specifically, stress management techniques, such as mindfulness, have been found to down-regulate amygdala activation (Cozolino, 2010). Such down-regulation of amygdala activation is related to decreased magnitude of stress response. Given that stress and the magnitude of the stress response will influence injury risk, this type of training might decrease this risk.

Another potential explanation for the effectiveness of the intervention could be that mindfulness and stress management practice have been related to functional changes in the brain's attention systems (Fox et al., 2006; Hölzel et al., 2011). These changes can lead to increased capacity to pay attention to relevant cues in the environment (Cozolino, 2010). Because previous research has found peripheral vision narrowing to be a predictor of sport injuries (Rogers & Landers, 2005), increased attentional abilities might decrease injury risk. The explanation for this suggestion may be that attention and executive functions are closely related with humans' abilities to select goal-directed behaviours through, for example, paying attention towards important information (Clacy et al., 2013). More appropriate selection of behaviours (e.g. move to avoid a tackle) that meet the demands for a specific situation might be associated with a decreased injury risk.

A third potential explanation is that different types of relaxation techniques as well as meditation, used in many of the included studies, are related to a reduction in anxiety levels (Manzoni et al., 2008). This might, in line with the suggestions in the model of stress and athletic injury (Williams & Andersen, 1998), decrease the risk of injury via decreased magnitude of stress responses.

In some of the interventions, imagery exercises have been included as a substantial part of the intervention programmes. Imagery training has, in various populations, been shown to increase muscle strength (Slimani et al., 2016). Muscle strength (and strength training) is, in turn, associated with a decreased risk of sport injuries (Zouita et al., 2016). Another explanations for the potential positive effects of imagery on injury prevention are via the development of adequate motor control strategies (Benjaminse et al., 2019) and decreased levels of anxiety symptoms (Holmes & Mathews, 2005).

Common factors

As outlined above, it is interesting that most studies have used different intervention programmes (e.g. cognitive-behavioural therapy, psychological skills training, mindfulness and acceptance training) but still generated similar results. Except the possible, more content-based, explanations presented so far in this chapter, there might be other, more general explanations, for the similarity in results between the different intervention studies.

First, research has shown that the specific techniques used in therapy do not account for much of the potential effects of the treatment. Several meta-syntheses, comparing results of meta-analyses from different psychotherapy perspectives (e.g. general psychotherapy, CBT, psychodynamic psychotherapy), have shown similar therapeutic effects between the various treatments (e.g. Wampold, 2015). Research has suggested that it is, instead, the common factors (e.g. the quality of the therapeutic relationship) that are present in all psychotherapy models that will probably have a substantial impact on outcomes (e.g. Mulder et al., 2017; Rogers, 1992; Wampold, 2015).

One of the factors that has gained the most attention in the literature is the quality of the relationship between the therapist and the client. If it is a high-quality, non-judgmental relationship where the client feels comfortable to talk about anything, it is more likely that the intervention will have an effect compared to a lower quality interpersonal relationship (e.g. Andersen & Ivarsson, 2016; Schore, 2014).

IF IT WORKS, WHY DO ATHLETES AND TEAMS NOT USE IT?

Despite most studies having shown that psychological-based training programmes can reduce the number of injuries within several different sports, there are few teams, clubs, or organizations that have included this type of training into their general injury prevention programmes (Gledhill & Forsdyke, 2018). There might be several reasons for the rather unsuccessful implementation of this type of content into general prevention practice.

One general barrier for implementation evidence-based injury preventive initiative, listed by sport coaches, is perceived lack of time (e.g. Saunders et al., 2010). This might, in comparison to other preventive techniques (e.g. strength training, FIFA 11+ etc.), be an even larger barrier for implementing psychological-based techniques. The reasons for these are (1) that most of the programmes tested have long sessions, and (2) none of the studies have integrated the interventions into the regular training sessions. These aspects together are likely to mean that coaches place less emphasis into activities that not are integrated into the regular practice.

Other potential barriers for the implementation of psychological intervention programmes might simply be that they are psychology-focussed. Research has, for example, shown that coaches and academy directors within soccer expressed six barriers related to the implementation of applied sport psychology (Pain & Harwood, 2004). The listed barriers were negative perceptions of psychology, lack of sport psychology knowledge, integrating with players and coaching staff, role and service clarity, practical constraints and perceived value of sport psychology. It is likely that these aspects might have negatively influenced the likelihood of implement psychological techniques for injury prevention. Also, sports medicine staff (e.g. physiotherapist, athletic trainers) are important gatekeepers when it comes to the implementation of psychological intervention programmes (Heaney, 2018). Even if sports medicine staff are aware of the potential benefits of including psychological techniques or intervention into the injury preventive work (e.g. Alexanders et al., 2015), such practice is underrepresented in the literature (Vriend et al., 2017). One explanation for the lack of implementation of psychological interventions is that the sport medicine staff feel insufficiently trained to run this type of intervention (Alexanders et al., 2015).

A final potential explanation for the lack of implementation might be, in comparison to other injury preventive initiative (e.g. FIFA 11+), related to the number of studies using small sample sizes, thus generating less convincing evidence for the potential effect. When coaches, directors, or sport medicine staff are selecting what to direct their time and money to, it is probably likely that they decide to go with the preventive initiatives that have the strongest evidence.

'WHERE DO WE GO FROM HERE'?

Methodological considerations and implications

In the published intervention studies, some methodological similarities run through most of the investigations. First, a majority of the studies have used quasi-experimental designs with control groups, meaning that the participants in the control group would not be offered any placebo or attentional treatment. In other words, in the attempt to control for potential confounders in the designs of intervention studies, RCT investigations with placebo/attentional control treatments should be conducted (Shadish et al., 2002).

Second, most studies have had small samples (e.g. Ivarsson et al., 2017). This might be problematic both from a statistical as well as generalizability perspective. From a statistical perspective, it is problematic because the statistics generated from the analyses (e.g. *p*-value, effect sizes) are all influenced by sample size (Ivarsson et al., 2013; Ivarsson et al., 2015a). Larger sample sizes are, therefore, warranted. Also, to improve the generalizability of results, studies with larger sample sizes are important.

Third, some of the studies have screened athletes before the intervention started to choose participants who fit at-risk profiles according the Williams and Andersen (1998) model of stress and athletic injury (e.g. Johnson et al., 2005). This screening for at-risk athletes has the advantage of delivering interventions to those who may most need them while not spending time and money on those who are not likely to become injured. The disadvantage is that some members of the team may feel left out of the special treatments others are receiving. Testing intervention programmes on the full range of athletes, from low to high risk, may also be a direction in which research designs should be further elaborated. To be able to show effects on all types of athletes may make it easier to promote a programme to coaches and administrators who hold the purse strings.

Applied considerations and implications

As previously discussed, one of the main challenges is to implement psychologically based prevention interventions into everyday injury prevention practice. To increase the likelihood of such implementation, the following aspects warrant attention.

First, more well-designed studies with larger sample size and control groups are necessary to establish stronger evidence for the potential effects of preventive initiatives on injury risk (Gledhill et al., 2018; Ivarsson et al., 2017). Also, when designing interventions, it is important to consider making them more integrated into current training practice. This will, hopefully, increase the likelihood of implementation.

Second, even though researchers have suggested that the interplay between physiological and psychosocial factors might increase the injury risk, no studies have, to our knowledge, tested a prevention programme based on both physiological as well as psychosocial techniques. It is therefore warranted to investigate if a prevention programme based on such a combination of approaches will be even more effective than regular prevention programmes in reducing injuries (Gledhill et al., 2018).

Third, and perhaps most important, is to, within the sport community, better promote the importance to also consider psychosocial factors in the injury prevention work. To get access to coaches and sport medicine staff in, for example, education can be one way to increase the knowledge of important gatekeepers.

Fourth, one way to integrate the psychological perspective can be to include routinely screening of the athletes into the screening procedures (Gledhill & Forsdyke, 2018) that already are conducted within many clubs and teams (especially on elite level). To screen for, for example, daily hassles, negative life events as well as cognitive and somatic stress responses might provide a basis for referral to a sport psychologist who can conduct the necessary intervention (Gledhill & Forsdyke, 2018). It is, therefore, important to include a sport psychologist within the sport medicine team.

Another aspect where psychology can be useful within the injury prevention work is via the use of behavioural theories to guide the implementation of different types of prevention programmes (Gabriel et al., 2019). To use theories, such as theory of planned behaviours, can, potentially, increase the likelihood of a successful implementation of a prevention programme due to the facilitation of behaviour change (Chan & Hagger, 2012).

THE CASE: IMPLEMENTING A PSYCHOLOGICAL INJURY PREVENTION PROGRAMME WITHIN A SOCCER ACADEMY

The town where you live is home to a soccer club with one large youth academy. You are contacted by one of the youth coaches that have found a research article about psychological perspective on injury prevention in sport very interesting. The coach now wants to integrate psychological techniques into their regular injury prevention routine within all youth teams in the club. To do that, the coach is scheduling a meeting with the academy director to convince this person about the positive aspects of including psychology. You are asked by the coach to argue for the importance of also focusing on psychological approaches for injury prevention. There is, however, short on time so you will only be able to raise three points.

Questions

1. What three aspects would your raise to convince the academy director to consider implementing the psychological programmes into their injury prevention work?

Great news! You have been successful in convincing the academy director to implement a psychological programme for injury prevention. You are now meeting with the coaches and sport medicine team to inform them about the practical procedures of the programme.

2. How would you designee the programme to (1) be effective in preventing injuries and (2) increase the chance of good adherence, both from coaches/sport medicine practitioners as well as from players?

After your talk for the coaches, you are asked to go to a players meeting to inform them about the programme and the practical issues. The ages of the players range between 15 and 19.

3. How would you approach the players to have them 'buy-in' to the program?

References

Alexanders, J., Anderson, A., & Henderson, S. (2015). Musculoskeletal physiotherapits' use of psychological interventions: A systematic review of therapists' perceptions and practice. *Physiotherapy, 101*, 95–102.

Almeida, P. H. G. L. D., Olmedilla, A., Rubio, V. J., & Palou, P. (2014). Psychology in the realm of sport injury: What it is all about. *Revista de Psicología del Deporte, 23*(2), 395–400.

Andersen, M. B., & Ivarsson, A. (2016). A methodology of loving kindness: How interpersonal neurobiology, compassion, and transference can inform researcher-participant encounters and storytelling. *Qualitative Research in Sport, Exercise and Health, 8*, 1–20. DOI: 10.1080/2159676X.2015.1056827.

Bahr, R. (2016). Why screening tests to predict injury do not work—and probably never will: A critical review. *British Journal of Sports Medicine, 50*(13), 776–780. DOI: 10.1136/bjsports-2016-096256.

Benjaminse, A., Webster, K. E., Klmp, A., Meijer, M., & Gokeler, A. (2019). Revised approach to the role of fatigue in anterior cruciate ligament injury prevention: A systematic review with meta-analyses. *Sports Medicine, 49*, 565–586.

Chan, D. K. C., & Hagger, M. (2012). Theoretical integration and the psychology of sport injury prevention. *Sports Medicine, 42*, 725–732.

Clacy, A. L., Sharman, R., & Lovell, G. P. (2013). Risk factors to sport-related concussion for junior athletes. *OA Sports Medicine, 1*, 4.

Cozolino, L. (2010). *The neuroscience of psychotherapy: Healing the social brain* (2nd ed.). Norton.

Davis, J. (1991). Sports injuries and stress management: An opportunity for research. *The Sport Psychologist, 5*, 75–182.

Edvardsson, A., Ivarsson, A., & Johnson, U. (2012). Is a cognitive-behavioural biofeedback intervention useful to reduce injury risk in junior football players? *Journal of Sport Science and Medicine, 11*, 331–338.

Fox, M. D., Corbetta, M., Snyder, A. Z., Vincent, J. L., & Raichle, M. E. (2006). Spontaneous neuronal activity distinguishes human dorsal and ventral attention systems. *Proceedings of the National Academy of Sciences of the United States of America, 103*, 10046–10051. DOI: 10.1073%2Fpnas.0604187103.

Gabriel, E. H., McCann, R. S., & Hoch, M. C. (2019). Use of social and behavioural theories in exercise-related injury prevention program research: A systematic review. *Sports Medicine, 49*, 1515–1528.

Gledhill, A., & Forsdyke, D. (2018). An ounce of prevention is better than a pound of cure: shouldn't we be doing EVERYTHING to reduce sports injury incidence and burden? *British Journal of Sports Medicine, 52*, 1292–1293.

Gledhill, A., Forsdyke, D., & Murray, E. (2018). Psychological interventions used to reduce sports injuries: A systematic review of real-world effectiveness. *British Journal of Sports Medicine, 52*, 967–971.

Heaney, C. (2018). What do sports medicine professionals working in football need to know about sport psychology? *Football Medicine & Performance, 26*, 18–20.

Holmes, E. A., & Mathews, A. (2005). Mental imagery and emotion: A special relationship? *Emotion, 5*, 489–497.

Hölzel, B. K., Lazar, S. W., Gard, T., Schumen-Oliver, Z., Vago, D. R., & Ott, U. (2011). How does mindfulness meditation work? Proposing mechanisms of action from a conceptual and neural perspective. *Perspectives on Psychological Science, 6*, 537–559. DOI: 10.1177/1745691611419671.

Ivarsson, A., Andersen, M. B., Johnson, U., & Lindwall, M. (2013). To adjust or not adjust: Nonparametric effect sizes, confidence intervals, and real-world meaning. *Psychology of Sport and Exercise, 14*, 97–102. DOI: 10.1016/j.psychsport.2012.07.007.

Ivarsson, A., Andersen, M. B., Stenling, A., Johnson, U., & Lindwall, M. (2015a). Things we still haven't learned (so far). *Journal of Sport & Exercise Psychology, 37*, 449–461. DOI: 10.1123/jsep.2015-0015.

Ivarsson, A., Johnson, U., Andersen, M. B., Fallby, J., & Altemyr, M. (2015b). It pays to pay attention: A mindfulness-based program for injury prevention with soccer players. *Journal of Applied Sport Psychology, 27*, 319–334.

Ivarsson, A., Johnson, U., Andersen, M. B., Tranaeus, U., Stenling, A., & Lindwall, M. (2017). Psychosocial factors and sport injuries: Meta-analyses for prediction and prevention. *Sports Medicine, 47*, 353–365.

Johnson, U., Ekengren, J., & Andersen, M. B. (2005). Injury prevention in Sweden: Helping soccer players at risk. *Journal of Sport & Exercise Psychology, 27*, 32–38.

Kerr, G., & Goss, J. (1996). The effects of a stress management program on injuries and stress levels. *Journal of Applied Sport Psychology, 8*, 109–117. DOI: 10.1080/10413209608406312.

Kolt, G. S., Hume, P. A., Smith, P., & Williams, M. M. (2004). Effects of a stress-management program on injury and stress of competitive gymnasts. *Perceptual and Motor Skills, 99*, 195–207.

Leppänen, M., Aaltonen, S., Parkkari, J., Heinonen, A., & Kujala, U. M. (2014). Interventions to prevent sports related injuries: A systematic review and meta-analysis of randomized controlled trials. *Sports Medicine, 44*, 473–486.

Maddison, R., & Prapavessis, H. (2005). A psychological approach to the prediction and prevention of athletic injury. *Journal of Sport & Exercise Psychology, 27*, 289–310.

Manzoni, G. M., Pagnini, F., Castelnuovo, G., & Molinari, E. (2008). Relaxation training for anxiety: A ten-years systematic review with meta-analysis. *BMC Psychiatry, 8*, 41.

Mulder, R., Murray, G., & Rucklidge, J. (2017). Common versus specific factors in psychotherapy: Opening the black box. *Lancet Psychiatry, 4*, 953–962.

Noh, Y-E., Morris, T., & Andersen, M. B. (2007). Psychological intervention programs for reduction of injury in ballet dancers. *Research in Sports Medicine, 15*, 13–32. DOI: 10.1080/15438620600987064.

Olmedilla-Zafra, A., Rubio, V. J., Ortega, E., & Garcia-Mas, A. (2017). Effectiveness of a stress management pilot program aimed at reducing the incidence of sports injuries in young football (soccer) players. *Physical Therapy in Sport, 24*, 53–59.

Pain, M. A., & Harwood, C. G. (2004). Knowledge and perceptions of sport psychology within English soccer. *Journal of Sports Sciences, 22*, 813–826.

Perna, F. M., Antoni, M. H., Baum, A., Gordon, P., & Schneiderman, N. (2003). Cognitive behavioral stress management effects on injury and illness among competitive athletes: A randomized controlled trial. *Annals of Behavioral Medicine, 25*, 66–73. DOI: 10.1207/S15324796ABM2501_09.

Rogers, C. R. (1992). The necessary and sufficient conditions of therapeutic personality change. *Journal of Consulting and Clinical Psychology, 60*, 827–832. DOI: 10.1037/0022-006X.60.6.827.

Rogers, T. M., & Landers, D. M. (2005). Mediating effects of peripheral vision in the life event stress/athletic injury relationship. *Journal of Sport and Exercise Psychology, 27*, 271–288.

Saunders, N., Otago, L., Romiti, M., Donaldson, A., White, P., & Finch, C. (2010). Coaches' perspective on implementing an evidence-informed injury prevention programme in junior community netball. *British Journal of Sports Medicine, 44*, 1128–1132.

Schore, A. N. (2014). The right brain is dominant in psychotherapy. *Psychotherapy, 51*, 388–397. DOI: 10.1037/a0037083.

Shadish, W. R., Cook, T. D., & Campell, D. T. (2002). *Experimental and quasiexperimental designs for generalized causal inference*. Cengage Learning.

Slimani, M., Tod, D., Chaabene, H., Miarka, B., & Chamari, K. (2016). Effects of mental imagery on muscular strength in healthy and patient participants: A systematic review. *Journal of Sports Science & Medicine, 15*, 434–450.

Soligard, T., Myklebust, G., Steffen, K., Holme, I., Silvers, H., Bizzini, M., & Andersen, T. E. (2008). Comprehensive warm-up programme to prevent injuries in young female footballers: Cluster randomised controlled trial. *British Medical Journal, 337*, a2469.

Thorborg, K., Krommes, K. K., Esteve, E., Clausen, M. B., Bartels, E. M., & Rathleff, M. S. (2017). Effect of specific exercise-based football injury prevention programmes on the overall injury rate in football: A systematicreview and meta-analysis of the FIFA 11 and 11+ programmes. *British Journal of Sports Medicine, 51*(7), 562–571. https://doi.org/10.1136/bjsports-2016-097066.

Tranaeus, U., Johnson, U., Engström, B., Skillgate, E., & Werner, S. (2015a). A psychological injury prevention group intervention in Swedish floorball. *Knee Surgery, Sports Traumatology, Arthroscopy, 23*, 3414–3420.

Tranaeus, U., Johnson, U., Ivarsson, A., Engström, B., Skillgate, E., & Werner, S. (2015b). Sports injury prevention in Swedish elite floorball players: Evaluation of two consecutive floorball seasons. *Knee Surgery, Sports Traumatology, Arthroscopy, 23*, 899–905.

Vriend, I., Gouttenbarge, V., Finch, C. F., van Mechelen, W., & Verhagen, E. A. L. M. (2017). Intervention strategies used in sport injury prevention studies: A systematic review identifying studies applying the Haddon Matrix. *Sports Medicine, 47*, 2027–2043.

Wampold, B. E. (2015). How important are the common factors in psychotherapy? An update. *World Psychiatry, 14*, 270–277.

Wiese-Bjornstal, D. M. (2010). Psychology and socioculture affect injury risk, response, and recovery in high-intensity athletes: A consensus statement. *Scandinavian Journal of Medicine and Science in Sports, 20*, 103–111. DOI: 10.1111/j.1600-0838.2010.01195.x.

Williams, J. M., & Andersen, M. B. (1998). Psychosocial antecedents of sport injury: Review and critique of the stress and injury model. *Journal of Applied Sport Psychology, 10*(1), 5–25. DOI: 10.1080/10413209808406375.

Zadeh, M. M., Ajilchi, B., Salman, Z., & Kisely, S. (2019). Effect of a mindfulness programme training to prevent the sport injury and improve the performance of semi-professional soccer players. *American Psychiatry*, 27, 589–595. DOI: 10.1177/1039856219859288.

Zouita, S., Zouita, A. B., Kebsi, W., Dupont, G., Ben Abderrahman, A., Ben Salah, F. Z., & Zouhal, H. (2016). Strength training reduces injury rate in elite young soccer players during one season. *Journal of Strength and Conditioning Research, 30*, 1295–1307.

Part II

PSYCHOLOGICAL RESPONSES TO SPORTS INJURY

Despite everybody's best efforts, sports injuries are an unfortunate consequence of recreational or competitive sport participation. We've long known that pre-injury factors can influence how an athlete responds to an injury (Wiese-Bjornstal, 2010), as can a multitude of different factors such as age, sex and sport socioculture. We also know that injury has historically been considered a solely negative experience for athletes that can have a number of implications on mental health. However, more recently, researchers and practitioners have begun to explore how injury can, under the correct conditions, become a more positive developmental experience for injured athletes.

In the first part of Part 2, Diane Wiese-Bjornstal will give you an insight into the different factors that can influence athletes' responses to injury. The chapter will begin by looking at different theoretical approaches to understanding responses to sports injury (e.g. Wiese-Bjornstal, 2010). Following this, Diane will discuss some of the different factors that can influence an athletes' response to injury, such as age, sex and sport socioculture. This understanding is crucial to those working with injured athletes, given that responses to injury can influence injury outcomes (Forsdyke et al., 2016).

Following Diane's chapter, Adam Gledhill will take a look at the downside of sports injury. We know there is a wealth of empirical and anecdotal evidence, which highlights the significant mental health challenges that injured athletes can face (e.g. Putukian, 2016). In particular, Adam will use this chapter to discuss mental health considerations such as chronic fear of reinjury and movement, anxiety, depression and suicidal ideations when managing injured athletes, as well as to highlight appropriate professional bodies and referral networks that you can access to seek further support.

Finally, in ending this section on a more positive note, Chris Hammer, Leslie Podlog and Adam Gledhill will take a look at the upside of sports injury and disability. There is a growing body of literature that has begun to focus on injury being viewed as a more developmental and positive experience. This body of work has often become termed 'sport injury-related growth' (e.g. Salim & Wadey, 2018). With the hope of supporting sports injury practitioners in working with their injured athletes to create a more positive injury experience, this chapter will provide evidence-informed examples of how injury responses can be shaped to be more positive. In doing so, not only are we more likely to protect the mental health of injured athletes, we are also potentially able to facilitate more positive injury outcomes.

References

Forsdyke, D., Smith, A., Jones, M., & Gledhill, A. (2016). Psychosocial factors associated with outcomes of sports injury rehabilitation in competitive athletes: A mixed studies systematic review *British Journal of Sports Medicine, 50*, 537–544.

Putukian, M. (2016). The psychological response to injury in student athletes: A narrative review with a focus on mental health. *British Journal of Sports Medicine, 50*, 145–148.

Salim, J., & Wadey, R. (2018). Can emotional disclosure promote sport injury-related growth? *Journal of Applied Sport Psychology, 30*, 367–387.

Wiese-Bjornstal, D. M. (2010). Psychology and socioculture affect injury risk, response, and recovery in high intensity athletes: A consensus statement. *Scandinavian Journal of Medicine and Science in Sports, 20*, 103–111.

3 PERSONAL AND SITUATIONAL FACTORS AFFECTING PSYCHOLOGICAL RESPONSE TO SPORT INJURIES

Diane M. Wiese-Bjornstal

Athletes are unique and complex individuals training and competing under varied conditions and circumstances. Because of this, research demonstrates that an idiographic approach towards understanding psychological response to sport injuries advantages consideration of the many personal and situational factors that interact to influence them over the course of injury onset, rehabilitation, and return to play. Distinctive athletes represent diverse individual differences such as injury histories as well as psychological, sociodemographic and physical/biological characteristics and are influenced by variable sport, social and rehabilitation situations or environments. As such, it is apparent that there is really no universal or predictable set of psychological responses to sport injuries, no one 'normal' response. The answer to how athletes respond psychologically to sport injuries is, 'it depends'. It depends on many pre-existing, relatively more stable personal and situational factors, which affect the emergent and more state-like or dynamic psychological responses specific to the sport injuries themselves across sport injury lifespans. In other words, normality in the context of psychological response to sport injuries is subjective and idiosyncratic.

INTRODUCTION

In order to illustrate research findings about these personal and situational factors affecting psychological response to sport injuries, the purpose of this chapter is to use the integrated model of psychological response to the sport injury and rehabilitation process (Wiese-Bjornstal et al., 1998) as a conceptual framework guiding the discussion. The first section of the chapter overviews basic concepts concerning psychological response to sport injuries and displays the conceptual model that guides the remainder of the chapter. The second section uses the conceptual model to list and illustrate via brief research examples many of the personal factors influencing psychological response to sport injuries, such as injury, psychological, sociodemographic and physical/biological factors. The third section of the chapter in a similar fashion discusses brief research examples illustrating many of the situational factors influencing psychological response to sport injuries, such as sport, social and environmental factors. The fourth section of the chapter concludes by drawing an illustration of how these research findings could translate into a professional practice application in contexts such as sport psychology, sport coaching and sports medicine care and provides a case study that provides an opportunity to apply chapter concepts.

PSYCHOLOGICAL RESPONSE TO SPORT INJURIES

Psychological response to sport injuries refers to psychological, psychiatric and social constructs and processes that are evident when athletes cope with and manage the short- and long-term consequences or outcomes associated with the challenges and stressors within sport injury situations (Wiese-Bjornstal et al., 2015). Psychological aspects include dynamic cycles of thoughts, feelings and actions related to sport injuries, such as perceptions of poor recovery status leading to frustration and poor rehabilitation adherence. Psychiatric aspects include the prevention, diagnosis and treatment of clinical mental health concerns associated with sport injuries, such as depression and anxiety disorders. Psychosocial aspects refer to intersections of the patient with the external physical or social environment (such as interpersonal communications with healthcare providers), and influences of the social climate or culture with respect to risks, healthcare and return to play (sociocultural aspects, such as the sport norm of playing hurt) (Wiese-Bjornstal et al., 2015).

With respect to these psychological responses, they are subjective and unique to each athlete, and the frequency, intensity, time (duration) and type (FITT) of the cognitive appraisals, emotional responses and behavioural responses seem to depend on a complex person by situation interaction that incorporates consideration of internal and external influences (Wiese-Bjornstal, 2014). These FITT dimensions perhaps serve as characteristics distinguishing between adaptive and maladaptive psychological responses. Athletes who cannot get past certain cognitions such as catastrophizing or ruminations about injuries, or work through affects such as reinjury anxieties or performance fears, will not successfully achieve the hoped for physical and psychological recoveries. One means of better understanding the psychological response to sport injuries is to consider the personal and situational factors influential in athletes' unique situations.

Factors influencing psychological response to sport injuries

The integrated model of psychological response to the sport injury and rehabilitation process (Wiese-Bjornstal et al., 1998) provided a framework for understanding the influence of personal and situational factors individual psychological response to sport injuries (see Figure 3.1). The development of

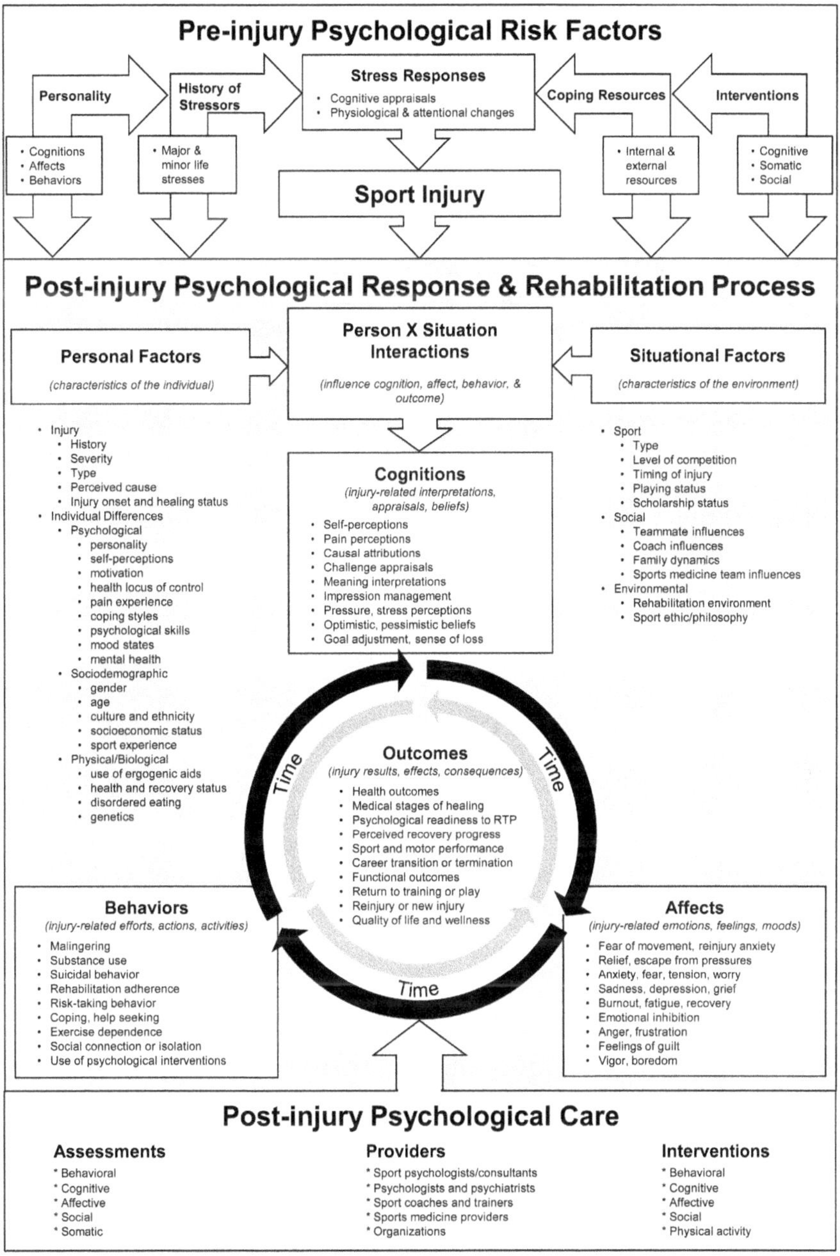

Figure 3.1 Integrated model of psychological response to the sport injury and rehabilitation process (Wiese-Bjornstal, 2019). Adapted from 'An integrated model of response to sport injury: Psychological and sociological dynamics', by D. M. Wiese-Bjornstal et al., 1998, *Journal of Applied Sport Psychology, 10*, p. 49. Copyright 1998 by the Association for Applied Sport Psychology

the model served both research and clinical practice functions, and research from a diverse array of studies and reviews has supported many of the predictions regarding psychological response to sport injuries (e.g. Forsdyke et al., 2016; te Wierike et al., 2013; Wiese-Bjornstal et al., 2012). Within this model, the core dynamic cycle of psychological response to the sport injury derives from the transactional theory of stress (Lazarus & Folkman, 1987). Fluid cycles of cognitions, affect and behaviour represent the psychological response to sport injuries that influence physical and psychological outcomes over the course of a sport injury lifespan (Wiese-Bjornstal et al., 2018).

Personal and situational factors depicted in centre postinjury psychological response and rehabilitation section of the model are the focus of the present chapter. These factors are conceptualized as pre-existing or concomitant factors that are not necessarily in and of themselves specific to the athlete's psychological response to sport injuries but rather as relatively stable factors that initially and throughout the sport injury lifespan influence dynamic responses. Wiese-Bjornstal et al. (1995) conceptualized that these factors would interact based on the dynamic field approach of Lewin (1939) to influence postinjury cognitions, affect, behaviour and outcomes. The remainder of this chapter discussed evidence regarding these interactions and influences of personal and situational factors on psychological response to sport injuries, beginning with personal factors.

PERSONAL FACTORS AFFECTING PSYCHOLOGICAL RESPONSE TO SPORT INJURIES

Personal factors refer characteristics of the individual athlete that might influence psychological response to sport injuries. These personal factors broadly include injury factors and individual differences, as shown in Figure 3.1. The following describe brief examples of research examining these personal factors.

Injury factors

Injury factors refer to characteristics such as an individual's sport injury history, the nature of the current injury situation and perceptions of injury causality and recovery status. The following examples illustrate research showing how injury factors relate to psychological response to sport injuries.

Injury history

Injury history has shown both positive and negative influences on subsequent psychological response to sport injury. Male and female university athletes reporting a history of three or more sport concussions, for example, reported significantly lower quality of life and more frequent headaches than those with two or less prior sport concussions (Kuehl et al., 2010). With respect to orthopedic injuries, Lam and Markbreiter (2019) reported lower health-related quality of life in areas such as physical, school and social functioning among adolescent athletes with a knee injury history compared to their peers with no such history. Collegiate athletes with an ankle sprain history displayed higher levels of fear than did healthy counterparts, especially evident among those with a history of recurrent sprains (Houston et al., 2018).

Injury type and severity

Two of the most studied sport injury types in terms of their influences on post-injury psychological response have been anterior cruciate ligament (ACL) injuries and sport-related concussions (SRC), which associate with slightly different responses. Injury severity based on time-loss has been shown to predict postinjury responses such as mood state among injured athletes (Smith et al., 1993). Athletes with severe injuries undergoing surgical intervention, such as ACL reconstruction (ACLR), have shown high fear of reinjury, high psychological distress, low self-efficacy, high external locus of control and low adherence to rehabilitation (Christino et al., 2015; Nordahl et al., 2014). Stein et al. (2016) showed that the most psychologically distressing aspect of SRC specifically was the loss of physical activity.

Perceived cause of injury

Perceptions of injury causality also have the potential to affect psychological distress associated with injury (Wiese-Bjornstal et al., 2014; Wiese-Bjornstal et al., 2015). Reel et al. (2018), for example, concluded based on their qualitative study of injury and disordered eating behaviour among female professional dancers that 'the dancers also personalized their injuries by taking full, individual responsibility for them; that is, blaming themselves for becoming injured and subsequently engaging in altered eating and exercise behaviors to compensate' (p. 376). A case study of a soccer player sustaining a serious knee injury highlighted the influence of his beliefs about injury causality on psychological response (McArdle, 2010). The athlete perceived that an opposing player deliberately hurt him and felt that his perceptions of intentional injury causality were supported by the observations of teammates and fans. His psychological response was to be angry at the opponent who tackled him, and to feel 'cheated' out of his season and even out of achieving future goals. McArdle reported that 'his anger toward his culpable opponent was so intense that he expressed a desire to injure the culpable party once he was playing competitive soccer again' (p. 74) and that the athlete exhibited signs of posttraumatic stress and depressed mood.

Injury onset and healing status

Injury onset and recovery status refer to the idea that athletes' perceptions and realities concerning their injury onset and recovery status affect psychological response to sport injuries across a sport injury lifespan (Wiese-Bjornstal et al., 2018). Russell and Wiese-Bjornstal (2015) found during the onset of microtrauma injury among novice marathon runners that the psychological narrative reflected two behavioural themes: self-diagnosis and self-treatment, and not taking time off. There appears to be an interval before athletes with microtrauma injuries recognize and acknowledge injury, occurring prior to them seeking treatment from sports medicine providers. Ruddock-Hudson et al. (2014) documented dynamic fluctuations in psychological response to injury in studies among male Australian Rules football players out of play from 9 weeks to 10 months. Their results showed that cognitive, affective and behavioural themes differed across three injury phases: reactions to injury, reactions to rehabilitation and reactions to return to play (Ruddock-Hudson et al., 2014).

Individual differences factors

Individual differences refer to psychological, sociodemographic and physical/biological factors that have been examined within the sport injury psychology literature. These represent some of the many areas of personal differences that make athletes unique and have at least preliminary evidence supporting their importance in understanding psychological response to sport injuries.

Psychological factors

These include factors such as personality, motivation and mental health that influence psychological response to sport injury (see Figure 3.1).

Personality

Several different aspects of personality traits or characteristics have been examined in the research literature, such as hardiness, neuroticism or perfectionism relative to psychological response to sport injuries such as symptom reports and coping strategies. Wadey et al. (2012) showed that adult-mixed sport athletes high in hardiness utilized a broad selection of problem- and emotion-focused coping strategies, whereas athletes low in hardiness used more avoidance coping. A study examining preinjury relationships between personality traits and self-reported postconcussion symptoms among intercollegiate athletes showed that higher neuroticism scores were associated with more symptoms, whereas higher agreeableness scores were associated with fewer symptoms (Merritt et al., 2015). The influence of perfectionism dimensions on the ways in which marathon runners coped with injury was examined by Jowett et al. (2018), who showed that specific subtypes of perfectionism related differentially to the use of problem-focused, emotion-focused and avoidance coping among these adult male and female runners.

Self-perceptions

A wide variety of self-perceptions, those descriptions or appraisals of ourselves and our identities within specific roles or contexts, influence psychological response to sport injuries. Bateman and Morgan (2019) looked at general self-efficacy as a possible mediator of post-traumatic stress disorder symptoms (i.e., thought intrusions, avoidance, hyperarousal) among male and female adult injured athletes from four different sports, suggesting that self-efficacy beliefs 'may be important to coping responses postinjury, while conceivably influencing other injury-related factors, such as injury duration, severity, and chronicity' (p. 149). In a postinjury context, Brewer et al. (2007) found that athletes with higher levels of athletic identity and lower optimism were more vulnerable to persistent negative moods for the first 42 days following surgery. In their mixed methods study of college athletes, Hilliard et al. (2017) concluded that 'personal factors such as athletic identity and situational factors such as athletic trainer influences may combine to influence rehabilitation behavior' (p. 216).

Motivation

Motivational characteristics of individuals, such as sport commitment, passion for one's sport, desire to return to play and burnout, are among the personal factors that influence thoughts, feelings and behaviours postinjury. Weiss (2011), for example, noted that differences in sport commitment types were related to rehabilitation behaviours such as effort and persistence. Iñigo et al. (2015) found that several specific aspects of sport commitment, such as sport enjoyment and social support, motivated athletes' returns to sport following severe sport injuries. In a qualitative study examining the reasons for attitudes and behaviours associated with playing when in pain or injured, Madrigal et al. (2015) observed that passion for the sport, composed of (a) love of the sport, (b) meaning of the sport, and (c) desire to be on the field, influenced rugby players to want to continue playing through pain and injury.

Health locus of control

Health locus of control refers to individuals' appraisals about the sources of control over their health and is important because they correlate with coping behaviours and health outcomes (Wiese-Bjornstal et al., 2018). Examining athletes following ACLR, for example, Nyland et al. (2013) observed that a greater reliance on an internal health locus of control was associated with higher level sport involvement and subjective knee function. Among a diverse sample of adult athletes and exercisers, Wiese-Bjornstal et al. (2018) found that religious or spiritual (R/S) individuals relied to a greater extent than no-R/S individuals on a God health locus of control and the use of active coping strategies while managing the challenges of sport injuries. No-R/S individuals relied to a greater extent than did R/S individuals on an internal health locus of control during sport injuries, such as believing that one's own behaviour had direct responsibility in determining rehabilitation and outcomes.

Pain experience

Anxious and catastrophic thoughts about and experiences with pain influence many bodily systems, such as neuromuscular, cardiovascular, immune and neuroendocrine (Campbell & Edwards, 2009), which can influence cognitions, affects and behaviours. Among recreational athletes, for example, Levy et al. (2009) observed through interviews that lack of motivation and confidence hindered home-based rehabilitation adherence behaviours, whereas ineffective pain coping and social support negatively affected clinic-based rehabilitation adherence. The qualitative work of Hunt and Day (2019) supports consideration of chronic pain and injury as an influence on current and future sports participation and performance. Athletes living with chronic pain and injury described feelings of imprisonment but also developed new coping strategies such as respecting their bodies more and adapting their sport participation engagement. Other research has suggested that pain coping and pain behaviours may differ based on interactions with gender and sport type (Madrigal et al., 2016; Meyers et al., 2015).

Coping style

Coping style refers to dispositional tendencies in the way athletes tolerate or adjust to stressful situations and is related to concepts such as resilience and mental toughness. Coping effectively with perceived major and minor life event stress, particularly negative life event stress, is important to health both before and after sport injury (Williams & Andersen, 1998). For athletes already experiencing significant levels of stress in their lives, sustaining a sport injury not only does not typically alleviate existing life event stress but also may compound and exacerbate perceptions of life event stress and a lack of sufficient coping resources (Wiese-Bjornstal et al., 2012). With respect to coping styles, although avoidance coping is often considered to be a maladaptive coping strategy, Carson and Polman (2010) found that avoidance coping had beneficial aspects among male professional rugby union players recovering from ACLR, such as by withdrawing temporarily from injury environments via the use of physical distraction techniques or developing alternate interests. Religious/spiritual coping showed largely positive influences on sport injury recoveries among religiously committed athletes in a study by Wiese-Bjornstal et al. (2018). Codonhato et al. (2018) found in their study of resilience, stress and injuries among elite rhythmic gymnasts that 'resilient athletes will overcome the unpleasant feelings and emotions following an injury and better deal with the negative psychological aspects of it' (p. 13).

Psychological skills

The inclusion of psychological skills as a personal factor refers to the preinjury or baseline competence of athletes in mental skills such as imagery, goal setting and stress management. However, there is somewhat limited research on the relationship between baseline psychological skill development, its transferability to a sport injury situation and the effects on postinjury psychological response. Milne et al. (2005) found that cognitive and motivational imagery were used by injured athletes more than was healing imagery, and cognitive imagery predicted task self-efficacy for rehabilitation, although it is not clear if imagery skill was in place prior to injury. In their qualitative study of female soccer players returning to play following ACLR, Johnson et al. (2016) found that the ability to set reasonable goals was one of the most important indicators of successful coping with rehabilitation.

Mood states

Mood states refer generally to positively or negatively valenced affective or feeling states that are relatively vague and vary in intensity, which, although transient, can be somewhat dispositional in nature. Early studies of psychological response to sport injuries tracked mood states from baseline through injury recovery (e.g. Morrey et al., 1999) and noted patterns in mood state response that reflected both dispositional and state-like aspects. For example, Wiese-Bjornstal et al. (2012) found that intercollegiate athletes who were injured were more likely to display higher negative mood states before, during and after injury than were their uninjured teammates. Kontos et al. (2019) reported on clinical characteristics and preliminary findings regarding several SRC clinical profiles, showing that one of these profiles, the anxiety/mood clinical profile, is related to personal and situational factors such as medical history, preinjury risk factors and injury information about the specific concussion injury.

Mental health

A significant number of athletes struggle with mental health concerns even prior to injury (Foskett & Longstaff, 2018; Pluhar et al., 2019). For athletes with pre-existing mental health conditions or concerns, recent position statements from key organizations have identified sport injuries as among those stressful sport situations that might trigger or exacerbate mental health concerns, which then affect postinjury psychological cognitions, affects and behaviours (Moesch et al., 2018; Neal et al., 2015; Schinke et al., 2018). In their systematic review, Rice et al. (2016) concluded that injury was a particularly risky triggering event for new or intensified mental health concerns, and Baum (2005) stated that injury was one of the major risk factors for suicide in athletes, particularly when compounded by pre-existing psychopathology.

Sociodemographic factors

These include factors such as gender, age, culture and ethnicity, socioeconomic status (SES), and sport experience. Sociodemographic factors have been shown to be related to psychological response to sport injuries, as illustrated by the following research examples.

Gender

Female and male athletes are relatively similar in cognitive and emotional response to injury, although a few studies do report modest gender differences (Wiese-Bjornstal et al., 2015). With respect to depression, for example, Kontos et al. (2012) found that concussed high school and college athletes experienced elevated depression scores for up to 2 weeks postinjury but showed no significant gender differences in these depression scores. Appaneal et al. (2009) assessed greater depression in injured female athletes based on clinical interviews but found no gender differences in postinjury depression based on athletes' self-reports. With respect to anxiety, Cassidy (2006) found that intercollegiate female athletes overall reported higher levels of sport injury anxiety, and in particular higher anxieties than males about being perceived as weak, experiencing pain, reinjury and impaired self-image.

Age

Sport injury psychology research to date has primarily focused on adolescent to early adult-aged competitive athletes, with limited research on child athletes, middle- to older-aged athletes or on participants from physical activity settings other than competitive sport (Wiese-Bjornstal et al., 2018). Beischer et al. (2019) found that 'adolescent athletes, especially females, perceived enhanced self-efficacy, had a higher return-to-sport rate, and were more motivated to reach their goals after ACL reconstruction compared with adults' (p. 1567). Lichtenstein et al. (2019) noted intersections between age and injury severity among exercisers, reporting that 'injured exercisers with symptoms of depression reported high stress levels and impaired daily functioning, were younger, and were more likely to have over 10 days injury-related work absence' (p. 46).

Culture and ethnicity

The influence of cultural and ethnic differences on psychological response to sport injuries is evident not only research examining populations from many countries around the world, but also in areas such as ethnic or racial differences within countries, religious beliefs and in individuals embracing the unique cultures of their own sports. Arvinen-Barrow et al. (2016) looked across three countries and two categories of sport types at athletes' expectations about sport injury rehabilitation, finding differing expectations of personal commitment to rehabilitation and facilitative conditions of the rehabilitation environment based on both variables. Another relevant aspect of athlete culture and ethnicity within injury contexts is religiosity (Wiese-Bjornstal, 2019).

Chamari et al. (2012), for example, observed that religious behaviours affected injury rates among Muslim professional soccer players competing in Tunisia during the commemoration of Ramadan. An illustration of how the culture of specific sports affects psychological response to sport injuries is evident in the ethnographic study of rhythmic gymnasts by Cavallerio et al. (2016) looking at how sport culture influenced athlete behaviour when dealing with overuse injuries.

Socioeconomic status

SES may directly or indirectly affect psychological response to sport injuries, such as directly or indirectly via attitudes, social interactions or financial constraints on access to high-quality healthcare. Druckman and Rothschild (2018) found among injured athletes that SES 'negatively correlates with perceptions of having a harder life and being tolerant of pain; moreover, those from lower classes are significantly more likely to believe that their family and friends will be disappointed should they be unable to play due to an injury' (Results section). Druckman et al. (2018) examined intersections between racial bias and SES in sports medicine contexts in terms of how this related to interactions with healthcare professionals. They concluded that college medical staff showed racial bias in pain perception and that 'this bias is mediated by socioeconomic status; people seem to assume that Blacks feel less pain but only if and when they assume Blacks have lower socioeconomic status' (Druckman et al., 2018, p. 727). Bejar and Butryn (2016) interviewed lower-to-middle class injured intercollegiate athletes about how SES and related factors (e.g. religion, cultural background, family values) influenced coping with sport injuries. The athletes' psychological response to injury (e.g. catastrophizing, positive reframing) related to their SES backgrounds, leading the authors to conclude that SES represented 'a relevant consideration when examining athletes' response to injury' (Bejar & Butryn, 2016, p. 360).

Sport experience

Socialization through sport experience can influence knowledge, attitudes and behaviours relative to playing through pain and injury. Nippert (2005), for example, found that older high school gymnasts were more likely to compete while injured than were younger high school gymnasts. Lasenby-Lessard and Morrongiello (2011) showed that high sensation seeking children with significant experience and expertise in their physical activities took more physical risks when wearing sport safety gear than when not wearing it. Sport specialization among younger athletes also raises concerns about implicit or explicit pressures from parents, coaches and others to play with and through injuries in ways that may lead to long-term health consequences, burnout and sport dropout (Jayanthi et al., 2013; Wiese-Bjornstal & Wood, 2018). Jayanthi et al. (2018) found that 'high-SES athletes reported more serious overuse injuries than low-SES athletes, potentially due to higher rates of sports specialization, more hours per week playing organized sports, higher ratio of weekly hours in organized sports to free play, and greater participation in individual sports' (p. 303), which may have led them to ignore early warning signs.

Physical/biological factors

Represented within the following research examples are the influences of physical and biological factors on psychological response to sport injuries. These include use of ergogenic aids, health and recovery status, disordered eating and genetics.

Use of ergogenic aids

Substances used to enhance performance, known as ergogenic aids, range from safe to harmful, and legal to illegal. One example is doping in sport, which refers to conscious decisions to consume banned substances for the purpose of enhancing performance through cheating. Whitaker et al. (2014) found among competitive adult athletes that suffering injury was the circumstance within which athletes were most willing to dope. Overbye et al. (2013) similarly found relationships between sport injuries and intended doping behaviour. They reported the results of their survey of elite American athletes from a variety of sports about hypothetical doping scenarios. Relative to incentives for adopting doping behaviours in response to sport injuries, their results showed that 'top incentives were related to…improved health or faster recovery from injury … and the threat [injury] posed to an elite career' (Overbye et al., 2013, p. 119). The use of opiates and analgesics as a means of increasing pain tolerance and the ability to play through pain and injuries, even though it may be legal, also represents a factor that influences psychological response to sport injuries (Wiese-Bjornstal, 2018).

Health and recovery status

Athlete's overall health status, and their general recovery status in terms of resting and recuperating physically and mentally from training and competition, has received significant research attention in the past 10 years in terms of its relationship to injuries (e.g. Lathlean et al., 2019). Lack of recovery refers to inadequate physical and mental recuperation from sport-related stressors associated with training and competition that is detrimental to athlete health and/or performance. Soligard et al. (2016) summarized concerns about lack of recovery as follows.

> We consider the relationship between load and health as a well-being continuum, with load and recovery as mutual counteragents. Sport and non-sport loads impose stress on athletes, shifting their physical and psychological well-being along a continuum that progresses from homeostasis through the stages of acute fatigue, functional and non-functional over-reaching, overtraining syndrome,

> subclinical tissue damage, clinical symptoms, time-loss injury or illness and—with continued loading—ultimately death (Soligard et al., 2016, p. 1030).

Van Der Does et al. (2017) found among team sport players that lower general recovery was associated with greater risk of acute injuries and lower sport recovery was associated with greater risk of overuse injuries. Relative to postinjury responses, the salient point is that there is not always a single demarcation point in 'when' an athlete is injured, as the onset of overuse injuries is insidious and diffuse.

Disordered eating

Sport injuries can trigger new, or exacerbate existing, unhealthy attitudes and behaviours that are associated with the disordered eating continuum. The disordered eating continuum refers to eating behaviours ranging from dieting to clinical eating disorders. Reel et al. (2018) found the following in a study of dancers.

> Many dancers revealed having an eating disorder history and expressed concern about a risk for relapse that could be triggered by having an injury. As Lizzie noted, eating disorders 'get heightened with injury'. Corrine commented that injured dancers 'start to get obsessed with what goes in [their] mouth', especially when they 'had trouble with an eating disorder in the past'. Raven echoed this dysfunctional relationship between eating disordered behaviour and injury, indicating that, following her injury, she started to 'slip back into [her] anorexia' (Reel et al., 2018, pp. 370–371).

Looking at distance runners, Busanich et al. (2014) found through narrative analysis that 'elite athletes who adhere solely to a performance narrative are at risk of using food and exercise primarily as tools to punish and shape the body, especially following periods of perceived performance and/or body failure' (p. 711), such as sport injury.

Genetics

Biopsychosocial approaches and integrative models of psychological, social and healing processes such as the sport injury lifespan and psychological sequelae model (Wiese-Bjornstal et al., 2018) reveal the complexity and interaction of biological, psychological and social influences on response to sport injuries. One study illustrated significant interrelationships between genetic markers and psychological factors (e.g. pain catastrophizing, depressive symptoms) relative to shoulder pain intensity, disability and duration following a 5-day exercise-induced pain protocol among healthy adult participants (George et al., 2014). Puthucheary et al. (2011), suggested that 'the role of genetic variation in determining psychological state and responses remains poorly understood; only recently have specific genes been implicated in motivational behaviour and maintenance of exercise' (p. 846). Within the context of the present discussion, these genetic influences on psychological state and responses could affect factors such as adherence to rehabilitative exercise.

These many personal factors, such as injury factors and individual difference factors, interact with situational factors to influence cognitions, affect, behaviour and outcomes following sport injuries. The next section reviews some of the situational factors affecting psychological response to sport injuries.

SITUATIONAL FACTORS AFFECTING PSYCHOLOGICAL RESPONSE TO SPORT INJURIES

Situational factors refer characteristics of the psychosocial or physical environment that might influence psychological response to sport injuries. These situational factors broadly include sport, social and environmental factors, as shown in Figure 3.1. The following describe brief examples of research examining these situational factors.

Sport factors

Sport factors include sport type, level of competition, timing of injury, playing status and scholarship status. These have all been found to influence psychological response to sport injuries.

Sport type

Sport injuries occur within diverse groups or sport types of physically active participants, including competitive and recreational athletes, exercisers, military trainees, dancers, and extreme or outdoor adventure sport participants of all ages and skill levels (Wiese-Bjornstal et al., 2018). The predominance of research on psychological response to sport injuries has focused on competitive athletes, but even within this category, there are various aspects of sport type that may affect these response, such as individual versus team sports or contact versus non-contact sports. Madrigal et al. (2016) compared female athletes from two contact sports, reporting that rugby athletes higher on mental toughness were more likely to play through injury, whereas roller derby athletes lower on mental toughness were more likely to play through. Further, injured roller derby athletes displayed more negative response to injury than did rugby athletes. Based on a survey of child and adolescent athletes from a sports injury prevention centre, Pluhar et al. (2019) showed that individual sport athletes reported higher levels of anxiety and depression than did team sport athletes and played more so for goal-oriented reasons, which are factors that could affect psychological response to injuries.

Level of competition

Level of play refers to the competitiveness and intensity of training and contests and typically reflects the time commitment allotted to sport as well. As an example of a finding relative to level of competition, athletes undergoing ACLR at higher competitive levels of play reported greater negative affect at return to sport transitions than those at lower levels of play (Morrey et al., 1999). McGannon et al. (2013) explored the media's coverage of the concussion of a high-profile National Hockey League player and uncovered themes illustrating how the normative culture of high level sport relates to concussion narratives. Themes revealed the physically risky and violent nature of professional ice hockey and athletes' acceptance of these risks. The prevailing ethos of toughness and negative effects on perceptions of masculinity if not playing hurt are among the many factors that influence elite athlete thoughts, feelings and actions surrounding sport concussions (McGannon et al., 2013; Wiese-Bjornstal et al., 2015).

Timing of injury

Gayman and Crossman (2003) provided one of the few studies looking explicitly at timing of injury relative to season, event (practice/training or competition) and point in career. They interviewed 20 varsity and recreational basketball players about how the timing of injury onset in hypothetical scenarios would be thought to influence their psychological response to sport injuries. Athletes in their study indicated that preseason injuries would be frustrating, upsetting and terrible, while midseason injuries would be disappointing for many reasons such as missing the social cohesion of playing and traveling with the team. End of season injuries seemed to influence motivation, while postseason injuries might leave athletes feeling devastated and angry. However, their findings strongly illustrated the complex interactions of time in season with related personal and situational factors such as playing status (e.g. starter versus substitute), time in career (e.g. year of eligibility) and injury severity (e.g. time loss) in understanding psychological response to sport injuries (Gayman & Crossman, 2003).

Playing status

Research on playing status, such as starter or substitute, or nonvarsity versus varsity, relative to psychological response to sport injuries also shows interactions with other personal and situational variables. Research on high school football players with knee injuries noted differences in return to play behaviours by playing status and time in season (Baker et al., 2018). Baker et al. found the following:

> Varsity athletes injured during the regular season remained significantly less likely to be out 1–3 weeks or more than three weeks compared with varsity athletes injured in the preseason. Players at the varsity level were returned to the field faster than nonvarsity athletes. Varsity athletes returned to play faster 'in season' than preseason and were also returned faster for injuries that occurred during competition. (pp. 631–632)

Scholarship status

Sport scholarships, such as intercollegiate athletic scholarships, influence athlete motivation, autonomy and behaviour. Cremades et al. (2012) discussed an example of how scholarship status among intercollegiate track and field athletes may influence athletes' psychological response to sport injuries, noting that it affected motivation, return to play decisions and behaviours. Speaking from a sport management and legal perspective, Root (2009) suggested that scholarship status can affect decisions related to athlete health, such as return to play decisions. He stated the following:

> The symbiotic relationship between student-athletes and their universities is ripe for exploitation of the student-athlete's health. The economic incentives associated with successful intercollegiate athletics tempt universities to sacrifice the long-term interests of student-athletes for immediate financial gain. Moreover, conflicts of interest arise when all three parties – the team physician, student-athlete and university – possess incentives to sacrifice the student-athlete's long-term health. Indeed, the significant financial stakes create a 'perfect storm' of conflicts that could compromise the athlete's long-term health. (Root, 2009, p. 287)

Social factors

Social factors refer to social influences, such as social pressure or support and interpersonal interactions. Research examining the influences of teammates, coaches, family and sports medicine team members is next described.

Teammate influences

Teammates are highly salient influences on injured athletes, contributing both social support and social pressure to recovery and return to play behaviours, such as found by Nippert (2005) among female high school gymnasts. Norlin et al. (2016) reported that coaches, teammates, family and sports medicine providers all influenced the psychological response of soccer players in their study. The following excerpts illustrate some of the teammate influences on postinjury response:

> One participant said that the support from the team was quite poor because they never met during the rehabilitation period. Another participant described a complete lack of support. 'I had not played soccer for almost a year. I had no support from the team. No support anywhere'. Many of them also felt that their teammates stopped caring when the rehabilitation took a long time. 'Half of the team disappeared during the first injury, and after the second operation no one was left. They did not wonder how the operation had gone or how I was feeling' (Norlin et al., 2016, p. 182).

Coach influences

Many sport coaches are very supportive to athletes when injured, but others pressure athletes concerning injury reporting and returns to play. Coaches, among others, were among several psychosocial determinants of intentions of high school athletes to report SRC (Register-Mihalik et al., 2013). Determinants predicting higher intentions to report SRC included positive attitudes towards reporting (e.g. perceiving it as important, valuable and beneficial), beliefs about whether others expect reporting (e.g. coaches, teammates, and athletic trainers) and perceived personal control over reporting behaviours. In a study on the causes of overuse injuries, 67% of coaches and athletes interviewed reported that coaches influenced the emergence of overuse injuries (Van Wilgen & Verhagen, 2012). Coach-athlete relationship factors such as poor communication, differing personalities, excessive demands and failure to account for injuries in training plans were among the negative influences perceived as contributing to the onset of overuse injuries.

Family dynamics

Families and family dynamics, such as parents, spouses and siblings, affect athletes' psychological response to injuries. Kroshus et al. (2015) examined pressures from several social sources on intercollegiate athletes' decisions to report injury and continue playing following head impacts. Male and female athletes from team and individual sports who reported feeling greater pressure from teammates, parents/guardians and fans to return to play following head impact were more likely to refrain from reporting their injuries. Podlog et al. (2012) found generally positive forms of social support provided by parents during injury rehabilitations among their children, such as gathering financial resources to fund-needed healthcare, providing transportation to medical appointments, performing rehabilitation exercises along with the patient, and providing positive encouragement and reassurance.

Sports medicine team influences

Athletic trainers, physical therapists and other healthcare providers influence psychological response to sport injuries. Using self-determination theory as a framework, Bejar et al. (2019) found in their qualitative study of rehabilitation experiences that athletic trainer behaviours influenced perceptions of needs satisfaction among athletes. Providing encouragement, soliciting athlete input and building rapport or relationship benefitted need satisfaction, which in turn improved athlete motivation during sport injury rehabilitation. Clement and Shannon (2011) reported that although social support from coaches and teammates was also important, social support from athletic trainers offered the most salient influence on athletes' rehabilitation and well-being. Gender intersections between athlete and athletic trainer affected perceptions of mastery or performance motivational climates in a study by Brinkman-Majewski and Weiss (2018), which in turn affected athletes' intrinsic motivation concerning rehabilitation.

Environmental factors

Environmental factors demonstrate some of the intersections between the social and physical environments surrounding sport. Two examples in this section include the rehabilitation environment and the influences of the sport ethic/ philosophy inherent across sport environments.

Rehabilitation environment

Both the social and physical environments associated with rehabilitation affect thoughts, feelings and behaviours following injury. Fisher and Hoisington (1993) reported that characteristics such as the psychosocial environment and physical accessibility of rehabilitation facilities influenced the psychological response of athletes to injury. They found the following: 'Factors deemed significant to rehabilitation adherence were: (a) good rapport and communication between athletic trainers and injured athletes, (b) support from athletic trainers and coaches, (c) self-motivation on the part of athletes, and (d) convenience, accessibility, and flexibility of the rehabilitation facility and staff' (Fisher & Hoisington, 1993, p. 48). Referencing similar factors, Doyle (2002) referred to this as the importance of cultivating the 'spirit' of the athletic training room in a way that invites, welcomes and includes athletes seeking care. Driediger et al. (2016) found that factors such as the comfort and emotional security of the rehabilitation environment, and the personal characteristics and qualities of the physical therapist, were very important to females high in social physique anxiety in determining their satisfaction with rehabilitation.

Sport ethic/philosophy

Conformity to the cultural expectations for taking risks and playing hurt, such as ignoring pain and proving one's toughness, is an environmental theme often intersecting with many of the personal and social influences (Wiese-Bjornstal, 2018). In their study of youth athletes, Whatman et al. (2018) found that 87% of players reported hiding an injury in order to play. Further, significant numbers of coaches and players had observed athletes playing hurt, while 50% reported witnessing athletes being pressured to play when injured. Among elite youth basketball players, Schneider et al. (2019) found that 6% of the athletes would still play even if medically banned from playing and also showed that the 'willingness to play while hurt, sick or in pain increases significantly with age' (p. 47), but with no gender differences evident. Noting interactions with other personal and situational factors, Mayer et al. (2018) concluded that among elite adolescent athletes, 'the group with the highest WCH [Willingness to Compete Hurt] were athletes from technical sports who have a coach with an autocratic leadership style' (p. 143).

In sum, these situational influences interact with personal factors to affect psychological response of athletes to sport injuries. Recognizing some of these intersections has the potential to benefit the work of sport psychologists, sport coaches and sports medicine providers by informing evidence-based practice through treating athletes holistically and with consideration for the many influences on their cognitive, affective and behavioural responses to sport injuries. The final section of this chapter provides brief examples through interview and case study of how these research findings might inform professional practice.

CONCLUSIONS

The primary conclusion is that personal and situational factors affect psychological response to sport injuries, affirming that although there may be some common patterns of response, normality is subjective in terms of understanding each unique athlete within his or her own distinctive context. These personal and situational factors do not act in isolation, but rather interact to influence psychological response over time. It is also the case, however, that there is a significant need for further research explicitly examining the influences of these factors. From an applied perspective, it is professionally relevant to consider how sport psychologists, sport coaches or sports medicine providers might use this knowledge to advantage their work. This final chapter section provides a brief example of a conversational or interview guide to illustrate an applied strategy derived from the findings outlined in this chapter and concludes with a case study example within which professionals can consider how information learned from this chapter can be relevant in real-life scenarios.

Practical implications

One of the practical implications is that perhaps professionals could utilize as part of the assessment and screening and consulting process a conversation or questionnaire that derives some background information about the personal and situational factors that might be influencing the injured athletes' psychological response to injuries. This would serve to help the professional better 'get to know' the athletes and understand potential influences on their response that may lead the practitioner to differential intervention strategies based on the person by situation interaction profile affecting response to injuries. Other general sport psychology intake interviews (e.g. Performance Interview Guide, PiNG; Aoyagi et al., 2017) and sport injury psychology-specific intake interviews (e.g. Emotional Responses of Athletes to Injury Questionnaire; Smith, 1999) reflected similar ideas about probing insights into factors such as athlete's goals, motivations, supports and pressures. As such, an example outlining some ideas for structuring a practitioner interview or conversation about personal and situational factors affecting athletes' psychological response to sport injuries is shown in Table 3.1.

Table 3.1 Ideas for constructing a practitioner interview or conversation about personal and situational factors affecting the athlete's psychological response to sport injuries:

Instructions: In order to help me better work with you during your injury recovery process, I'd like to ask you if you are willing to share a little bit about yourself and your situation concerning some areas related to me helping you cope with this injury.

No.	*Factor*	*Sample ideas for provider interview or conversation questions*
Personal factors: Characteristics of you as a unique individual		
1.	Injury	a. Tell me a little bit about your history of sport injuries b. What would you like me to know about your current injury, such as the type or severity? c. What do you think was the cause of your injury? d. Where would you say you are at in your recovery process from this current injury?
2.	Individual differences – psychological	a. How would you describe your personality? b. How invested in sport are you, and how motivated are you to return to that same sport? c. What types of coping strategies generally work best for you? d. Does managing pain normally pose any problems for you? e. What do you think is your current mood state, are you feeling mentally strong or are you worried about how you are feeling?
3.	Individual differences – sociodemographic	a. Tell me anything you'd like to about yourself that you think will affect how you cope with this injury, such as your gender identity, age or ethnicity/culture b. Do you have any concerns about your financial situation and how that might affect your healthcare? c. Have you had any prior experiences in sport, or sport injuries, which you think might help or hurt your ability to deal with this current injury?
4.	Individual differences – physical/biological	a. Are you using any substances that you think might affect your ability to recover from this injury? b. How was your physical health status prior to sustaining this injury? Do you feel that your recovery status was good or were you feeling run down? c. Tell me a little bit about your nutritional status, do you feel like you are eating well?
Situational factors: Characteristics of your sport and social environment		
5.	Sport	a. Tell me a little bit about the sport you were playing in when this injury happened, such as the sport type, level of play or time in season b. What was your current playing status on that team, were you a starter, which positions, were you on scholarship, do you plan to return to that sport following recovery? c. Did the injury happen during practice or a game, and what were you doing when it happened?

(*Continued*)

Table 3.1 Ideas for constructing a practitioner interview or conversation about personal and situational factors affecting the athlete's psychological response to sport injuries:

Instructions: In order to help me better work with you during your injury recovery process, I'd like to ask you if you are willing to share a little bit about yourself and your situation concerning some areas related to me helping you cope with this injury. (*Continued*)

No.	*Factor*	*Sample ideas for provider interview or conversation questions*
6.	Social	a. Tell me a little bit about your teammates or training partners, do you think they will affect your sport injury recovery? b. Which kinds of support do you think you can expect from your coaches or sports medicine providers? c. Do you feel any pressure to return to sport quickly or any guilt for not being able to play right now?
7.	Environmental	a. Tell me a little bit about how comfortable you feel going into the athletic training room or other rehabilitation environments? b. Do you feel that you have good access to high-quality rehabilitation services, or are there some barriers preventing you from getting the help and care that you need? c. What do you think the professionals working with you during injury recovery can do to make your rehabilitation a success?

Note: Not all questions are ethically appropriate for all professionals to ask of athletes and so it is important for all providers to stay within their scope of practice, ethics and personal level of comfort asking these types of questions. These sample questions are meant to illustrate that interviews or informal conversations can help providers better understand each athlete as a unique individual in ways that help them understand athletes thoughts, feelings and actions surrounding the rehabilitation process and advantage their ability to provide effective service within their professional roles in benefitting athlete recoveries from sport injuries

Case study

The following case study provides an opportunity to apply concepts learned in this chapter.

Case scenario. Nicole was a 17-year-old senior starter and captain on her high school varsity softball team, hoping to receive an offer of a university sports scholarship before her May graduation. She was driven to excel, a perfectionist and high achiever in academics and music as well as in sports, and she considered herself 'absolutely' an athlete. She was a bit overtrained, burned out and under-recovered as she was simultaneously competing with a premier league youth soccer club. During the regional high school softball championships, with university scouts in the stands and a chance to earn a spot in the state championship playoffs on the line, the unexpected happened. While covering 3rd base for the tag, the baserunner intentionally slid in high with spikes up into Nicole's leg plant leg, causing her ankle to twist awkwardly. She attempted to stand and walk it off, but the ankle was unstable and she fell back to the ground where she was tended to by sports medicine staff. It immediately began to swell, and diagnosis confirmed that Nicole had sustained a grade 2 ankle sprain that would keep her out of sports for an estimated 4–8 weeks. She was worried about telling her father, who was counting on her receiving an athletic scholarship to pay for school since the family did not have the financial resources to support her university tuition. The high school athletic training room was understaffed and so it was difficult to get much personal help or care during rehabilitation, although she was given some treatment and a list of exercises to do at home. Unfortunately her family did not have sufficient medical insurance to pay for additional rehabilitation sessions at a hospital or clinic, and further, it was very difficult to get access to this care because she lived in a rural area where the nearest hospital or clinic was 20 mi away. Nicole's senior softball season was over, her club soccer play was on hold with an uncertain date of return and her chance at a university scholarship was in jeopardy.

Questions to consider

1. Using the integrated model of psychological response to the sport injury and rehabilitation process (Figure 3.1) as a guide and some of the specific examples discussed in this chapter, respond to the following.
   a. What personal factors are evident in Nicole's case that might affect her psychological response to her ankle sprain?
      i. Injury characteristics
      ii. Individual differences – psychological
      iii. Individual differences – sociodemographic
      iv. Individual differences – physical/biological
   b. What situational factors are evident in Nicole's case that might affect her psychological response to the ankle sprain?
      i. Sport
      ii. Social
      iii. Environmental
2. How do you think these personal and situational factors might interact and, as a result, what might you predict to be Nicole's psychological response to the ankle sprain?
   a. Interactions between personal and situational factors
   b. Cognitions
   c. Affects
   d. Behaviours
3. How do you think these personal and situational factors, and the associated psychological response (cognition, affect, behaviour), would influence Nicole's mental and physical recovery outcomes?
4. Looking at the bottom of Figure 3.1 concerning postinjury psychological care, and at Table 3.1 for some ideas about possible interview or conversational questions, how could you use this information about Nicole's personal and situational factors influencing her

psychological response to the ankle sprain to guide practice within the professional role of your choice (e.g. sport psychology consultant, sport coach, sports medicine provider)?

References

Aoyagi, M., Poczwardowski, A., Statler, T., Shapiro, J., Cohen, A., & Brown, R. T. (2017). The performance interview guide: Recommendations for initial consultations in sport and performance psychology. *Professional Psychology: Research and Practice*, *48*, 352–360. https://psycnet.apa.org/doi/10.1037/pro0000121.

Appaneal, R. N., Levine, B. R., Perna, F. M., & Roh, J. L. (2009). Measuring postinjury depression among male and female competitive athletes. *Journal of Sport & Exercise Psychology*, *31*, 60–76. https://www.ncbi.nlm.nih.gov/pubmed/19325188.

Arvinen-Barrow, M., Clement, D., Hamson-Utley, J., Kamphoff, C., Zakrajsek, R., Lee, S., Hemmings, B., Lintunen, T., & Martin, S. (2016). Athletes' expectations about sport-injury rehabilitation: A cross-cultural study. *Journal of Sport Rehabilitation*, *25*, 338–347. http://dx.doi.org/10.1123/jsr.2015-0018.

Baker, C., Browning, S., Charnigo, R., Bunn, T., & Sanderson, W. (2018). Factors related to return to play after knee injury in high school football athletes. *Annals of Epidemiology*, *28*, 629–634. https://doi.org/10.1016/j.annepidem.2018.06.008.

Bateman, A., & Morgan, K. A. D. (2019). The postinjury psychological sequelae of high-level Jamaican athletes: Exploration of a posttraumatic stress disorder–self-efficacy conceptualization. *Journal of Sport Rehabilitation*, *28*, 144–152. https://doi.org/10.1123/jsr.2017-0140.

Baum, A. L. (2005). Suicide in athletes: A review and commentary. *Clinics in Sports Medicine*, *24*(4), 853–869.

Beischer, S., Hamrin Senorski, E., Thomeé, C., Samuelsson, K., & Thomeé, R. (2019). How is psychological outcome related to knee function and return to sport among adolescent athletes after anterior cruciate ligament reconstruction? *American Journal of Sports Medicine*, *47*, 1567–1575. https://doi.org/10.1177/0363546519843073.

Bejar, M. P., & Butryn, T. M. (2016). Experiences of coping with injury in NCAA Division I athletes from low-to-middle socioeconomic status backgrounds. *Journal of Sport Behavior*, *39*, 345–371.

Bejar, M. P., Raabe, J., Zakrajsek, R. A., Fisher, L. A., & Clement, D. (2019). Athletic trainers' influence on national collegiate athletic association division i athletes' basic psychological needs during sport injury rehabilitation. *Journal of Athletic Training*, *54*, 245–254. DOI: 10.4085/1062-6050-112-18.

Brewer, B. W., Cornelius, A. E., Sklar, J. H., Van Raalte, J. L., Tennen, H., Armeli, S., Corsetti, J. R., & Brickner, J. C. (2007). Pain and negative mood during rehabilitation after anterior cruciate ligament reconstruction: A daily process analysis. *Scandinavian Journal of Medicine & Science in Sports*, *17*, 520–529. DOI: 10.1111/j.1600-0838.2006.00601.x.

Brinkman-Majewski, R. E., & Weiss, W. M. (2018). The motivational climate and intrinsic motivation in the rehabilitation setting. *Journal of Sport Rehabilitation*, *27*, 460–468. https://doi.org/10.1123/jsr.2016-0228.

Busanich, R., McGannon, K. R., & Schinke, R. J. (2014). Comparing elite male and female distance runner's experiences of disordered eating through narrative analysis. *Psychology of Sport & Exercise*, *15*, 705–712. http://dx.doi.org/10.1016/j.psychsport.2013.10.002.

Campbell, C. M., & Edwards, R. R. (2009). Mind-body interactions in pain: The neurophysiology of anxious and catastrophic pain-related thoughts. *Translational Research, 153*, 97–101. https://doi.org/10.1016/j.trsl.2008.12.002.

Carson, F., & Polman, R. C. J. (2010). The facilitative nature of avoidance coping within sports injury rehabilitation. *Scandinavian Journal of Medicine & Science in Sports, 20*, 235–240. https://psycnet.apa.org/doi/10.1111/j.1600-0838.2009.00890.x.

Cassidy, C. M. (2006). *Development of a measure of sport injury anxiety: The Sport Injury Appraisal Scale*. Unpublished doctoral dissertation, University of Tennessee. https://trace.tennessee.edu/cgi/viewcontent.cgi?article=3169&context=utk_graddiss.

Cavallerio, F., Wadey, R., & Wagstaff, C. R. D. (2016). Understanding overuse injuries in rhythmic gymnastics: A 12-month ethnographic study. *Psychology of Sport & Exercise, 25*, 100–109. http://dx.doi.org/10.1016/j.psychsport.2016.05.002.

Chamari, K., Haddad, M., Wong, D. P., Dellal, A., & Chaouachi, A. (2012). Injury rates in professional soccer players during Ramadan. *Journal of Sports Sciences, 30*, 93–102. DOI: 10.1080/02640414.2012.696674.

Clement, D., & Shannon, V. R. (2011). Injured athletes' perceptions about social support. *Journal of Sport Rehabilitation, 20*, 457–470. PMID 22012499.

Codonhato, R., Resende, C., Pujals, C., & Fiorese, L. (2018). Resilience, stress and injuries in the context of the Brazilian elite rhythmic gymnastics. *PLoS One, 13*(12), E0210174. https://doi.org/10.1371/journal.pone.0210174.

Cremades, J. G., Flournoy, B., & Gomez, C. B. (2012). Scholarship status and gender differences in motivation among U. S. collegiate track and field athletes. *International Journal of Sports Science & Coaching, 7*, 333–344. https://journals.sagepub.com/doi/10.1260/1747-9541.7.2.333.

Christino, M. A., Fantry, A. J., & Vopat, B. G. (2015). Psychological aspects of recovery following anterior cruciate ligament reconstruction. *Journal of the American Academy of Orthopaedic Surgeons, 23*, 501–509. https://doi.org/10.5435/JAAOS-D-14-00173.

Doyle, M. (2002). A new dimension for the athletic training room: The spirit of the room. *Athletic Therapy Today, 7*(1), 34–35. https://doi.org/10.1123/att.7.1.34.

Driediger, M. V., McKay, C. D., Hall, C. R., & Echlin, P. S. (2016). A qualitative examination of women's self-presentation and social physique anxiety during injury rehabilitation. *Physiotherapy, 102*, 371–376. https://doi.org/10.1016/j.physio.2015.10.001.

Druckman, J. N., & Rothschild, J. E. (2018). Playing with pain: Social class and pain reporting among college student-athletes. *Sport Journal*, 1–8. http://thesportjournal.org/article/playing-with-pain-social-class-and-pain-reporting-among-college-student-athletes/

Druckman, J. N., Trawalter, S., Montes, I., Fredendall, A., Kanter, N., & Rubenstein, A. P. (2018). Racial bias in sport medical staff's perceptions of others' pain. *Journal of Social Psychology, 158*, 721–729. https://doi.org/10.1080/00224545.2017.1409188.

Fisher, A., & Hoisington, L. (1993). Injured athletes' attitudes and judgments toward rehabilitation adherence. *Journal of Athletic Training, 28*, 48–54.

Forsdyke, D., Smith, A., Jones, M., & Gledhill, A. (2016). Psychosocial factors associated with outcomes of sports injury rehabilitation in competitive athletes: A mixed studies systematic review. *British Journal of Sports Medicine, 50*, 537–544. DOI: 10.1136/bjsports-2015-094850.

Foskett, R. L., & Longstaff, F. (2018). The mental health of elite athletes in the United Kingdom. *Journal of Science & Medicine in Sport, 21*, 765–770. https://doi-org.ezp3.lib.umn.edu/10.1016/j.jsams.2017.11.016.

Gayman, A. M., & Crossman, J. (2003). A qualitative analysis of how the timing of the onset of sports injuries influences athlete reactions. *Journal of Sport Behavior, 26*, 255–271.

George, S. Z., Parr, J. J., Wallace, M. R., Wu, S. S., Borsa, P. A., Dai, Y., & Fillingim, R. B. (2014). Biopsychosocial influence on exercise-induced injury: Genetic and psychological combinations are predictive of shoulder pain phenotypes. *The Journal of Pain, 15*, 68–80. DOI: 10.1016/j.jpain.2013.09.012.

Hilliard, R. C., Blom, L., Hankemeier, D., & Bolin, J. (2017). Exploring the relationship between athletic identity and beliefs about rehabilitation overadherence in college athletes. *Journal of Sport Rehabilitation, 26*, 208–220. http://dx.doi.org/10.1123/jsr.2015-0134.

Houston, M. N., Hoch, J. M., & Hoch, M. C. (2018). College athletes with ankle sprain history exhibit greater fear-avoidance beliefs. *Journal of Sport Rehabilitation, 27*, 419–423. https://doi.org/10.1123/jsr.2017-0075.

Hunt, E. R., & Day, M. C. (2019). Narratives of chronic pain in sport. *Journal of Clinical Sport Psychology, 13*, 1–16. https://doi.org/10.1123/jcsp.2017-0003.

Iñigo, M. M., Podlog, L., & Hall, M. S. (2015). Why do athletes remain committed to sport after severe injury? An examination of the sport commitment model. *The Sport Psychologist, 29*, 143–155. http://dx.doi.org/10.1123/tsp.2014-0086.

Jayanthi, N. A., Holt, D. B., LaBella, C. R., & Dugas, L. R. (2018). Socioeconomic factors for sports specialization and injury in youth athletes. *Sports Health: A Multidisciplinary Approach, 10*, 303–310. https://doi.org/10.1177/1941738118778510.

Jayanthi, N., Pinkham, C., Dugas, L., Patrick, B., & LaBella, C. (2013). Sports specialization in young athletes: Evidence-based recommendations. *Sports Health: A Multidisciplinary Approach, 5*, 251–257. DOI: 10.1177/1941738112464626.

Johnson, U., Ivarsson, A., Karlsson, J., Hägglund, M., Waldén, M., & Börjesson, M. (2016). Rehabilitation after first-time anterior cruciate ligament injury and reconstruction in female football players: A study of resilience factors. *BMC Sports Science, Medicine & Rehabilitation, 8*, 1–8. DOI: 10.1186/s13102-016-0046-9.

Jowett, G. E., Hill, A. P., Forsdyke, D., & Gledhill, A. (2018). Perfectionism and coping with injury in marathon runners: A test of the 2 × 2 model of perfectionism. *Psychology of Sport & Exercise, 37*, 26–32. https://doi.org/10.1016/j.psychsport.2018.04.003.

Kontos, A. P., Covassin, T., Elbin, R. J., & Parker, T. (2012). Depression and neurocognitive performance after concussion among male and female high school and collegiate athletes. *Archives of Physical Medicine and Rehabilitation, 93*, 1751–1756. DOI: 10.1016/j.apmr.2012.03.032.

Kontos, A. P., Sufrinko, A., Collins, M. W., Sandel, N., & Kouros, E. (2019). Sport-related concussion clinical profiles: Clinical characteristics, targeted treatments, and preliminary evidence. *Current Sports Medicine Reports, 18*, 82–92. https://doi.org/10.1249/JSR.0000000000000573.

Kroshus, E., Garnett, B., Hawrilenko, M., Baugh, C. M., & Calzo, J. P. (2015). Concussion under-reporting and pressure from coaches, teammates, fans, and parents. *Social Science & Medicine, 134*, 66–75. DOI: 10.1016/j. socscimed.2015.04.011.

Kuehl, M. D., Snyder, A. R., Erickson, S. E., & McLeod, T. C. (2010). Impact of prior concussions on health-related quality of life in collegiate athletes. *Clinical Journal of Sport Medicine, 20,* 86–91. DOI: 10.1097/JSM.0b013e3181cf4534.

Lam, K. C., & Markbreiter, J. G. (2019). The impact of knee injury history on health-related quality of life in adolescent athletes. *Journal of Sport Rehabilitation, 28,* 115–119. https://doi.org/10.1123/jsr.2017-0226.

Lasenby-Lessard, J., & Morrongiello, B. A. (2011). Understanding risk compensation in children: Experience with the activity and level of sensation seeking play a role. *Accident Analysis & Prevention, 43,* 1341–1347. http://dx.doi.org/10.1016/j.aap.2011.02.006.

Lathlean, T. J. H., Gastin, P. B., Newstead, S. V., & Finch, C. F. (2019). A prospective cohort study of load and wellness (sleep, fatigue, soreness, stress, and mood) in elite junior Australian Football players. *International Journal of Sports Physiology & Performance, 14,* 839–840. https://doi.org/10.1123/ijspp,2018-0372.

Lazarus, R. S., & Folkman, S. (1987). Transactional theory and research on emotions and coping. *European Journal of Personality, 1,* 141–169. DOI: 10.1002/per.2410010304.

Levy, A. R., Polman, R. C. J., Nicholls, A. R., & Marchant, D. C. (2009). Sport injury rehabilitation adherence: Perspectives of recreational athletes. *International Journal of Sport & Exercise Psychology, 7,* 212–229. https://psycnet.apa.org/doi/10.1080/1612197X.2009.9671901.

Lewin, K. (1939). Field theory and experiment in social psychology: Concepts and methods. *American Journal of Sociology, 44,* 868–896.

Lichtenstein, M. B., Gudex, C., Andersen, K., Bojesen, A. B., & Jørgensen, U. (2019). Do exercisers with musculoskeletal injuries report symptoms of depression and stress? *Journal of Sport Rehabilitation, 28,* 46–51. https://doi.org/10.1123/jsr.2017-0103.

Madrigal, L., Robbins, J., Gill, D. L., & Wurst, K. (2015). A pilot study investigating the reasons for playing through pain and injury: Emerging themes in men's and women's collegiate rugby. *The Sport Psychologist, 29,* 310–318. http://dx.doi.org/10.1123/tsp.2014-0139.

Madrigal, L., Wurst, K., & Gill, D. L. (2016). The role of mental toughness in coping and injury response in female roller derby and rugby athletes. *Journal of Clinical Sport Psychology, 10,* 137–154. http://dx.doi.org/10.1123/JCSP.2015-0021.

Mayer, J., Giel, K. E., Malcolm, D., Schneider, S., Diehl, K., Zipfel, S., & Thiel, A. (2018). Compete or rest? Willingness to compete hurt among adolescent elite athletes. *Psychology of Sport & Exercise, 25,* 143–150. https://doi.org/10.1016/j.psychsport.2017.12.004.

McArdle, S. (2010). Psychological rehabilitation from anterior cruciate ligament-medial collateral ligament reconstructive surgery: A case study. *Sports Health, 2,* 73–77. https://dx.doi.org/10.1177%2F1941738109357173.

McGannon, K. R., Cunningham, S. M., & Schinke, R. J. (2013). Understanding concussion in socio-cultural context: A media analysis of a National Hockey League star's concussion. *Psychology of Sport & Exercise, 14,* 891–899. DOI: 10.1016/j.psychsport.2013.08.003.

Merritt, V. C., Rabinowitz, A. R., & Arnett, P. A. (2015). Personality factors and symptom reporting at baseline in collegiate athletes. *Developmental Neuropsychology, 40,* 45–50. https://psycnet.apa.org/doi/10.1080/87565641.2014.979928.

Meyers, M. C., Higgs, R., LeUnes, A. D., Bourgeois, A. E., & Matthew Laurent, C. (2015). Pain-coping traits of nontraditional women athletes: Relevance to optimal treatment and rehabilitation. *Journal of Athletic Training, 50,* 1034–1041. DOI: 10.4085/1062-6050-50.8.04.

Milne, M., Hall, C., & Forwell, L. (2005). Self-efficacy, imagery use, and adherence to rehabilitation by injured athletes. *Journal of Sport Rehabilitation, 14*, 150–167. https://psycnet.apa.org/record/2005-05674-001.

Moesch, K., Kenttä, G., Kleinert, J., Quignon-Fleuret, C., Cecil, S., & Bertollo, M. (2018). FEPSAC position statement: Mental health disorders in elite athletes and models of service provision. *Psychology of Sport & Exercise, 38*, 61–71. http://dx.doi.org/10.1016/j.psychsport.2018.05.013.

Morrey, M. A., Stuart, M. J., Smith, A. M., & Wiese-Bjornstal, D. M. (1999). A longitudinal examination of athletes' emotional and cognitive response to anterior cruciate ligament injury. *Clinical Journal of Sports Medicine, 9*(2), 63–69. https://www.ncbi.nlm.nih.gov/pubmed/10442619.

Neal, T. L., Diamond, A. B., Goldman, S., Liedtka, K. D., Mathis, K., Morse, E., & Quandt, E. (2015). Interassociation recommendations for developing a plan to recognize and refer student-athletes with psychological concerns at the secondary school level: A consensus statement. *Journal of Athletic Training, 50*, 231–249. https://dx.doi.org/10.4085%2F1062-6050-50.3.03.

Nippert, A. H. (2005). *"I have four months to compete, eight months to heal". The sport ethic and girls' interscholastic gymnastics participation: What does it mean to play through pain.* Doctoral dissertation. Retrieved from ProQuest Dissertations and Theses Database (ATT 3167684).

Nordahl, B., Sjöström, R., Westin, M., Werne, S., & Alricsson, M. (2014). Experiences of returning to elite alpine skiing after ACL injury and ACL reconstruction. *International Journal of Adolescent Medicine and Health, 26*, 69–77. https://doi.org/10.1515/ijamh-2012-0114.

Norlin, T., Fitzgerald, U. T., & Alricsson, M. (2016). Barriers to and possibilities of returning to play after a severe soccer injury: A qualitative study. *European Journal of Physiotherapy, 18*, 179–184. http://dx.doi.org/10.3109/21679169.2016.1174296.

Nyland, J., Mauser, N., & Caborn, D. (2013). Sports involvement following ACL reconstruction is related to lower extremity neuromuscular adaptations, subjective knee function and health locus of control. *Knee Surgery, Sports Traumatology, Arthroscopy, 21*, 2019–2028. DOI: 10.1007/s00167-013-2366-6.

Overbye, M. L., Knudsen, M., & Pfister, G. (2013). To dope or not to dope: Elite athletes' perceptions of doping deterrents and incentives. *Performance Enhancement and Health, 2*, 119–134. DOI: 10.1016/j.peh.2013.07.001.

Pluhar, E., McCracken, C., Griffith, K. L., Christino, M. A., Sugimoto, D., & Meehan III, W. P. (2019). Team sport athletes may be less likely to suffer anxiety or depression than individual sport athletes. *Journal of Sports Science & Medicine, 18*, 490–496. http://www.jssm.org/

Podlog, L., Kleinert, J., Dimmock, J., Miller, J., & Shipherd, A. (2012). A parental perspective on adolescent injury rehabilitation and return to sport experiences. *Journal of Applied Sport Psychology, 24*, 175–190. DOI: 10.1080/10413200.2011.608102.

Puthucheary, Z., Skipworth, J. R. A., Rawal, J., Loosemore, M., Van Someren, K., & Montgomery, H. E. (2011). Genetic influences in sport and physical performance. *Sports Medicine, 41*, 845–859. DOI: 10.2165/11593200-000000000-00000.

Rabinowitz, A.R., Li, X., & Levin, H.S. (2014). Sport and nonsport etiologies of mild traumatic brain injury: Similarities and differences. *Annual Review of Psychology, 65*, 301–331. DOI: 10.1146/annurev-psych-010213-115103.

Reel, J. J., Podlog, L., Hamilton, L., Greviskes, L., Voelker, D. K., & Gray, C. (2018). Injury and disordered eating behaviors: What is the connection for female professional dancers? *Journal of Clinical Sport Psychology, 12*, 365–381. https://doi.org/10.1123/jcsp.2017-0007.

Register-Mihalik, J. K., Linnan, L. A., Marshall, S. W., Valovich McLeod, T. C., Mueller, F. O., & Guskiewicz, K. M. (2013). Using theory to understand high school aged athletes' intentions to report sport-related concussion: Implications for concussion education initiatives. *Brain Injury, 27*, 878–886. DOI: 10.3109/02699052.2013.775508.

Rice, S., Purcell, R., Silva, S., Mawren, D., McGorry, P., & Parker, A. (2016). The mental health of elite athletes: A narrative systematic review. *Sports Medicine, 46*, 1333–1353. DOI: 10.1007/s40279-016-0492-2.

Root, B. C. (2009). How the promises of riches in collegiate athletics lead to the compromised long-term health of student-athletes: Why and how the NCAA should protect its student-athletes' health. *Health Matrix: Journal of Law-Medicine, 19*, 279–315. http://scholarlycommons.law.case.edu/healthmatrix.

Ruddock-Hudson, M., O'Halloran, P., & Murphy, G. (2014). The psychological impact of long-term injury on Australian Football League players. *Journal of Applied Sport Psychology, 26*, 377–394. DOI: 10.1080/10413200.2014.897269.

Russell, H. C., & Wiese-Bjornstal, D. M. (2015). Narratives of psychological response to microtrauma injury among long-distance runners. *Sports, 3*, 159–177. DOI: 10.3390/sports3030159.

Schinke, R. J., Stambulova, N. B., Si, G., & Moore, Z. (2018). International society of sport psychology position stand: Athletes' mental health, performance, and development. *International Journal of Sport and Exercise Psychology, 16*, 632–639. https://doi.org/10.1080/1612197X.2017.1295557.

Schneider, S., Sauer, J., Berrsche, G., Löbel, C., & Schmitt, H. (2019). "Playing hurt": Competitive sport despite being injured or in pain. *German Journal of Sports Medicine, 70*, 43–52. DOI: 10.5960/dzsm.2019.365.

Smith, A. M. (1999). Assessing athletes through individual interview. In R. Ray & D. M. Wiese-Bjornstal (Eds.), *Counseling in sports medicine* (pp. 75–91). Human Kinetics.

Smith, A. M., Stuart, M. J., Wiese-Bjornstal, D. M., Milliner, E. K., O'Fallon, W. M., & Crowson, C. S. (1993). Competitive athletes: Preinjury and postinjury mood state and self-esteem. *Mayo Clinic Proceedings, 68*, 939–947. https://doi.org/10.1016/s0025-6196(12)62265-4.

Soligard, T., Schwellnus, M., Alonso, J., Bahr, R., Clarsen, B., Dijkstra, H. P., Gabbett, T., Gleeson, M., Hägglund, M., Hutchinson, M. R., van Rensburg, C. J., Khan, K. M., Meeusen, R., Orchard, J. W., Pluim, B. M., Raftery, M., Budgett, R., & Engebretsen, L. (2016). How much is too much? (Part 1): International Olympic Committee consensus statement on load in sport and risk of injury. *British Journal of Sports Medicine, 50*, 1030–1041. DOI: 10.1136/bjsports-2016-096581.

Stein, C., MacDougall, R., Quatman-Yates, C., Myer, G., Sugimoto, D., Dennison, R., & Meehan, W. (2016). Young athletes' concerns about sport-related concussion: The patient's perspective. *Clinical Journal of Sport Medicine, 26*, 386–390. DOI: 10.1097/JSM.0000000000000268.

te Wierike, S. C. M., van der Sluid, A., van den Akker-Scheek, L., Elferink-Gemser, M. T., & Visscher, C. (2013). Psychological factors influencing the recovery of athletes with anterior cruciate ligament injury: A systematic review. *Scandinavian Journal of Sports Medicine, 23*, 527–540. DOI: 10.1111/sms.12010.

Van Der Does, H., Brink, M., Otter, R., Visscher, C., & Lemmink, K. (2017). Injury risk is increased by changes in perceived recovery of team sport players. *Clinical Journal of Sport Medicine, 27*, 46–51. DOI: 10.1097/JSM.0000000000000306.

Van Wilgen, C. P., & Verhagen, E. A. L. M. (2012). A qualitative study on overuse injuries: The beliefs of athletes and coaches. *Journal of Science & Medicine in Sport, 15*, 116–121. https://doi.org/10.1016/j.jsams.2011.11.253.

Wadey, R., Evans, L., Hanton, S., & Neil, R. (2012). An examination of hardiness throughout the sport-injury process: A qualitative follow-up study. *British Journal of Health Psychology, 17*, 872–893. DOI: 10.1111/j.2044-8287.2011.02025.x.

Weiss, W. M. (2011). Longitudinal analysis of sport commitment types: Does injury play a role? *International Journal of Sport Psychology, 42*, 565–585. http://www.ijsp-online.com/abstract/view/42/565.

Whatman, C., Walters, S., & Schluter, P. (2018). Coach and player attitudes to injury in youth sport. *Physical Therapy in Sport, 32*, 1–6. https://doi.org/10.1016/j.ptsp.2018.01.011.

Whitaker, L., Long, J., Petroczi, A., & Backhouse, S. (2014). Using the prototype willingness model to predict doping in sport. *Scandinavian Journal of Medicine & Science in Sports, 24*, 398–405. DOI: 10.1111/sms.12148.

Wiese-Bjornstal, D. M. (2014). Sport injury psychology. In A. Ivarsson & U. Johnson (Eds.), *Psychological bases of sport injuries* (4th ed.). FIT Publishing.

Wiese-Bjornstal, D. M. (2018). Sociocultural aspects of sport injury and recovery. In *Oxford research encyclopedia of psychology*. Oxford University Press. http://dx.doi.org/10.1093/acrefore/9780190236557.013.174.

Wiese-Bjornstal, D. M. (2019). Christian beliefs and behaviours as health protective, resilience, and intervention factors in the context of sport injuries. In B. Hemmings, N. J. Watson, & A. Parker (Eds.), *Sport psychology and Christianity: Welfare, performance and consultancy* (pp. 54–70). Routledge.

Wiese-Bjornstal, D. M., Albinson, C. B., Henert, S. E., Arendt, E. A., Schwenz, S. J., Myers, S. S., & Gardetto-Heller, D. M. (2012). Evaluating the dynamic model of psychological response to sport injury and rehabilitation. In J. H. Bastos & A. C. Silva (Eds.), *Athlete performance and injuries* (pp. 79–98). Nova Science Publishers.

Wiese-Bjornstal, D. M., Franklin, A. N., Dooley, T. N., Foster, M. A., & Winges, J. B. (2015). Observations about sports injury surveillance and sports medicine psychology among female athletes. *Women in Sport and Physical Activity Journal, 23*, 64–73. http://dx.doi.org/10.1123/wspaj.2014-0042.

Wiese-Bjornstal, D. M., Smith, A. M., & LaMott, E. E. (1995). A model of psychologic response to athletic injury and rehabilitation. *Athletic Training: Sports Health Care Perspectives, 1*(1), 16–30.

Wiese-Bjornstal, D. M., Smith, A. M., Shaffer, S. M., & Morrey, M. A. (1998). An integrated model of response to sport injury: Psychological and sociological dynamics. *Journal of Applied Sport Psychology, 10*, 46–69. https://doi.org/10.1080/10413209808406377.

Wiese-Bjornstal, D. M., White, A. C., Russell, H. C., & Smith, A. M. (2015). Psychology of sport concussions. *Kinesiology Review, 4*, 169–189. http://dx.doi.org/10.1123/kr.2015-0012.

Wiese-Bjornstal, D. M., White, A. C., Wood, K. N., & Russell, H. C. (2018). Sports medicine psychology. In T. S. Horn & A. L. Smith (Eds.), *Advances in sport and exercise psychology* (4th ed.) (pp. 387–408). Human Kinetics.

Wiese-Bjornstal, D. M., & Wood, K. N. (2018). Sport injuries among female children and youth. In *2018 Report of the Tucker Center for Research on Girls & Women in Sport, Developing physically active girls: An evidence-based multidisciplinary approach* (pp. 73–98). University of Minnesota. https://www.cehd.umn.edu/tuckercenter/library/docs/research/2018-Tucker-Center-Research-Report_Developing-Physically-Active-Girls_Full-Report.pdf.

Wiese-Bjornstal, D. M., Wood, K. N., & Kronzer, J. R. (2018). Sport injuries and psychological sequelae. In G. Tennenbaum & R. Eklund (Eds.), *Handbook of sport psychology* (4th ed., Vol. 1) (pp. xx–xx). Wiley.

Wiese-Bjornstal, D. M., Wood, K. N., White, A. C., Wambach, A. J., & Rubio, V. J. (2018). Exploring religiosity and spirituality in coping with sport injuries. *Journal of Clinical Sport Psychology*, Advance online publication, 1–35. https://doi.org/10.1123/jcsp.2018-0009.

Williams, J. M., & Andersen, M. B. (1998). Psychosocial antecedents of sport injury: Review and critique of the stress and injury model. *Journal of Applied Sport Psychology, 10*, 5–25. http://dx.doi.org/10.1080/10413209808406375.

4 THE DOWNSIDE OF SPORTS INJURY

POOR MENTAL HEALTH IN INJURED ATHLETES

Dr Adam Gledhill

Despite the oft superhuman persona, athletes are not immune to poor mental health (Gorczynski et al., 2019). There are many reasons that athletes might experience poor mental health and let's not sugar coat this: but for a few specific examples, sport injury – especially severe sports injury – is something that athletes don't want to go through. Whilst it is possible for athletes to experience growth as a result of their injury and the associated experiences, a sport injury is something that athletes would rather avoid. Many athletes interpret severe sports injury as a major negative life event (Chang et al., 2020; Gouttebarge et al., 2019; Putukian, 2016; Souter et al., 2018), with experts viewing sudden and prolonged sports injury as a contributor to poor mental health in athletes (Gorczynski et al., 2019).

Whilst responses to such sports injuries are relatively individual in nature (e.g. Wiese-Bjornstal et al., 1998), they can be categorized under one of two broad categories: (1) typical responses (also referred to as normal responses) and (2) problematic or negative responses. These two broad categories refer to the notions that there are certain responses to a sports injury that can be reasonably expected as a natural part of the injury process (i.e. are quite typical or normal and, crucially, they subside), with examples of these including sadness, perceived isolation, anger, frustration, decreased motivation and altered sleep patterns (Forsdyke et al., 2016; Putukian, 2016). Conversely, more problematic responses to sports injuries are those which maintain (i.e. they do not subside), worsen over time, or where the severity of the symptoms seems excessive (Putukian, 2016). These responses can manifest at different stages of the sports injury, starting with the immediate response to injury and if not appropriately monitored and addressed, can remain after an athlete has returned to performance (e.g. Gledhill et al., 2020) and can negatively impact on rehabilitation outcomes (Forsdyke et al., 2016). Despite recognition of these views, support for athletes to manage these problematic responses to injury, or athletes who engage in help-seeking behaviours, is still stigmatized in certain environments and can be restrictive to athletes accessing this support (e.g. Gouttebarge et al., 2016).

Just as an athlete's physical health is one of their significant occupational resources (i.e. physically healthier athletes can perform better), so is their mental health. Indeed, the World Health Organization defines mental health as 'a state of wellbeing in which every individual realizes her or his own potential, can cope with the normal stresses of life, can work productively and fruitfully, and is able to make a contribution to her or his community' (WHO, 2014). It stands to reason, therefore, that an athlete's mental health is a resource that could help them perform well, deal with stress and contribute to achieving team and individual goals. In the context of sports injury, this could mean they are better able to manage injury-related setbacks and work diligently towards achieving rehabilitation goals. However, an athlete's progress towards and subsequent return to physical health tends to be the prime focus of injury rehabilitation, with less attention afforded to mental health (Gouttebarge et al., 2016, 2019). Therefore, enhancing mental health literacy (MHL) (e.g. Gorczynski et al., 2019; Jorm et al., 1997) as pertains to the context of sports injury is an important function of this chapter.

Consequently, the purposes of this chapter are to (1) summarize knowledge on poor mental health, symptoms and disorders associated with sports injury; (2) discuss barriers and facilitators to help-seeking behaviours in sport; (3) provide evidence-informed strategies for improving mental health in injured athletes and (4) present an applied case study for consideration. Consistent with current expert and consensus statements (e.g. Castaldelli-Maia et al., 2019; Gorczynski et al., 2019), the terms 'poor mental health' and 'mental health symptoms and disorders' will be used throughout this chapter.

MENTAL HEALTH SYMPTOMS AND DISORDERS IN INJURED ATHLETES

The relationship between sports injuries and different mental health symptoms and disorders is well established across sports and populations (Gouttebarge et al., 2015, 2016, 2019; Putukian, 2016; Reardon et al., 2019). This section of the chapter will summarize the key relationships with this body of research, to demonstrate the scale of the problem and form the foundations of understanding the need for increased mental health support for athletes. The foci within this chapter will be on depression, fear, anxiety, post-traumatic stress disorder (PTSD), their associated symptoms, links to rehabilitation outcomes and their relationships to other maladaptive behaviours in injured athletes.

DEPRESSION AND DEPRESSIVE SYMPTOMS

Sports injury is a prominent risk factor for depression that has been reported and discussed across different contexts, including student athletes (Putukian, 2016), elite athletes (Gouttebarge et al., 2019), men athletes (Souter et al., 2018), men soccer players (Gouttebarge et al., 2015, 2016) and NFL players (e.g. Didebahni et al., 2013). As well as being problematic in and of itself, depression contributes to other responses (e.g. sleep disturbance, adverse alcohol and substance misuse; suicidal ideations) in athletic populations. These additional responses can be triggered by a sense of loss following severe injury, or not being able to play or train following injury, and can have subsequent further injury risk. For example, according to the Biopsychosocial Model of Athletic Injury and Health (Appaneal & Perna, 2014), sleep disturbance is a risk factor for both illness and injury.

Reviewing literature into depression in student athlete populations, Putukian (2016) offered stark observations between depression, injury and suicide. When discussing Smith and Milliner's (1994) work examining suicide in student athletes, Putukian (2016, p. 146) summarized five common factors of people who completed suicide: (1) considerable success before injury, (2) serious injury requiring suicide, (3) long rehabilitation with restriction from play, (4) inability to return to pre-injury levels of performance and (5) being replaced in their position by a team mate.

FEAR OF RE-INJURY

Fear of re-injury is considered to be a biological response to the danger posed by sports injury (Walker et al., 2010). It is one of the most frequently investigated and reported negative responses to injury (e.g. Forsdyke et al., 2016; Truong et al., 2020). It is experienced by both adolescent and adult athletes (Forsdyke et al., 2016) and has been noted as a standalone (Ross et al., 2017) and contributory (Tjong et al., 2013) factor for poorer rehabilitation outcomes. Fear of re-injury can subsequently increase the risk of re-injury because of avoidance or reduced effort (Bateman & Morgan, 2019). Athletes experiencing fear of re-injury may be hesitant to fully engage within rehabilitation activities, with this lack of engagement contributing to reduced rehabilitation progress and recovery rates (Forsdyke et al., 2016; Hsu et al., 2017). For example, athletes with high levels of self-reported fear of re-injury (measured using the Tampa Scale of Kinesiophobia) were four times more likely to report lower levels of activity and those with high levels of self-reported fear were up to 13 times more likely to suffer a second ACL injury after ACL reconstruction (Paterno et al., 2018).

Appropriate psychological interventions can be used to reduce fear of re-injury (Hsu et al., 2017; Rodriguez et al., 2019). Hsu et al. (2017) summarized existing evidence on psychosocial interventions and their impact on sports injury, noting that education, goal setting, imagery, self-talk, social support and relaxation activities can all be used to manage fear of re-injury. Education can improve an athlete's knowledge of their injury and expected progress, which can reduce fear through a greater awareness and perceived control. Goal setting can provide direction and increase perceptions of treatment efficacy. Imagery can enhance sport and injury-related confidence, as well as reducing stress hormone secretion. Self-talk can help athletes to recognize and change negative thoughts. Social support is multifaceted but generally can increase an athlete's perceived connectedness to others as well as enhancing their feelings of being informationally supported. Finally, relaxation can be used to reduce tension and fear-related symptoms. As can be seen, there are different options that can be used to reduce fear of re-injury, as well as any concurrent re-injury anxiety (Gledhill, 2016; Gledhill et al., 2020; Hsu et al., 2017; Rodriguez et al., 2019).

ANXIETY

Anxiety is a prominent consideration with injured athletes (Forsdyke et al., 2016). Injured athletes report more severe generalized anxiety disorder symptoms than non-injured athletes (Reardon et al., 2019). Moreover, re-injury anxiety is a negative emotional response to injury with cognitive and somatic symptoms that manifest themselves due to the chances of injury recurrence, of the same type as the original injury (Walker & Thatcher, 2011). Re-injury anxiety can be caused by surgery, the timing of the surgery following injury, the requirement to perform under the same circumstances that elicited the injury, a lack of confidence in the injured body part and concerns over rehabilitation setbacks (Ardern et al., 2013; Forsdyke et al., 2016). It has been identified as a factor in reduced chances of successful return to sport (Forsdyke et al., 2016).

POST-TRAUMATIC STRESS DISORDER

PTSD is an exposure to trauma followed by at least 1 month of mental health symptoms, can be experienced by athletes as a result of sports injury (Reardon et al., 2019). Sport-related musculo-skeletal injury is associated with elevated PTSD symptomology (Bateman & Morgan, 2019; Padaki et al., 2018). PTSD symptoms – specifically avoidance, intrusion and hyperarousal – were recorded in patients who had suffered ACL injuries, with athletes in the 15–21 age range and those with higher levels of athletic identity displaying symptoms to a greater degree (Padaki et al., 2018). However, the elevated symptoms in the higher athletic identity group did not reach statistical significance.

Athletes who have experienced sport-related concussion also demonstrate PTSD symptomology (e.g. Brassil & Salvatore, 2018). Specifically, post-concussion athletes reported symptoms including struggling to get thoughts about the incident out of their head and having flashbacks.

Symptomology of PTSD can occur at any time, but particularly during situations similar to the original injury-inciting event (Bateman & Morgan, 2019). Trauma-related symptoms include avoiding physical and psychological reminders of the injury, re-experiencing symptoms (e.g. nightmares, flashbacks, intrusive thoughts), dissociation and irritability (Reardon et al., 2019). Trauma-related complaints may also include poorer rehabilitation progress, decreased sport performance and somatic complaints without any evident injury/re-injury (e.g. Gledhill, 2016; Reardon et al., 2019; Wenzel & Zhu, 2013). Poorer rehabilitation progress may be influenced by poorer immune functioning that can slow the healing process or as a result of the injured athletes' reluctance to engage with their rehabilitation activities fully (Aron et al., 2019). Finally, trauma-related complaints may contribute to athletes adopting maladaptive health behaviours such as substance misuse and disordered eating (Reardon et al., 2019; Wenzel & Zhu, 2013).

BARRIERS TO HELP-SEEKING BEHAVIOURS

It is common that athletes won't seek support with enhancing their mental health and there are many reasons for this (Castaldelli-Maia et al., 2019; Gorczynski et al., 2019; Gouttebarge et al., 2015; Stillman et al., 2019; Reardon et al., 2019).

As a result of this tendency to avoid seeking support, athletes may also then consequently place themselves at greater risk of poor mental health (Putukian, 2016). In order to develop strategies aimed at enhancing mental health in injured athletes, it is first important to understand the reasons that athletes may not seek support with improving mental health. These reasons extend from athletes' reporting time constraints and scheduling demands as a barrier (e.g. Watson, 2006), through to themes of MHL, sport culture and stigma (Castaldelli-Maia et al., 2019; Putukian, 2016; Reardon et al., 2019; Stillman et al., 2019).

MENTAL HEALTH LITERACY

MHL aims to (1) enhance knowledge of mental health problems, including risk factors and causes, symptom recognition, and self-care practice; (2) improve attitudes toward poor mental health and help-seeking behaviours and (3) increase intentions, and knowledge of how, to seek help (Gorczynski et al., 2019). A lack or low levels of MHL is considered a barrier in different levels of sport (Beauchemin, 2014; Biggin et al., 2017; Gulliver et al., 2012a). Athletes may not always know who to approach for support to improve their mental health (Coyle et al., 2017). Further, even in instances where athletes do know who to approach, they are less likely to seek that help (Stillman et al., 2019). Athletes have fewer positive attitudes to support with mental health than the general population (Barnard, 2016; Stillman et al., 2019) and are less willing to seek support as a result.

Education to increase knowledge about the most prevalent mental health symptoms and disorders (e.g. anxiety, sleep disorders, depression, eating disorders, and alcohol or substance misuse) is important for enhancing athletes' MHL (Castaldelli-Maia et al., 2019). Moreover, having easy access to appropriate mental health support (e.g. within the geographical locality and practitioners with an understanding of the nuances of sports injury) is likely to increase athletes' tendencies for help-seeking behaviours (Castaldelli-Maia et al., 2019).

SPORT CULTURE

The culture within sport also appears to be an important barrier to help-seeking behaviours, and the coach and teammates appear to be important cultural architects in this regard. For example, the world of professional football is typically closed off and can be dependent on support from within that world (Gouttebarge et al., 2015). In sport more broadly, it is not uncommon that athletes will be viewed as weak if they seek support (Putukian, 2016), which is a challenge in an environment that celebrates perceptions of toughness and belies a hypermasculine, pain-tolerant culture (Gorczynski et al., 2017; Putukian, 2016; Stillman et al., 2019). Furthermore, perhaps as a consequence of the sport culture, athletes may be afraid to disclose any mental health symptoms (Putukian, 2016). Moreover, athletes have concerns over selection if they seek support with improving their mental health, along with broader concerns over how they will be perceived by teammates and coaches should they seek support (Biggin et al., 2017; Delenardo & Terrion, 2014; Green et al., 2012).

STIGMA

Stigma is the most consistently reported barrier to help-seeking behaviours, evident across 18 studies included in a recent systematic review (Castaldelli-Maia et al., 2019). This stigma relates to both public stigma (stigma endorsed by the general public) and self-stigma (individuals' own stigmatized attitudes related to internalization of public stigma), and differences are evident in different levels of athletes, and between athletes and non-athletes. For example, Castaldelli-Maia and colleagues reviewed that elite athletes demonstrate greater levels of stigma, public stigma and self-stigma than non-athletes. Of all of the barriers to help-seeking behaviours, stigma is considered to be the most important (Putukian, 2016); therefore, ways of reducing stigma will likely be central to the success of any attempts to provide mental health support for athletes.

In summary, the main barriers to support-seeking behaviours in athletes are commonly related to stigma, low MHL, negative past experiences with seeking mental health support and scheduling or time demands (Castaldelli-Maia et al., 2019; Gorczynski et al., 2019; Stillman et al., 2019). Understanding these findings can support practitioners in designing interventions (e.g. stigma-reducing interventions) and developing effective climates for supporting support-seeking behaviours in athletes. Brief anti-stigma interventions, whilst not evidencing long-term change in mental health, do demonstrate promising initial results in overcoming barriers related to stigma (Castaldelli-Maia et al., 2019).

FACILITATORS TO HELP-SEEKING BEHAVIOUR AND IMPROVING MENTAL HEALTH

As with barriers to help-seeking behaviours, there are also many reported facilitators, each of which can be linked to the different barriers outlined above. Some of these facilitators are linked to the broader cultural considerations. For example, as professional football belies a closed-off approach, a major facilitator for help-seeking behaviours might be to have the support services coming from within football (Gouttebarge et al., 2015). Irrespective of the levels or types of sport, the approaches to facilitating mental health improvements following sports injury can be generally grouped under (1) evaluation and diagnosis, (2) goals and (3) treatments/interventions (Gouttebarge et al., 2019; Putukian, 2016; Stillman et al., 2019).

EVALUATION AND DIAGNOSIS

Understanding any barriers to help-seeking behaviours is an integral part of supporting athletes. Understanding these barriers can then form the basis of psychoeducation. This psychoeducation could include the athlete and those around the athlete (e.g. coach, agents, family members etc.) and should include education around the symptoms of poor mental health, as well as the benefits of engaging with a programme of support (Gulliver et al., 2012a and b; Putukian, 2016; Reardon et al., 2019; Stillman et al., 2019). Early diagnosis can be an important step in facilitating help-seeking behaviours, as it can raise awareness of both symptoms and benefits for the athlete earlier (Gouttebarge et al., 2019).

Owing to the aforementioned reluctance for athletes to engage with support due to the stigmas attached with poor mental health, it may be important for the support work to be reframed as performance support (Stillman et al., 2019). It is also important to note, as part of the early stages of education, how the support will benefit both performance and quality of life (Gouttebarge et al., 2019). As sports injuries, particularly severe injuries, can elicit a perceived lack of control within athletes where they can feel like they are unable to keep developing as an athlete (Forsdyke et al., 2016), this multi-function approach of health and performance enhancement may be particularly beneficial for restoring a sense of control in injured athletes.

Exploring the multi- or interdisciplinary support opportunities, which include stakeholders from within the sport as well as outside it, may also form an important part of the initial evaluation and diagnosis (Putukian, 2016; Stillman et al., 2019). As athletes may be reluctant to disclose information, this wider support could be valuable in gaining information. Moreover, it can create a perception of a collaborative working alliance which could be important for enhancing an athlete's sense of social connectedness and the support from significant others may also facilitate adherence to mental health support strategies (Gouttebarge et al., 2015; Gulliver et al., 2012a and b; Putukian, 2016; Stillman et al., 2019). Where other stakeholders (e.g. coaches, agents, family members) are involved, maintaining client confidentiality is an important consideration. Agreeing limits of information sharing from the outset can be an important part of establishing productive working patterns (e.g. Gledhill et al., 2020).

GOALS

After the initial diagnosis, evaluation and needs analysis have been completed, it is important to establish clear goals (Stillman et al., 2019). Aside from the benefits of directing the mental health support for the athlete, having a collaborative approach to scoping and setting between the athlete and the support provider can create a sense of shared goal commitment within the therapeutic relationship. This is important as perceived shared goal commitment and working alliance are important common factors in the success of psychotherapeutic interventions (Wampold, 2015). Goals could be related to specific aspects of mental health symptoms and disorders (e.g. changes to substance misuse, improvements in sleep behaviours, engaging with CBT) or could also be related to rehabilitation goals.

TREATMENTS/INTERVENTIONS

Typically, interventions based on self-management are likely to be beneficial and can serve to empower the injured athlete towards sustainable health, functioning and quality of life (Gouttebarge et al., 2015). Individual approaches to supporting mental health in injured athletes include Cognitive Behavioural Techniques and Motivational Enhancement Techniques (Stillman et al., 2019). Whilst the available trial-based evidence for these techniques in injury specific contexts is sparse, there are case examples where these techniques have been used to help athletes understand and reappraise their injury-related thoughts using CBT-based approaches, and to help injured athletes identify and resolve their ambivalence to injury-related change through motivational interviewing (e.g. Gledhill et al., 2020). Internet-based support interventions have been positively perceived and demonstrate promise in encouraging help-seeking behaviours (e.g. Gulliver et al., 2012b).

Support-based interventions with injured athletes can also serve to improve injured athletes' mental health (Podlog & Dionigi, 2010; Putukian, 2016; Stillman et al., 2019). Support-based interventions allow injured athletes to draw on their support networks to express their thoughts, experience empathy and a sense of social connectedness (Forsdyke et al., 2016; Putukian, 2016; Stillman et al., 2019). Furthermore, there is evidence that the support relationship can be beneficial for the support receiver and provider (Brown et al., 2018). As well as showing effectiveness as a treatment for anxiety and depression related symptoms in athletes, improving social networks within sport is also suggested as a complementary method alongside other treatments for potentially reducing the risk of suicide (Rao et al., 2015).

The International Olympic Committee consensus statement on mental health in elite athletes (Reardon et al., 2019) provides further guidelines for practitioners to overcome some common obstacles that can interfere with psychotherapy in elite athletes. These suggestions include that a practitioner should be flexible about timings of sessions (whilst being cognizant of avoiding repeated cancellations) and that practitioners should be supportive of or encourage couples or family sessions when relational issues impact on performance. Further guidelines also relate to the use of pharmacological therapy and treatments for substance misuse (see Reardon et al., 2019).

Collectively, all of these points are likely to create a sense of a more psychologically safe, supportive and developmental environments for athletes, which can be important in improving mental health (Putukian, 2016; Reardon et al., 2019; Stillman et al., 2019). As well as improving the injured athlete's mental health (e.g. by reducing anxiety/depression symptoms, increasing perceptions of social connectedness), creating this type of environment may also reduce the risk of further injury in athletes. By creating a safe and supportive environment, the athlete's experience of life stress will likely reduce, as will the magnitude of their stress response. Both of these are risk factors for sports injury (Ivarsson et al., 2017). However, future research is needed to explore the causal and sequencing of the relationship between mental health symptoms and disorders and subsequent injury risk (Gouttebarge et al., 2016).

EXISTING STUDY LIMITATIONS

Whilst the insights into mental health symptoms and disorders as a result of sports injury have experienced steady growth over the past 10 years, some limitations remain. For example, the body of research is awash with cross-section/correlational research, but longitudinal research is less evident (Gouttebarge et al., 2019). Furthermore, many of the scales used within the body of research were not originally validated for use with elite athletic populations (Gouttebarge et al., 2019; Reardon et al., 2019), so there may be a need for further scale development specific for this sporting population or further consideration given more generally to mental health screening in sport (Reardon et al., 2019). Moreover, further examination of the efficacy or effectiveness of interventions specifically within injured athlete populations is warranted, to examine their impact on help-seeking behaviours, including any cultural influences on the support available for athletes (Reardon et al., 2019). For further detailed research applied directions arising from the recent International Olympic Committee Consensus Statement, see Reardon et al. (2019).

CONCLUSION

Sports injuries, particularly severe or recurrent sports injuries, are considered major negative life events for athletes and a significant downside of sports injuries is that can elicit problematic mental health symptoms and disorders in injured athletes. Despite this and the general need for intervention to support improvements in mental health, athletes are often reluctant to adopt help-seeking behaviours, with the stigma attached to mental health being the most significant barrier. However, appropriate support from key people within the athlete entourage (e.g. partner, family members, coach or agent) can serve to reduce these barriers and support to facilitate the athlete's engagement with strategies to improve their mental health.

Case study

Jamal is a 17-year-old academy football player, registered with the league one (third tier of English football) club in England. He has ruptured his Anterior Cruciate Ligament in training, suffering a non-contact injury that required surgical repair 6 weeks ago. His parents have contacted you as the sport psychologist for the club as they have some concerns about him following his surgery.

Jamal's mother shares with you that he keeps waking up during the night, sometimes, he will be screaming audibly, whereas other times he wakes up having had nightmares about his injury. Jamal has told his mother that he keeps 'seeing himself getting injured like he's watching on a video' when he is asleep and that he wakes up when he 'hears the pop'. Jamal has shared with his parents that he is concerned about his future in football, because he doesn't have any confidence that he won't get injured again. His mother tells you that he is really scared he will get injured again, but he doesn't want to admit that he is scared as he doesn't want 'the lads at the club to rip him' for it [colloquialism for constant banter and making jokes at his expense]. He also said that he doesn't really understand any of the information that the consultant has provided, but he didn't want to look silly by asking any questions. When she asked him how long he had felt like this, Jamal said 'since it happened and I had the op'.

When Jamal's mother asked him if he had spoken to anybody at the club, he said that he hadn't because he didn't want to look soft and he is worried that, if he does have to ask for help, his coach might think he isn't tough enough to be a football player. Jamal is one of the youngest players in his age group and the decisions regarding whether youth players will be released or retained are going to be made in four months' time.

1. What are the major factors influencing Jamal's health and are indicators of poor mental health?
2. What are the indicators of barriers to help-seeking behaviour?
3. How could you best facilitate Jamal in seeking help and what support would he benefit from?

References

Ardern, C., Taylor, N., Feller, J. A., & Webster, K. (2013). A systematic review of the psychological factors associated with returning to sport following injury. *British Journal of Sports Medicine, 47*, 1120–1126.

Aron, C. M., Harvey, S., Hainline, B., Hitchcock, M. E., & Reardon, C. L. (2019). Post-traumatic stress disorder (PTSD) and other trauma-related mental disorders in elite athletes: A narrative review. *British Journal of Sports Medicine, 53*, 779–784.

Appaneal, R., & Perna, F. (2014). Biopsychosocial model of injury. In R. Eklund & G. Tenenbaum (Eds.), Encyclopedia of sport and exercise psychology (pp. 74–76). Sage Publications, Inc.

Barnard, J. D. (2016). Student-athletes' perceptions of mental illness and attitudes towards help-seeking. *Journal of College Student Psychotherapy, 30*, 161–175.

Bateman, A., & Morgan, K. A. D. (2019). The post-injury psychological sequelae of high-level Jamaican athletes: Exploration of posttraumatic stress disorder-self-efficacy conceptualisation. *Journal of Sport Rehabilitation, 28*, 144–152.

Beauchemin, J. (2014). College student-athlete wellness: An integrative outreach model. *College Student Journal, 48*, 268–280.

Biggin, I. J. R., Burns, J. H., & Uphill, M. (2017). An investigation of athletes' and coaches' perceptions of mental ill-health in elite athletes. *Journal of Clinical Sport Psychology, 11*, 126–147.

Brassil, H. E., & Salvatore, A. P. (2018). The frequency of post-traumatic stress disorder symptoms in athletes with and without sports related concussion. *Clinical Translational Medicine, 7*, 25.

Brown, C. J., Webb, T. L., Robinson, M. A., & Cotgreave, R. (2018). Athletes' experiences of social support in their transition out of elite sport: An interpretive phenomenological analysis. *Psychology of Sport and Exercise, 36*, 71–80.

Castaldelli-Maia, J. M., Gallinaro, J. G. M., Falcão, R. S., Gouttebarge, V., Hitchcock, M. E., Hainline, B., Reardon, C. L., Stull, T. (2019). Mental health symptoms and disorders in elite athletes: A systematic review on cultural influencers and barriers to athletes seeking treatment. *British Journal of Sports Medicine, 53*, 707–721.

Chang, C., Putukian, M., Aerni, G., Diamond, A., Hong, G., Ingram, Y., & Wolanin, A. (2020). Mental health issues and psychological factors in athletes: Detection, management, effect on performance and prevention: American Medical Society for Sports Medicine position statement – Executive summary. *British Journal of Sports Medicine, 54*, 216–220.

Coyle, M., Gorczynski, P., & Gibson, K. (2017). "You have to be mental to jump off a. board anyway": Elite divers' conceptualisations of mental health. *Psychology of Sport and Exercise, 29*, 10–18.

Delenardo, S., & Terrion, J. L. (2014). Suck it up: Opinions and attitudes about mental illness stigma and help-seeking behaviour of male varsity football players. *Canadian Journal of Community Mental Health, 33*, 43–56.

Didebahni, N., Cullum, C., Mansinghani, S., Conover, H., & Hart, J Jr. (2013). Depressive symptoms and concussion in aging retired NFL players. *Archives of Clinical Neuropsychology, 28*, 418–424.

Forsdyke, D., Smith, A., Jones, M., & Gledhill, A. (2016). Psychosocial factors associated with outcomes of sports injury rehabilitation in competitive athletes: A mixed-studies systematic review. *British Journal of Sports Medicine, 50*, 537–544.

Gledhill, A. (2016). "I can't return to play" – When fear of re-injury dominates after ACL reconstruction. *British Medical Journal Talk Medicine* [audio podcast]. Retrieved from: https://soundcloud.com/bmjpodcasts/i-can't-return-to-play-when-fear-of-reinjury-dominates-after-acl-reconstruction-adam-gledhill.

Gledhill, A. Ahmed, O. H., & Forsdyke, D. (2020). Effectively managing anterior cruciate ligament injury and return to performance in elite women's soccer. In J. Dixon, J. Barker, R. Thelwell, and I. Mitchell (eds.). *The Psychology of Soccer*. Routledge.

Gorczynski, P., Coyle, M., & Gibson, K. (2017). Depressive symptoms in high-performance athletes and non-athletes: A comparative meta-analysis. *British Journal of Sports Medicine, 51*, 1348–1354.

Gorczynski, P., Gibson, K., Thelwell, R., Papathomas, A., Harwood, C., & Kinnafick, F. (2019). The BASES expert statement on mental health literacy in elite sport. *The Sport and Exercise Scientists, 59*, 6–7.

Gouttebarge, V., Aoki, H., Ekstrand, J., Verhagen, E. A. L. M., & Kerkoffs, G. M. M. J. (2016). Are severe musculoskeletal injuries associated with symptoms of common mental disorders among male European professional footballers? *Knee Surgery, Sports Traumtology and Arthroscopy, 24*, 3934–3942.

Gouttebarge, V., Castaldelli-Maia, J. M., Gorczynski, P., Hainline, B., Hitchcock, M. E., Kerkhoffs, G. M., Rice, S. M., Reardon, C. L. (2019). Occurrence of mental health symptoms and disorders in current and former elite athletes: A systematic review. *British Journal of Sports Medicine, 53*, 700–707.

Gouttebarge, V., Frings-Dresen, M. H. W., & Sluiter, J. K. (2015). Mental and psychosocial health among current and former professional football players. *Occupational Medicine, 65*, 190–196.

Green, M., Morgan, G., & Manley, A. (2012). Elite rugby players' attitudes toward sport psychology consulting. *Sport, Exercise Psychology Review, 8*, 32–44.

Gulliver, A., Griffiths, K. M., & Christensen, H. (2012a). Barriers and facilitators to mental health help-seeking for young athletes: A qualitative study. *BMC Psychiatry, 12*, 157.

Gulliver, A., Griffiths, K. M., Christsen, H., Mackinnon, A., Calear, A. L., Parsons, A, & Stanimirovic, R. (2012b). Internet-based interventions to promote mental health help-seeking in elite athletes: an exploratory randomised controlled trial. *Medical Internet Research, 14*, e69.

Hsu, C-J., Meierbachtol, A., George, S. Z., & Chmielewski, T. L. (2017). Fear of re-injury in athletes: Implications for rehabilitation. *Sports Health, 9*, 162–167.

Ivarsson, A., Johnson, U., Andersen, M. B., Tranaeus, U., Stenling, A., & Lindwall, M. (2017). Psychosocial factors and sport injuries: Meta-analyses for prediction and prevention. *Sports Medicine, 47*, 353–365.

Jorm, A. F., Korten, A. E., Jacomb, P. A., Christensen, H., Rodgers, B., Pollitt, P. (1997). "Mental health literacy": A survey of the public's ability to recognise mental disorders and their beliefs about the effectiveness of treatment. *Medical Journal of Australia, 166*, 182–186.

Padaki, A. S., Noticewala, M. S., & Levine, W. N. (2018). Prevalence of posttraumatic stress disorder symptoms among young athletes after anterior cruciate ligament rupture. *Orthopaedic Journal of Sports Medicine, 6*, 2325967118787159.

Paterno, M. V., Flynn, K., Thomas, S., & Schmitt, L. C. (2018). Self-reported fear predicts functional performance and second ACL injury after ACL reconstruction and return to sport: A pilot study. *Sports Health, 10*, 228–233.

Podlog, L., & Dionigi, R. (2010). Coach strategies for addressing psychosocial challenges during the return to sport from injury. *Journal of Sports Sciences, 28*, 1197–1208.

Putukian, M. (2016). The psychological response to injury in student athletes: A narrative review with a focus on mental health. *British Journal of Sports Medicine, 50*, 145–148.

Rao, A. L., Asif, I. M., Drezner, J. A., (2015). Suicide in National Collegiate Athletic Association (NCAA) athletes: A 9-year analysis of the NCAA resolutions database. *Sports Health, 7*, 452–457.

Reardon, C. L., Hainline, B., Aron, C. M., Baron, D., Baum, A. L., Bindra, A, & Engerbretson, L. (2019). Mental health in elite athletes: International Olympic Committee consensus statement (2019). *British Journal of Sports Medicine, 53*, 667–699.

Rodriguez, R. M., Marroquin, A., & Cosby, N. (2019). Reducing fear of reinjury and pain perception in athletes with first time anterior cruciate ligament reconstructions by implementing imagery training. *Journal of Sport Rehabilitation, 28*, 385–389.

Ross, C. A., Clifford, A., & Louw, Q. Q. (2017). Factors informing the fear of re-injury after anterior cruciate ligament reconstruction. *Physiotherapy Therapy and Practice, 33*, 103–114.

Smith, A. M., & Milliner, E. K. (1994). Injured athletes and the risk of suicide. *Journal of Athletic Training, 29*, 337–341.

Souter, G., Lewis, R., & Serrant, L. (2018). Men, mental health and elite sport: A narrative review. *Sports Medicine – Open, 4*, 57.

Stillman, M. A., Glick, I. D., McDuff, D., Reardon, C. L., Hitchcock, M. E., Fitch, V. M., & Hainline, B. (2019). Psychotherapy for mental health symptoms and disorders in elite athletes: A narrative review. *British Journal of Sports Medicine, 53*, 767–771.

Tjong, V. K., Murnaghan, L., Nyhof-Young, J. M., & Ogilvie-Harris, D. J. (2013). A qualitative investigation of the decision to return to sport after anterior cruciate ligament reconstruction. *American Journal of Sports Medicine, 42*, 336–342.

Truong, L. K., Mosewich, A. D., Holt, C. J., Lee, C. Y., Miciack, M., & Whittaker, J. (2020). Psychological, social and contextual factors across recovery stages following a sport-related knee injury: A scoping review. *British Journal of Sports Medicine*. Epub ahead of print. DOI: 10.1136/bjsports-2019-101206.

Walker, N., & Thatcher, J. (2011). The emotional response to athletic injury: Re-injury anxiety. In J. Thatcher, M. Jones & D. Lavallee (Eds.), *Coping and emotion in sport* (2nd ed., pp. 236–260). Routledge.

Walker, N., Thatcher, J., & Lavallee, D. (2010). A preliminary development of the reinjury anxiety inventory (RIAI). *Physical Therapy in Sport*, 11, 23–29.

Wampold, B. E. (2015). How important are the common factors in psychotherapy? An update. *World Psychiatry, 14*, 270–277.

Watson, J. C. (2006). College student athletes' attitudes toward help-seeking behaviour and expectations of counselling service. *Journal of College Student Development, 46*, 442–449.

Wenzel, T., & Zhu, I. J. (2013). Posttraumatic stress in athletes. In D. A. Baron, C. Reardon., & S. H. Baron (Eds.), *Clinical sport psychiatry: An international perspective* (pp. 102–114). Wiley.

Wiese-Bjornstal, D. M., Smith, A. M., Shaffer, S. M., & Morrey, M. A. (1998). An integrated model of response to sport injury: Psychological and sociological dynamics. *Journal of Applied Sport Psychology, 10*, 46–69

World Health Organisation WHO (2014). Mental health: a state of wellbeing. Available from: www.who.int/features/factfiles/mental_health/en.

5 THE UPSIDE OF SPORTS INJURY AND DISABILITY

PERSONAL GROWTH FOLLOWING ADVERSITY

Dr Chris Hammer, Dr Leslie Podlog and Dr Adam Gledhill

CHAPTER OVERVIEW

A growing body of evidence demonstrates the positive implications of sports injury or physically disabling events. Drawing from psychological research on sport injury and disability, this chapter will consider the ways in which injury – even severe life-altering ones – can be a learning opportunity enabling positive developmental experiences, self-exploration and greater sporting prowess. While terms such as benefit finding, stress-related growth or posttraumatic growth have all been used to connote notions of personal development following injury, in the current chapter, we employ the term 'personal growth' to capture growth experiences among individuals sustaining injuries of a greater or lesser severity. We first discuss the implications of injury – both positive and negative (Section 1) – followed by discussion of research examining the nature of growth as well as factors facilitating its development (Section 2). In the third section, we articulate practitioner-based strategies focused on facilitating personal growth with injured athletes and para sport athletes. We conclude the chapter (Section 4) with a case study exemplifying the notion of growth in the injury aftermath.

THE IMPLICATIONS OF INJURY

One of the most profound challenges facing an athlete is injury. Injury presents athletes with an onslaught of challenges from the moment of injury inception until resumption of competitive activities – or in the case of some athletes, adjustment to altered competitive activities or career termination (Clement et al., 2015; Leddy et al., 1994; Podlog & Eklund, 2006; Putukian, 2016; Tracey, 2003). Prominent issues following injury occurrence include challenges with pain management, heightened negative affect and difficulties accepting one's new incapacitations (Tracey, 2003). During the rehabilitation phase, other psychological challenges commonly emerge, such as a loss of confidence in one's physical capabilities, feelings of social isolation, a loss of athletic identity and inadequate social support (Ruddock-Hudson et al., 2012; Tracey, 2003). As the return to competitive activities draws near, enthusiasm about resuming self-defining activities may be diminished by re-injury apprehensions, perseverating thoughts about regaining previous competitive levels and worries regarding the impact of injury on skill execution (Podlog & Dionigi, 2010; Podlog & Eklund, 2006). Finally, returning athletes might also worry about meeting internal and external performance expectations, self-presentational concerns about appearing athletically incompetent and doubts over one's level of physical fitness (Evans et al., 2000; Podlog & Eklund, 2006; Walker et al., 2010).

The aforementioned impacts of injury may be all the more profound in the case of traumatic injuries resulting in permanent physical disability (Livneh & Antonak, 2005). Tasks taken-for-granted prior to impairment may subsequently require detailed consideration (e.g. bathing, using the stairs), while the psychological consequences can result in the fracturing of one's social life (Crawford et al., 2014; Day, 2013; Gallagher & MacLachlan, 2001). For these reasons, adjusting to a disability can be an extremely arduous and long-term process (Day, 2013; Gallagher & MacLachlan, 2001). For some, positive adjustment may never occur (Lucas, 2007). Problems of a clinical nature such as depression or even suicidal ideation may be pronounced among those experiencing a poor adjustment to disability (Crawford et al., 2014; Day, 2013).

Despite the prevalence of deleterious experiences often associated with sport injury or acquired disability, mounting evidence suggests that injury may not be an entirely negative experience. Rather, positive adjustments, constructive life changes, benefits or personal development may ensue in the injury aftermath (e.g. Dibb et al., 2014; McMillen & Cook, 2003; Udry et al., 1997; Unwin et al., 2009; Wadey et al., 2016). A range of positive adaptations have been reported in a sport injury context, for example physical (e.g. strengthening weaker body parts, improved fitness), social (e.g. opportunities to engage with non-sport peers), psychological (e.g. enhanced mental toughness, greater determination to reach goals) and technical/tactical ones (e.g. improved game strategy or tactical awareness) (Bianco et al., 1999; Day & Wadey, 2016; Hurley et al., 2007). Similarly, some individuals experiencing traumatic events such as loss of a limb or vision report positive experiences, such as greater appreciation for life, strengthened social relationships and enhanced life meanings (Chun & Lee, 2008; Crawford et al., 2014). Such findings indicate that there may be a 'silver lining' to the injury experience.

WHAT IS GROWTH AFTER INJURY AND WHAT FACTORS FACILITATE ITS DEVELOPMENT?

In an effort to capture benefits or positive adaptations following injury and disability, researchers have employed various terms, for example stress-related growth, posttraumatic growth, adversarial growth and benefit finding (Park & Lechner, 2006). As indicated, our use of the term 'personal growth' is used in the broadest sense to capture growth experiences among individuals sustaining injuries of a greater or lesser severity. Such verbiage is consistent with arguments advanced by Rubio et al. (2020) who recently suggested that research on growth following sport-related injuries is plagued with conceptual confusion, interchangeable use of terms that may or may not be similar in nature and a lack of clear consensus on the domains of growth. Building on arguments advanced by Wadey et al. (2011), Rubio et al. (2020) suggested that researchers have on occasion used the term posttraumatic growth to examine phenomena that may not be 'traumatic' in nature. Wadey et al. (2011) argued that use of the term posttraumatic growth should be reserved for individuals experiencing life-altering events (e.g. loss of a loved one, a near fatal accident, wartime experiences), rather than those of a lesser severity (e.g. a sport injury). Moreover, Rubio et al. (2020) suggested that discrepancies exist regarding the number of growth domains or benefits reported across sport injury studies, with some identifying as few as 3 overarching domains (Salim et al., 2015) and others reporting as many as 19 factors (Wadey et al., 2011).

In an attempt to clarify existing dimensions and develop a novel, consensually agreed upon multidimensional model, Rubio et al. (2020) employed an e-Delphi method, in which 24 psychology of sport injury experts provided insights into the domains of growth following a severe (4 weeks or more) sport injury. The process led to the development of a five-dimension model capable of describing athletes' experiences of personal growth following a severe sports-related injury. These included personal strength, improved social life, health benefits, sport benefits, and social support and recognition. Table 5.1 presents items from each of the five dimensions that emerged from the expert panel responses.

In addition to research examining the nature of the construct of growth and its dimensions, researchers have sought to uncover the intra-individual and external/environmental factors facilitating growth following sport injury and/or disabling life events. One key intra-individual factor that has been the focus of inquiry relates to an individual's reaction to a precipitating event, for example a sport injury or loss of a limb. Researchers have suggested a distinction be made between a precipitating event and one's reaction to the event, for it is the reaction which dictates whether or not a growth response is even a possibility. That is, if one does not have perceptions of helplessness, uncontrollability, life threat or other deleterious cognitions, then the growth response is not likely to take place (Joseph & Linley, 2005; Linley & Joseph, 2004; Tedeschi & Calhoun, 2004). In other words, negative thoughts and emotions appear to be a prerequisite for the occurrence of growth experiences. These negative perceptions, however, are not in and of themselves sufficient to guarantee a growth outcome. Rather, such perceptions set the stage for the necessary cognitive processing that *may* lead to subsequent growth.

Researchers in this area often refer to these initial deleterious perceptions as a challenge to one's core beliefs or a shattering of one's assumptive world – that is, an experience akin to an existential crisis (Janoff-Bulman, 1992). Said differently, the new information prompted by adversity causes one to question the world and their place in it. The processing of this information is necessary to relieve distress and reconstruct a coherent world view (Janoff-Bulman, 1992). Researchers have conceptualized this cognitive processing, characterized

Table 5.1 Items reflecting dimensions of sport-injury related growth

Items
Personal strength
I have become a more empathic person
I have transcended my own limits by rising above adversity
I have re-defined my identity beyond sport
I have understood that sport-related social recognition is transitory
I have developed mental toughness
I have found the time to develop non-sport related interests
I have become aware of my limits
I have challenged myself, both mentally and physically
I have learned to appreciate the small things in life
I have enhanced my spiritual strength
I have had the opportunity to think about what is important in my life
I have learned to interpret my injury as a sign that it's time to move on from sport before something more severe happens
Improved social life
I have a greater understanding of the importance of the people close to me
I have had time to foster personal relationships, including those outside of sport (e.g. family, friends)
I have had time to socialize and hang out with friends outside of my sport
I have learned to trust others more than before
My relationships with teammates and/or coaches have improved
My awareness of belonging to my group/team has grown
I have developed relationships with other (former or currently) injured athletes
I have learned to appreciate other people's contributions inside and outside of sport
I have realized who I can really count on
Health-related benefits
My appreciation for medical and healthcare professionals has deepened
I have identified support systems and resources that I can now rely on
My ability to manage physical pain in the future has improved
I have learned to avoid high-risk behaviours and/or to develop injury prevention measures
I have become more appreciative of maintaining good health and living free from injury
I have broadened my knowledge of my injury, my body and/or health guidelines (e.g. nutrition, rest)
My body has had the chance to recover from training and competition

(*Continued*)

Table 5.1 Items reflecting dimensions of sport-injury related growth (*Continued*)

Sport-related benefits
I have become a role model for other athletes (e.g. peers, young people)
I have learned to act as referee or coach
I have engaged in different roles supporting my team (e.g. stats keeping)
I have found a more valuable role within my team
I have gained a new perspective on sport
I have learned to appreciate opportunities for playing sports rather than taking them for granted
I have developed mental skills that are applicable to sports
I have been able to work on fitness, strength, endurance and flexibility
I have had the opportunity to work on technical aspects of sport, strategy and/or tactical awareness
I have improved my ability to handle pressure and/or to deal with competitive stress
I have furthered my commitment, motivation and passion for sport
My ability to differentiate between pain from practicing sport and injury-related pain has improved
Social support and recognition
I have seen that others value me as a person and not just as an athlete
I have received support for daily needs and responsibilities
I have received encouragement and/or emotional support
I have received attention and/or care from significant others
I have earned recognition and praise for my efforts during my rehabilitation
I have earned the respect of others for having sacrificed my body for sport

by its repetitive nature, in terms of intrusive rumination – that is, unsolicited, unwanted thoughts – and deliberate rumination, namely, purposeful meaning-making thoughts (Calhoun & Tedeschi, 1998, 2006; Cann et al., 2011; Tedeschi & Calhoun, 2004). While these two forms of rumination are conceptually different, they both play a role in the facilitation of growth. Specifically, research demonstrates that, in order for growth to be achieved, intrusive ruminations must eventually lead to and give way to deliberate ruminations (Hammer et al., 2020). The transition between intrusive and deliberate rumination is critical, as persisting intrusive ruminations can lead to a host of adverse consequences (Cann et al., 2010, 2011). In addition to leading to lower levels of growth (Hammer et al., 2020; Stockton et al., 2011), consequences of ongoing intrusive ruminations may include greater distress (Hammer et al., 2020), posttraumatic depreciation (Cann et al., 2011) and an inability to move to more constructive coping strategies (Cann et al., 2011).

The notion of cognitive processing and its role in the experience of personal growth has been examined in a variety of populations, from cancer patients

(Wilson et al., 2014), earthquake survivors (Taku et al., 2015) and even college students who reported stressful events (Cann et al., 2011). In a study involving para sport athletes with acquired physical disabilities, Hammer et al. (2020) sought to understand the process through which growth is experienced, as well as the role that para sport participation may play. Serial mediation analyses revealed that the experience of growth was achieved through ruminative processes. More specifically, several different ruminative paths from the initial challenge to one's core beliefs to current growth were evident. For example, initial challenges to one's core beliefs led to intrusive rumination occurring soon after the trauma, which subsequently predicted intrusive ruminations brought about by para sport participation. These intrusive ruminations, in turn, led to deliberate ruminations brought about by para sport participation, which ultimately translated to higher levels of current growth. Another path to growth bypassed intrusive rumination altogether, as the indirect effect of core belief challenge on growth existed solely through deliberate rumination soon after the trauma. A caveat to such findings was that all paths must eventually travel through deliberate rumination in order for growth to be achieved. Conversely, paths that *only* included intrusive rumination ultimately predicted not only lower levels of growth but also greater levels of current distress. The study also provided preliminary evidence that para sport participation could facilitate growth for some by prompting deliberate rumination.

In their grounded theory of sport injury related growth, Roy-Davis et al. (2017) noted a number of additional intra-individual factors, which, according to athletes, enabled them to experience personal growth in the injury aftermath. These included personality traits, coping styles, knowledge and prior experiences. Personality factors referred to important personal qualities (i.e. confidence, creativity, resilience, social intelligence, openness to experience, extraversion, optimism, reflexivity and emotional intelligence) that were perceived to elicit different forms of growth. These forms included a greater understanding of and ability to express emotions, being creative with maximizing one's free time and how one approached problems, being open to and acting upon opportunities in the environment, remaining resilient and confident in overcoming adversity and eliciting positive benefits and understanding the importance of 'give and take' in relationships. Athletes coping styles also impacted their self-reported likelihood of growth. In particular, those utilizing emotion-focused (e.g. meaning making, emotional venting, seeking support for emotional reasons and/or turning to religion) and problem-focused strategies (e.g. planning, active coping and seeking support for instrumental reasons) reported experiences of growth. In addition, perceived social support was suggested to be instrumental in helping injured athletes learn who in their support network could or would help if needed. Athletes reported that reflection on the availability of support helped them rationalize and control their thinking by reassuring them that they had the resources to cope, by instilling positive emotions (e.g. optimism and confidence) and by fostering facilitative responses (e.g. sustained effort to adhere to the rehabilitation regimen). Finally, knowledge and prior experiences enabled athletes to recognize that injury was part-and-parcel of the sport experience. It also assisted them to imagine how things could be worse, by comparing their sport injury to other stressful life events perceived as more 'traumatic'. Finally, knowledge and prior experiences instilled a sense of confidence that one could return to sport, physically and mentally stronger by drawing on previous growth-related experiences. Past experiences could pertain to sport (e.g. injury, illness and losing major championships) or non-sport critical incidents (e.g. death of a loved one, relationship breakup). Athletes also reported that previous experiences had occurred either directly to them or vicariously (e.g. witnessing a teammate overcome an injury).

In addition to various intra-individual factors, evidence suggests that one's external environment may also play a role in promoting personal growth following injury. According to the organismic valuing theory of growth through adversity (Joseph & Linley, 2005), one's ability to accommodate the trauma in a positive direction (i.e. growth) is contingent on one's social environment. If the social environment is supportive of the fundamental psychological needs of autonomy (perceptions of volitional engagement, the ability to choose one's course of action), competence (the belief that one is proficient and capable in interactions with environmental stimuli) and relatedness (perceptions of a secure relational base, connectedness with others and social support), the likelihood that the individual will be able to constructively cognitively process the trauma is enhanced. On the other hand, within organismic valuing theory, it is posited that thwarting of one's psychological needs is likely to impede growth processes.

Research in this domain has revealed some support for the role of need's support in the development of personal growth after adversity. In a qualitative study of para sport athletes with acquired disabilities, Hammer et al. (2019b) found that para sport helped to facilitate growth by providing meaningful social experiences (i.e. relatedness), opportunities to overcome challenges (i.e. competence) and becoming empowered such as gaining control over one's body and life (i.e. autonomy). Similarly, Podlog et al. (2010) found that support for injured athletes' needs facilitated enhanced well-being and positive return-to-sport outcomes. In particular, mediation analysis revealed that high perceptions of competence and autonomy need support during injured athletes' rehabilitation increased positive affect, which, in turn, augmented the likelihood of a 'renewed perspective on sport' (e.g. 'my appreciation of sport has been greater', 'my motivation for sport success has been greater', 'my mental toughness has been better').

Given the theoretical underpinnings of the organismic valuing theory as well as empirical evidence of the role of need satisfaction and cognitive processing in the development of personal growth, Hammer et al. (2019a) sought to understand how cognitive processing *and* need satisfaction interact to facilitate growth among para sport athletes with acquired disabilities. Specifically, the authors hypothesized that the extent to which one's needs were satisfied through their para sport participation would moderate the indirect effect of challenged core beliefs on growth through deliberate rumination. While both needs satisfaction and deliberate rumination were separately predictive of growth, the hypothesized interaction was not significant. Nonetheless, the study provided further support for the role of purposeful cognitive processing and need satisfaction in the development of growth.

Roy-Davis et al. (2017) highlighted a number of additional external/environmental factors influencing growth, namely, cultural scripts, physical resources, time and *received* social support. Cultural Scripts referred to narratives embedded in injured athletes' sport culture and reflected notions of 'triumph over adversity'. Such narratives could come in the form of televised events (e.g. Paralympic Games), films (e.g. Rocky), drama series (e.g. Friday Night Lights), celebrity autobiographies (e.g. Kelly Holmes, Black, White and Gold) and accounts of former athletes' successful recovery outcomes. Injured athletes utilized these stories of 'success-against-the-odds' to help identify and act upon opportunities, as sources of inspiration and as vehicles to channel their negative emotions in an adaptive manner. Physical resources (e.g. transport, Internet, TV, medical care and conditioning/rehabilitation equipment) could also be mobilized to help athletes rationalize strain responses, instil and heighten positive emotions and promote facilitative responses. Athletes also articulated the value of receiving social support in promoting growth, in particular, emotional support (e.g. listening, encouragement, sympathy and challenge) and tangible support (e.g. partners completing household chores, providing transport to medical appointments). Such forms of support were believed to help athletes reappraise the meaning of their injury, provide uplifting experiences throughout rehabilitation, and instil and maintain positive emotions through social exchanges that conveyed gratitude and inspiration. Finally, athletes spoke about the benefits of having more time to engage in non-sport-related hobbies and to socialize with their family and friends outside sport. Such opportunities helped gain a sense of perspective and calm, during an otherwise mentally challenging time period. A sense of calm was deemed invaluable in giving injured athletes the opportunity to contemplate the meaning of their injury experience and to help them see the benefits of the injury experience. In articulating the internal and external resources described above, Roy-Davis et al. (2017) noted that not all athletes demonstrated or used these different resources all of the time. Rather, they drew on different resources at various points, depending upon their needs at the time.

STRATEGIES FOR FACILITATING GROWTH

Based on the empirical findings highlighted above, we offer a number of practical strategies that practitioners and sport medicine providers can use to facilitate growth. In doing so, we recognize that growth may not be the only desirable outcome following injury and that practitioners should avoid employing strategies that extend beyond their expertise. As such, the suggestions below are intended as guides or heuristics that could likely be incorporated into conversations with athletes during physiotherapy sessions or in interactions between athletes and treatment team members (sport medicine physicians, physiotherapists, sport psychologists).

1. As discussed, the disruption to one's core beliefs caused by a sport injury or an acquired physical disability is not only a natural experience, but also

a necessary antecedent to personal growth. Consequently, rehabilitation practitioners ought to normalize these types of challenges when working with rehabilitating individuals. One avenue through which this may be achieved is by sharing narratives or stories of others who have faced similar setbacks and experienced similar disruption to their core beliefs. Practitioners can also inform athletes that there is no one *correct* sequence through which growth is achieved and that not all individuals will cognitively process an event in a similar fashion.

2. Practitioners may facilitate growth outcomes by encouraging individuals to deliberately ruminate about their acquired disability. That is, practitioners can help those with acquired disability to seek meaning and understanding about their disability or the precipitating event. One means to encourage deliberate rumination is through use of emotional disclosure exercises. For example, Salim and Wadey (2018) investigated the efficacy of a four-session emotional disclosure intervention, by comparing outcomes across three conditions: a written disclosure group (i.e. writing about one's deepest thoughts and feelings regarding a recent sports injury), a verbal disclosure group (i.e. talking about one's deepest thoughts and feelings regarding a recent sports injury) and a control condition (writing facts about one's daily life). Both the written and verbal disclosure groups experienced improved positive emotions; however, only the verbal disclosure group demonstrated growth. Practitioners may employ a variety of questions in an attempt to facilitate verbal disclosure and subsequent growth: (1) What implications, if any, might the injury have for you? (2) What can you learn from this injury? (3) How can this injury help you better understand your personal capabilities? (4) How can this injury help you progress in your sporting career or life outside sport? (5) How might this experience help you better cope with future challenges? (6) In what ways might this injury hold positive implications for your personal relationships? In asking such questions, practitioners should be careful to avoid re-traumatization. As indicated, referral to those with psychological training is advocated in circumstances where it may be evident that further guidance is needed.
3. Efforts to promote growth may also be facilitated by practitioner support for individuals' basic psychological needs. Specifically, injured performers should be given the opportunity to demonstrate physical competence (e.g. assign rehabilitation activities that provide a challenge, yet are attainable), make meaningful relationships (e.g. provide opportunities for group rehabilitation sessions or establish mentorship programs wherein individuals with more recent disabilities can be mentored by those with greater disability experience) and feel a sense of volitional control over their rehabilitation or para sport participation (e.g. provide options of rehabilitation exercises for the individual to choose from and rationales for prescribed exercises).
4. Another empirically validated strategy for facilitating growth is the promotion of gratitude. Salim and Wadey (2019) provided guidance for how practitioners might employ a gratitude exercise with injured individuals.

In particular, the researchers gave participants in the experimental condition time to write and read aloud a letter of gratitude to someone who had been particularly kind to them during their rehabilitation, but who had not been properly thanked or acknowledged (cf. Seligman et al., 2005). Results showed that athletes in the experimental condition reported a greater ability to relate to others – a key dimension of growth – in comparison to those in a control condition who had not had the benefit of such an exercise. These findings suggest that simple exercises may help athletes to better connect with practitioners who may be instrumental in influencing the quality and effectiveness of athletes' rehabilitation.

CONCLUSION

Adversity in the form of a sport injury or a disabling life event is often accompanied by a plethora of deleterious consequences. Conversely, researchers have also demonstrated that individuals can emerge more psychologically robust in the injury aftermath, that is, they can experience personal growth. Growth, however, is not a guaranteed outcome of having endured adversity. Rather, extant findings indicate that a number of intra-individual and environmental factors play a key role in the facilitation of growth. While research in this area is not without its limitations (e.g. lack of replication studies, issues with statistical power), the work on growth to date is providing guidance into the means by which growth may be cultivated (Salim & Wadey, 2018, 2019). Such insights may help turn injury into a transformative experience for the better.

Case study

Dan is a 25-year-old computer programmer and an active participant in a variety of recreational sports, such as softball, golf and triathlon. Though he never competed in any sport at an elite level, Dan always considered an active lifestyle, physical fitness and his athletic prowess to be a fundamental component of his identity. Many of Dan's friendships have developed through his sport participation – relationships he prizes and which add meaning to his life. Unfortunately, during a work sponsored ski trip, Dan crashed into a tree and suffered a traumatic brachial plexus injury to his dominant arm. The accident damaged the complex network of nerves in Dan's upper arm and neck region, which control the motions of Dan's hand, wrist and arm. The resulting injury left Dan with an inability to control, move or even feel his arm. The injury was debilitating to the point where his entire arm was left hanging limply. To date, extensive physical therapy has only enabled a minute improvement in feeling and control and the prognosis is that Dan will never regain more than 10–15% of his pre-accident functionality. As the accident occurred during a sanctioned event for Dan's work, medical bills are completely covered by the company, and Dan is provided further paid leave until he is well enough to return to work. After several weeks, however, Dan is still daunted by the prospect of having to learn to operate in a world where he is unable to use his dominant arm. Depressive thoughts bombard Dan day and night, as he cannot help but think about the accident and his resulting situation. As even small tasks such as putting toothpaste on his toothbrush seem insurmountable, Dan agonizes over how he will be able to function at his job, which requires typing all day on a computer. Moreover, while Dan's brother has moved in to help temporarily, Dan is worried that he will now permanently become dependent on other people for help performing simple tasks that once required no extra consideration. What's even more devastating to Dan is his belief that he will no longer be as physically active as he was previously. Dan worries that without his ability to participate in sports, he will lose his friends, his social life and ultimately his identity as an athletic, physically fit individual. Dan has always considered himself to be a resilient individual, but with his world shaken, he finds himself completely lost.

Questions

1. Does Dan's initial reaction of fear, anxiety and worry indicate that Dan is destined to a long-term prognosis of distress?
2. What sort of cognitive processing is Dan currently engaged in? What strategies might Dan employ to move towards a more constructive form of cognitive processing?
3. In what ways has Dan's psychological needs satisfaction been thwarted? What strategies might be used to facilitate satisfaction of these needs?
4. What resources might Dan drawn on to facilitate an experience of growth?

References

Bianco, T., Malo, S., & Orlick, T. (1999). Sport injury and illness: Elite skiers describe their experiences. *Research Quarterly for Exercise and Sport, 70*, 157–169.

Calhoun, L. G., & Tedeschi, R. G. (1998). Posttraumatic growth: Future directions. In R. G. Tedeschi, C. L. Park, & L. G. Calhoun (Eds.), *Posttraumatic growth: Positive changes in the aftermath of crisis* (pp. 215–238). Erlbaum.

Calhoun, L. G., & Tedeschi, R. G. (2006). *Handbook of posttraumatic growth: Research and practice*. Erlbaum.

Cann, A., Calhoun, L. G., Tedeschi, R. G., & Solomon, D. T. (2010). Posttraumatic growth and depreciation as independent experiences and predictors of well-being. *Journal of Loss and Trauma, 15*, 151–166. https://doi.org/10.1080/15325020903375826.

Cann, A., Calhoun, L. G., Tedeschi, R. G., Triplett, K. N., Vishnevsky, T., & Lindstrom, C. M. (2011). Assessing posttraumatic cognitive processes: The event related rumination inventory. *Anxiety, Stress, & Coping, 24*(2), 137–156. https://doi.org/10.1080/10615806.2010.529901.

Chun, S., & Lee, Y. (2008). The experience of posttraumatic growth for people with spinal cord injury. *Qualitative Health Research, 18*(7), 877–890.

Clement, D., Arvinen-Barrow, M., & Fetty, T. (2015). Psychosocial responses during different phases of sport-injury rehabilitation: A qualitative study. *Journal of Athletic Training, 50*, 95–104.

Crawford, J. J., Gayman, A. M., & Tracey, J. (2014). An examination of post-traumatic growth in Canadian and American ParaSport athletes with acquired spinal cord injury. *Psychology of Sport and Exercise, 15*(4), 399–406. https://doi.org/10.1016/j.psychsport.2014.03.008.

Day, M. C. (2013). The role of initial physical activity experiences in promoting posttraumatic growth in paralympic athletes with an acquired disability. *Disability and Rehabilitation, 35*(24), 2064–2072. https://doi.org/10.3109/09638288.2013.805822.

Day, M. C., & Wadey, R. (2016). Narratives of trauma, recovery, and growth: The complex role of sport following permanent acquired disability. *Psychology of Sport and Exercise, 22*, 131–138.

Dibb, B., Ellis-Hill, C., Donovan-Hall, M., Burridge, J., & Rushton, D. (2014). Exploring positive adjustment in people with spinal cord injury. *Journal of Health Psychology, 19*(8), 1043–1054. https://doi.org/10.1177/1359105313483158.

Evans, L., Hardy, L., & Fleming, S. (2000). Intervention strategies with injured athletes: An action research study. *The Sport Psychologist, 14*, 188–206. https://doi.org/10.1123/tsp.14.2.188.

Gallagher, P., & MacLachlan, M. (2001). Adjustment to an artificial limb: A qualitative perspective. *Journal of Health Psychology, 6*(1), 85–100.

Hammer, C., Podlog, L., Wadey, R., Galli, N., Forber-Pratt, A. J., & Newton, M. (2020). Cognitive processing following acquired disability for para sport athletes: A serial mediation model. *Disability and Rehabilitation, 42*(17), 2492–2500. https://doi.org/10.1080/09638288.2018.1563639.

Hammer, C., Podlog, L., Wadey, R., Galli, N., Forber-Pratt, A. J., & Newton, M. (2019a). From core belief challenge to posttraumatic growth in para sport athletes: Moderated mediation by needs satisfaction and deliberate rumination. *Disability and Rehabilitation, 41*(20), 2403–2411. https://doi.org/10.1080/09638288.2018.1466203.

Hammer, C., Podlog, L., Wadey, R., Galli, N., Forber-Pratt, A. J., Newton, M., Greviskes, L. E., & Hall, M. S. (2019b). Understanding posttraumatic growth of para sport athletes with acquired disability. *Disability and Rehabilitation, 41*(6), 674–682. https://doi.org/10.1080/09638288.2017.1402961.

Hurley, O. A., Moran, A., & Guerin, S. (2007). Exploring athletes' experiences of their injuries: A qualitative investigation. *Sport and Exercise Psychology Review, 3*, 14–22.

Janoff-Bulman, R. (1992). *Shattered assumptions: Towards a new psychology of trauma*. Free Press.

Joseph, S., & Linley, P. A. (2005). Positive adjustment to threatening events: An organismic valuing theory of growth through adversity. *Review of General Psychology, 9*(3), 262–280. https://doi.org/10.1037/1089-2680.9.3.262.

Leddy, M. H., Lambert, M. J., & Ogles, B. M. (1994). Psychological consequences of athletic injury among high-level competitors. *Research Quarterly for Exercise and Sport, 65*, 347–354.

Linley, P. A., & Joseph, S. (2004). Positive change following trauma and adversity: A review. *Journal of Traumatic Stress, 17*(1), 11–21.

Livneh, H., & Antonak, R. F. (2005). Psychosocial adaptation to chronic illness and disability: A primer for counselors. *Journal of Counseling & Development, 83*, 12–20.

Lucas, R. E. (2007). Long-term disability is associated with lasting changes in subjective well-being: Evidence from two nationally representative longitudinal studies. *Journal of Personality and Social Psychology, 92*(4), 717–730.

McMillen, J. C., & Cook, C. L. (2003). The positive by-products of spinal cord injury and their correlates. *Publication Psychology, 48*(2), 77–85.

Park, C. L., & Lechner, S. C. (2006). Measurement issues in assessing growth following stressful life experiences. In L. G. Calhoun, & R. G. Tedeschi (Eds.), *Handbook of posttraumatic growth: Research & practice* (pp. 47–67). Lawrence Erlbaum Associates Publishers.

Podlog, L., & Dionigi, R. (2010). Coach strategies for addressing psychosocial challenges during the return to sport from injury. *Journal of Sports Sciences, 28*, 1197–1208. https://doi.org/10.1080/02640414.2010.487873.

Podlog, L., & Eklund, R. C. (2006). A longitudinal investigation of competitive athletes' return to sport following serious injury. *Journal of Applied Sport Psychology, 18*, 44–68.

Podlog, L., Lochbaum, M., & Stevens, T. (2010). Need satisfaction, well-being and perceived return-to-sport outcomes among injured athletes. *Journal of Applied Sport Psychology, 22*, 167–182.

Putukian, M. (2016). The psychological response to injury in student athletes: A narrative review with a focus on mental health. *British Journal of Sports Medicine, 50*, 145–148.

Roy-Davis, K., Wadey, R., & Evans, L. (2017). A grounded theory of sport injury-related growth. *Sport, Exercise, and Performance Psychology, 6*(1), 35–52.

Rubio, V. J., Quartiroli, A., Podlog, L., & Olmedilla, A. (2020). Understanding the dimensions of personal growth following a severe sport injury: A DELPHI method approach. *PLOS One, 15*(6). https://doi.org/10.1371/journal.pone.0235149.

Ruddock-Hudson, M., O'Halloran, P., & Murphy, G. (2012). Exploring psychological reactions to injury in the Australian Football League (AFL). *Journal of Applied Sport Psychology, 24*, 375–390.

Salim, J., & Wadey, R. (2018). Can emotional disclosure promote sport injury-related growth? *Journal of Applied Sport Psychology, 30*, 367–387.

Salim, J., & Wadey, R. (2019). Using gratitude to promote sport injury-related growth. *Journal of Applied Sport Psychology*. https://doi.org/10.1080/10413200.2019.1626515.

Salim, J., Wadey, R., & Diss, C. (2015). Examining hardiness, coping and stress-related growth following sport injury. *Journal of Applied Sport Psychology, 28*, 154–169.

Seligman, M. E. P., Steen, T. A., Park, N., & Peterson, C. (2005). Positive psychology progress: Empirical validation of interventions. *American Psychologist, 60*, 410–421.

Stockton, H., Hunt, N., & Joseph, S. (2011). Cognitive processing, rumination, and posttraumatic growth. *Journal of Traumatic Stress, 24*(1), 85–92. https://doi.org/10.1002/jts.20606.

Taku, K., Cann, A., Tedeschi, R. G., & Calhoun, L. G. (2015). Core beliefs shaken by an earthquake correlate with posttraumatic growth. *Psychological Trauma: Theory, Research, Practice, and Policy, 7*(6), 563–569. https://doi.org/10.1037/tra0000054.

Tedeschi, R. G., & Calhoun, L. G. (2004). Posttraumatic growth: Conceptual foundations and empirical evidence. *Psychological Inquiry, 15*(1), 1–18. https://doi.org/10.1207/s15327965pli1501_01.

Tracey, J. (2003). The emotional response to the injury and rehabilitation process. *Journal of Applied Sport Psychology*, *15*(4), 279–293.

Udry, E., Gould, D., Bridges, D., & Beck, L. (1997). Down but not out: Athlete responses to season-ending injuries. *Journal of Sport and Exercise Psychology*, *19*(3), 229–248.

Unwin, J., Kacperek, L., & Clarke, C. (2009). A prospective study of positive adjustment to lower limb amputation. *Clinical Rehabilitation*, *23*, 1044–1050. https://doi.org/10.1177/0269215509339001.

Wadey, R., Evans, L., Evans, K., & Mitchell, I. (2011). Perceived benefits following sport injury: A qualitative examination of their antecedents and underlying mechanisms. *Journal of Applied Sport Psychology*, *23*, 142–158.

Wadey, R., Podlog, L., Galli, N., & Mellalieu, S. D. (2016). Stress-related growth following sport injury: Examining the applicability of the organismic valuing theory. *Scandinavian Journal of Medicine & Science in Sports*, *26*(10), 1132–1139.

Walker, N., Thatcher, J., & Lavellee, D. (2010). A preliminary development of the Re-Injury Anxiety Inventory (RIAI). *Physical Therapy in Sport*, *11*, 23–29. https://doi.org/10.1016/j.ptsp.2009.09.003.

Wilson, B., Morris, B. A., & Chambers, S. (2014). A structural equation model of posttraumatic growth after prostate cancer. *Psycho-Oncology*, *23*, 1212–1219. https://doi.org/10.1002/pon.3546.

Part III

ENHANCING SPORTS INJURY REHABILITATION EXPERIENCES WITH INJURED ATHLETES

As you learned through Part 2 of the book, there are many factors that can influence the way an athlete responds to injury. Part 3 of the book builds on this by going through the next stage of the injury journey, their rehabilitation. During injury rehabilitation, athletes can experience psychosocial stress, anxiety, emotional disturbance; their emotional integrity can be compromised; and they can struggle to make rational decisions about rehabilitation activities (Gledhill et al., in press). Consequently, Part 3 of this book looks at ways we can work with athletes to improve their rehabilitation experiences, with the intention of feeding this forward into return to sport outcomes.

In the first chapter, Adam Gledhill and Andreas Ivarsson take on one of the major challenges facing sports injury practitioners by looking at factors influencing athletes' rehabilitation adherence. An athlete's adherence to prescribed rehabilitation is typically poor and this can have a detrimental impact on rehabilitation outcomes (Ivarsson et al., 2017). Therefore, understanding the factors that can impact on rehabilitation adherence and the ways that it can be enhanced are central concerns for sports injury practitioners (Gledhill et al., in press).

Following the work on rehabilitation adherence, Dale Forsdyke considers the role of social support as one of the most powerful ways of enhancing an athlete's injury experience. Dale will look at the influence of social support and the roles that different social support providers can play in enhancing athletes' injury experiences. After discussing the different types of social support, Dale will then provide several practical suggestions for providing social support to injured athletes.

Adam Gledhill will then close Part 3 of the book by looking at different psychological intervention strategies that can be used during injury rehabilitation. As you have learned in previous sections and despite the best efforts of all involved, the injury experience is one that can be of detriment to an athlete in many ways. It can affect their confidence, create self-doubt, negatively impact on their mental health or can create just a general sense of tension and an inability to relax. With these considerations in mind, Adam closes Part 3 by providing evidence informed, applied suggestions that can serve to improve each of these different challenges faced by injured athletes. Given the strength of evidence suggesting that psychological interventions can reduce the risk of injury, reduce injury time-loss and reduce re-injury risk (Gledhill et al., 2018), Adam will specifically explore the role of imagery training and mindfulness-based approaches within sport injury rehabilitation.

References

Gledhill, A., Forsdyke, D., & Goom, T. (in press). "I'm asking you to believe—not in my ability to create change, but in yours.": Four strategies to enhance patients' rehabilitation adherence. *British Journal of Sports Medicine.*

Gledhill, A., Forsdyke, D., & Murray, E. (2018). Psychological interventions used to reduce sports injuries: A systematic review of real-world effectiveness. *British Journal of Sports Medicine*, 52, 967–971.

Ivarsson, A., Tranaeus, U., Johnson, U., Stenling, A. (2017). Negative psychological responses of injury and rehabilitation adherence effects on return to play in competitive athletes: A systematic review and meta-analysis. *Open Access Journal of Sports Medicine*, *8*, 27–32.

6 BELIEVE IN YOUR ABILITY TO CREATE CHANGE

PSYCHOSOCIAL FACTORS INFLUENCING SPORTS INJURY REHABILITATION ADHERENCE

Dr Adam Gledhill and Dr Andreas Ivarsson

Sports injuries present a serious burden for athletes and teams (Bahr et al., 2018), causing injury practitioners to question how we might best reduce sports injury burden (Gledhill & Forsdyke, 2018a). Not least of which, this burden is in part caused by the fact that sports injury is often a time where athletes can experience psychosocial stress, anxiety and emotional disturbance as negative responses to injury, and their ability to make rational decisions about rehabilitation activities can be compromised (Forsdyke et al., 2016; Gledhill et al., 2020). A central concern associated with an athlete's ability to make rational decisions is how this might impact on their choices about clinic-based and home-based rehabilitation behaviours, specifically how well an athlete adheres to their rehabilitation programme (Gledhill et al., 2020).

Drawing on the above, through this chapter we will (1) discuss the context and meaning of rehabilitation and rehabilitation adherence (RA), (2) discuss the scale of the RA problem and the methods of measuring RA, (3) discuss psychosocial considerations that positively and negatively influence injury RA, (4) highlight ways that athletes can improve their RA and (5) will close with an applied case study. Within this chapter, we acknowledge that athletes can often attend rehabilitation with the expectation that their injury practitioner will 'fix' them, but we ascribe to the notion that athletes are the centre of their rehabilitation process and should be active engagers with the process. In essence, drawing on the words of former US President Barrack Obama, Gledhill et al. (2020) acknowledge the importance of athletes believing not in their injury practitioners' ability to create change, but the athlete's own ability to do so.

THE CONTEXT AND MEANING OF REHABILITATION AND REHABILITATION ADHERENCE

In setting the landscape for this chapter, understanding key terminology is important. 'Rehabilitation' is the process that athletes go through from the point of injury, through to the hopefully pre-injury levels of performance. We appreciate this may be viewed as overly simplistic by some and the lens through which you view the sports injury experience may create a different perspective on what constitutes rehabilitation. For example, for a sports injury practitioner, an athlete remaining injury free after they return to sport might be an important criterion for successful rehabilitation, whereas an athlete or coach might determine that a faster return to sport has been more successful rehabilitation, whilst a parent, friend or spouse might view successful rehabilitation as the athlete being in a state of wellbeing, irrespective of sport performance (Gledhill, 2020). However, given that more often than not – and under ideal circumstances – athletes' and other key stakeholders' injury outcome goal will be that the athlete returns to at least pre-injury levels of performance (e.g. Ardern et al., 2016), we consider this to be the ideal endpoint of the rehabilitation process.

Whilst the terms 'adherence' and 'compliance' are used almost interchangeably within this body of research (Gledhill et al., 2018), they are different. The notion of adherence is characterized by athletes being actively, voluntarily and collaboratively involved in a mutually acceptable course of behaviour to produce a desired outcome (Meichenbaum & Turk, 1987). This is different to compliance, which connotes a much more passive role for the athletes, whereby they follow instructions from their sports injury practitioner without question or a great deal of input (Gledhill et al., 2018). In the context of this chapter, we consider sports injury RA to be athletes appropriately engaging with rehabilitation behaviours (e.g. exercise-based rehabilitation, functional training, psychological skills training, sleep, rest), in an attempt to return to at least pre-injury levels of performance.

THE SCALE OF REHABILITATION NON-ADHERENCE AND IMPACT OF SPORTS INJURY

Given that sports injuries do present such significant burden for athletes and teams, one could be forgiven for thinking that athletes of all levels will naturally and automatically adhere to their rehabilitation programme, in an attempt to make a swift return to sport. After all, the question of 'how fast can I be back?' is often one that athletes will pre-occupy themselves with, from the outset of their injury (Gledhill & Forsdyke, 2018b). Unfortunately, such an assumption would be incorrect: non-adherence rates are high, extending to almost 100% non-adherence at times and being viewed as a major challenge by sports injury practitioners (e.g. Granquist et al., 2014).

High non-adherence rates cause problems for athletes, teams and injury practitioners. Injury rehabilitation non-adherence is associated with poorer rehabilitation progress (Forsdyke et al., 2016) and reduced chance of return to sport post-injury (Ivarsson et al., 2017). Both of these scenarios (i.e. unnecessarily prolonged rehabilitation periods and poor return to sport outcomes) have a number of negative consequences. Sports injury, particularly severe or recurrent sports injury, puts athletes at increased risk of a number of mental health complaints, including anxiety disorder, disordered eating, depression and suicidal ideations (Putukian, 2016). Sports injuries are also a leading cause of career termination/retirement for top-level athletes (Ristolainen et al., 2012). Increased occurrence of injury is associated with less successful performance on the pitch, with fewer competitions won by teams who suffer more injuries (Hägglund et al., 2013). Injuries also have significant impact off the pitch, with injuries estimated as costing between €500,000 per month for each month out with an injury for an elite football player (Ekstrand, 2013), through to a total estimated cost of £45 million per season due to injury-related performance deficits in the English Premier League (Eliakim et al., 2020). To sum up, whether you're more focused on athletes' health, competitive advantages or economic health, sports injuries are a major concern (Gledhill & Ivarsson, 2020). Combining this with the fact that increased RA predicts more successful return to sport outcomes (Ivarsson et al., 2017) leads researchers and practitioners to conclude that understanding factors affecting RA and the ways in which we might best enhance RA holds multi-faceted importance for all involved with injury rehabilitation (Gledhill, 2020).

METHODS OF MEASURING REHABILITATION ADHERENCE

How we best measure RA has become a topic of debate in and of itself. These 'measurements' inevitably contain indications of rehabilitation session attendance and injury practitioner observations of appropriate engagement with activities, as well as self-reports of home-based RA. There are, however, also established scales that athletes and injury practitioners can use to get more of an objective measure of adherence. The three most relevant within the scope of this chapter are the Sports Injury RA Scale (SIRAS; Brewer et al., 2000b), the RA Measure for Athletic Training (RAdMAT; Granquist et al., 2010) and the Rehabilitation Overadherence Questionnaire (ROAQ; Podlog et al., 2013). Below, we provide a brief overview of these scales, their uses and the populations validated/used with and invite the reader to visit the original studies for more detailed information about each scale.

SPORTS INJURY REHABILITATION ADHERENCE SCALE

SIRAS (Brewer et al., 2000) is arguably the most widely used measure of RA within this body of literature. It is designed to specifically measure clinic-based adherence and can be adopted for use with specific rehabilitation sessions or for rehabilitation activities more broadly (Brewer et al., 2000; Kolt et al., 2007). SIRAS has predominantly been used in adult populations and is a brief measure with three items: (1) the injured athlete's intensity of rehabilitation activity completion, (2) the injured athlete's frequency of following instructions and advice and (3) the injured athlete's receptiveness to changes in the rehabilitation plan. Each of these subscales is measured on a five-point Likert scale that, when the scores are combined, gives an overall adherence score in the range of 3–15, with a higher score indicating higher levels of adherence to the rehabilitation activities. SIRAS is considered to have high levels of inter-rater reliability, as well as high levels of discriminant validity (i.e. the ability to discriminate between low, moderate and high levels of adherence; Kolt et al., 2007).

Despite being widely used to measure adherence, there has been debate as to whether SIRAS is more a measure of compliance (Bollen et al., 2014). Given that it involves the injured athlete being observed by the injury practitioner, the athlete may feel a sense of being compelled to complete activities in a predetermined manner and be complicit with instruction when they know they are being observed; hence, this would be more in tune with established definitions of compliance as opposed to adherence (Bollen et al., 2014).

REHABILITATION ADHERENCE MEASURE FOR ATHLETIC TRAINING

As with SIRAS, RAdMAT (Granquist et al., 2010) has been predominantly used with adult populations and was originally designed for use within the athletic training environment. It is a 16-item measure that allows the sports injury practitioner to measure clinic-based adherence. It gives a total score in the range of 16–64, with a higher score showing an indication of higher levels of RA. RAdMAT measures three subscales deemed to indicate adherence: (1) attendance and participation, (2) communication and (3) attitude and effort.

REHABILITATION OVERADHERENCE QUESTIONNAIRE

The ROAQ (Podlog et al., 2013) is a 10-item questionnaire with two subscales and is designed to measure the athletes' beliefs about their rehabilitation overadherence. The two subscales are (1) ignore practitioner recommendations (IPR) and (2) attempt at expedited rehabilitation (AER). The IPR subscale measures the athlete's willingness to rehabilitate irrespective of the advice given by their injury practitioner, whereas the AER subscale measures the athlete's desire to return to sport more quickly than would be considered normal (Podlog et al., 2013). Collectively, the two subscales provide an indication of rehabilitation over adherence and have been largely used to measure over adherence within high school and college level athletes (e.g. Hilliard et al., 2017; Podlog et al., 2013).

PSYCHOSOCIAL FACTORS INFLUENCING REHABILITATION ADHERENCE

Recently, two systematic reviews have been completed (Goddard et al., 2020; Ivarsson et al., 2017) that have investigated the relationships between psychosocial factors and RA. We shall first outline these two systematic reviews, before adopting principles of best evidence synthesis (e.g. Gledhill et al., 2018) to examine psychosocial factors that have gained particular prominence in more detail.

Many systematic reviews (e.g. Forsdyke et al., 2016) that have sought to explain the relationships between psychosocial factors and rehabilitation outcomes in competitive athletes have seemingly restricted their discussions to the direct relationships. Recognizing this limitation and the long-held recognition that RA might mediate the relationship between psychosocial factors and rehabilitation outcomes (e.g. Brewer et al., 2002; Wiese-Bjornstal et al., 1998) Ivarsson et al. (2017) sought to investigate the indirect effect of negative affective responses (e.g. fear of reinjury, self-presentation concerns) on return to play through RA. In their systematic review and meta-analysis of negative psychological responses of injury and rehabilitation effects on return to play in competitive athletes, Ivarsson and colleagues noted that negative affective responses had a small and statistically insignificant effect on RA. However, their path analysis also showed that 36% of variance in return to play outcomes was explained by negative affective responses to injury and RA.

Whilst Ivarsson and colleagues' work does incrementally shift the trajectory of this area of research by considering the mediating role of RA, the work isn't without limitation. The small number of included studies and effect sizes creates concern over the statistical power of the relationships. Also, the saturated model specified makes it impossible to assess model fit. Only having return to play as the target outcome variable may also be viewed as overly simplistic. However, in keeping with the ethos of this chapter and recognizing Ivarsson and colleagues' desire to report a concrete outcome for athletes, research and practitioners, we prefer to escalate and report the real-world value of the outcome as opposed to focus on the statistical limitations.

In a more recent systematic review, Goddard et al. (2020) combined findings of 17 studies to reflect the idea that factors influencing RA can be classified as either personal or situational factors. Unlike Ivarsson et al. (2017), Goddard and colleagues did not restrict study inclusion to specific study designs, thus providing a broader understanding of the research area (cf. Gledhill et al., 2018). Unlike previous related systematic reviews that have restricted inclusion to competitive athletes to provide more focused applied recommendations (e.g. Forsdyke et al., 2016; Ivarsson et al., 2017), Goddard and colleagues included studies of all levels of sport population. They reported that personal factors influencing RA included the impact of the injury, justification for adherence, motivation, confidence, self-efficacy, coping, social support, locus of control, cognitive appraisal, coping and psychological skills. The reported situational characteristics included the characteristics, strategies and effectiveness of the sports injury practitioner and treatment efficacy.

Whilst not a complete overview of the research area given the small number of included databases and the high number of omitted studies, Goddard and colleagues offer an initial and partially systematic insight into the research area as a whole. They provide descriptions of themes intended to guide researchers and practitioners moving forward. In doing so, they provide, in an introductory manner, a platform for future development of the area as a whole.

Another important contribution of the two aforementioned systematic reviews is the reflection that the majority of the work investigating factors influencing RA is correlational. As such, through the next section of this chapter, we will discuss some of the key psychosocial factors that are associated with greater RA. Broadly speaking, we'll discuss these under the headings of personal, cognitive, emotional, social and contextual and demographic factors.

Personal factors

Whilst the list of personal factors that are associated with higher levels of RA is extensive (e.g. agreeableness, conscientiousness, mental toughness, openness to experience, pain tolerance and many more), two personal factors which have garnered a fair amount of attention and support are athletic identity and self-motivation.

Of the different personal factors, athletic identity is one of the most established factors within this body of research (e.g. Brewer et al., 2003; Hilliard et al., 2017; Podlog et al., 2013). Higher levels of athletic identity are associated with higher levels of RA (e.g. Brewer et al., 2003) but are also associated with an increased likelihood of rehabilitation overadherence (Hilliard et al., 2017). Specifically, increased athletic identity increases the likelihood that an athlete will attempt an expedited rehabilitation (Hilliard et al., 2017). It is likely that this is due to personal and social considerations that influence athletic identity in athletes (Stephan & Brewer, 2007). For example, being socially connected with teammates, receiving recognition from coaches and being recognized as a high level athlete can all contribute to athletic identity. Injury disrupts each of these things; therefore, it is likely that an athlete might try to expedite their return to sport as a result. However, it is also likely that athletic identity does not increase the likelihood of an injured athlete ignoring the advice of their sports injury practitioners, as they are often viewed as the people who will 'fix' the athlete (i.e. contribute to restoration of athletic identity), thus their advice has value to the athlete. Athletes with high levels of athletic identity might also feel the need to meet ideals that are consistent with their roles as an athlete, such as training through pain or masking or not reporting pain (Murphy & Waddington, 2007; Tasiemski & Brewer, 2011). Moreover, athletes who are high in athletic identity may experience more worry over losing their place in the team/squad (Podlog et al., 2013) and are more susceptible to depression as a response to injury (Brewer et al., 1993). Collectively, these points illustrate the importance of understanding athletic identity and the impact it can have on RA.

Self-motivation is a generalized, non-specific tendency to persist in the long-term pursuit of behavioural goals, irrespective of extrinsic reinforcement or situational influences (Dishman & Ickles, 1981). It is another established personal factor linked to RA. Levy et al. (2008b) noted that self-motivation is specifically linked to clinic-based rehabilitation and attendance, but not home-based rehabilitation. Moreover, Brewer et al. (2003) noted that age moderated the relationship between self-motivation and RA, whereby self-motivation only significantly predicted home-based RA in older athletes.

Cognitive factors

Cognition consists of the mental activities associated with what we think and know and includes the ways in which our thoughts are organized, what a person is thinking about and how people think (Gledhill, 2020). Of the cognitive factors that have been investigated in sports injury RA contexts, the most prominent are having higher self-confidence and self-efficacy, perceived self-determined motivation and a stronger intention to complete their rehabilitation programme appropriately.

Self-efficacy – a situation-specific version of self-confidence – is predictive of clinic-based rehabilitation and attendance at rehabilitation sessions, but not of home-based rehabilitation (Levy et al., 2008b). Moreover, task self-efficacy is predictive of rehabilitation exercise completion and also appears to be influenced by the number of injuries that an athlete has experienced, with athletes who have experienced more injuries demonstrating greater confidence in their ability to perform their rehabilitation exercises (Milne et al., 2005). It is likely that the experience of previous injuries and the associated rehabilitation will reduce the level of uncertainty associated with rehabilitation and will provide injured athletes with tangible evidence of their ability to effectively complete rehabilitation activities (Forsdyke et al., 2016). It is also likely that low confidence will have more of an impact on home-based RA than clinic-based RA, particularly in instances where injured athletes are unsure of how to perform rehabilitation exercises correctly (Levy et al., 2009).

Injured athletes who perceive higher levels of self-determined motivation are more likely to adhere to their rehabilitation programme (Chan et al., 2009; Truong et al., 2020). It is likely that self-determined motivation has this influence due to higher levels of perceived control over the injury experience, greater perceptions of social connectedness and increased confidence in one's ability to appropriately complete rehabilitation exercises (Chan & Hagger, 2012; Forsdyke et al., 2016; Truong et al., 2020). Consequently, these can result in greater intention to complete rehabilitation activities and improved levels of RA (e.g. Carson & Polman, 2017; Chan & Hagger, 2012).

Emotional factors

Unsurprisingly, injury can be a time of significant emotional upheaval for athletes where their mood state can decrease (Forsdyke et al., 2016). Whilst significant attention to different emotional responses (e.g. fear, anxiety, anger) and their role in return to sport is evident (e.g. Truong et al., 2020), mood disturbance is the most overarching emotional response included in specific RA research (e.g. Daly et al., 1995). Athletes with higher levels of mood disturbance typically display lower levels of RA in comparison to those athletes who experience lower levels of mood disturbance. Emotional responses can be improved by increased perceptions of autonomy support (Carson & Polman, 2017).

Social and contextual factors

Typically, the type of support experienced and the environment in which rehabilitation is completed are virtually consistently associated with RA (e.g. Hildingsson et al., 2018; Johnson et al., 2016; Levy et al., 2008b; Poget et al., 2019). Perceived social support can increase an athlete's sense of feeling cared for, increase a sense of shared goal commitment and being in it together, and enhance their goal directed behaviour towards rehabilitation (e.g. Hildingsson et al., 2018; Poget et al., 2019). Having interaction with significant others is interpreted as especially important during severe injuries (Johnson et al., 2016). Moreover, an environment that facilitates group-based rehabilitation is seen as helpful in enhancing RA (Poget et al., 2019), whilst having an autonomy supportive injury therapist is predictive of RA (Levy et al., 2008b). A sport context where a hypermasculine culture, validating pain, downplaying injuries, social pressure from peers and an enacted culture of risk taking are independently or collectively evident is likely to increase the risk of rehabilitation non-adherence (Truong et al., 2020).

Demographic factors

Currently, only age has been related to differing levels of RA. In identifying a direct relationship between age and RA, Levy et al. (2008a) noted that younger athletes were better adherers to their rehabilitation programmes than older athletes. As well as this direct relationship, age is also recognized as a moderator between other psychological variables and RA, whereby age moderates the relationship between athletic identity and home exercise completion, social support and home exercise completion, self-motivation and home exercise completion, and athletic identity and home cryotherapy completion (Brewer et al., 2003).

ENHANCING REHABILITATION ADHERENCE

Given the importance of RA, one could be forgiven that there is a wealth of sport-based evidence investigating ways in which RA could be improved. Unfortunately, this isn't the case and there exists a paucity of evidence investigating this in sport (Goddard et al., 2020). However, the topic has been investigated more widely outside of the sport context. Thus, this section will draw on evidence from both sport and health contexts to provide suggestions for enhancing RA. The strategies available to date have largely targeted improving motivation, self-efficacy/confidence, improving coping skills and increasing social connectedness.

Self-determination theory (SDT; Deci & Ryan, 2000) provides a framework to explain why several of these factors can increase adherence and, in turn, improve rehabilitation outcomes. Within the SDT humans are suggested to have basic psychological needs that are essential nutrients for effective functioning and well-being. These are the need for autonomy (feeling volitional and free to engage in a behaviour), competence (feeling effective) and relatedness (feeling safe and cared for in interpersonal relationships). When these needs are satisfied, injured athletes will participate in treatment autonomously, that is, their motivation will be characterized by willingness to participate and perceiving valued benefits of participation. Satisfaction of the basic psychological needs is largely determined by the social context (i.e. interactions with other people) surrounding an individual. When these needs are satisfied, it is more likely that individuals will regulate their behaviour more autonomously, which in turn increases the likelihood of lasting behaviour change (Ng et al., 2012). Healthcare practitioners (e.g. physiotherapists) can, based on this assumption, satisfy or thwart the basic psychological needs of their patients depending on the type of communication style they use. A need-supportive communication style will satisfy the patient's basic psychological needs that, in turn, will lead to more autonomous motivation to treatment adherence and health-related behaviours

(Lonsdale et al., 2012, 2017). A need-supportive communication style involves strategies that satisfy the basic psychological needs. SDT outlines three dimensions of communication strategies: autonomy support, competence support and relatedness support (Ntoumanis, 2012). Autonomy support is provided when the practitioner takes the patients perspective, provides relevant choices and information, acknowledges negative feelings and encourages the patient to accept personal responsibility for the health behaviour while minimizing, coercion, demands and pressure (Lonsdale et al., 2012). Competence support/structure involves providing clear and understandable guidelines and expectations, instilling a sense of competence in the injured athletes and providing relevant feedback (Ryan et al., 2008). Relatedness support/involvement is displayed when the practitioner communicates a genuine interest in the injured athlete and his/her well-being and spends considerable time, energy and resources on them (Ryan et al., 2008). These three dimensions are often described as part of a need-supportive communication style that satisfies patients' basic psychological needs (Ntoumanis, 2012). In contrast, a need-thwarting style (also called controlling style) is evident when the practitioner trivializes the injured athletes opinions and feelings, imposes pressure and guilt-inducing language, uses pre- and proscriptions and prohibits a sense of volitional engagement (Ntoumanis, 2012). Although a need-supportive style is preferred and has been related to need satisfaction, autonomous motivation, patient well-being and long-term behaviour adherence (Ng et al., 2012), there is evidence suggesting that healthcare practitioners often adopt a need-thwarting approach (Braddock et al., 1999; Holden et al., 2009; Slade et al., 2009).

Several intervention studies have been conducted to evaluate the effectiveness of communication skills training in healthcare practitioners. The findings from several of these studies suggest that interventions, based on SDT, can increase patient adherence across a range of conditions, such as physical activity (Gourlan et al., 2016) and smoking cessation (Williams et al., 2016). Recent findings from a cluster Randomised Controlled Trial (RCT) focusing specifically on physiotherapists working with chronic low back pain showed that an SDT-based communication skills training (CONNECT; Lonsdale et al., 2012) for physiotherapists increased their need-supportive behaviours towards patients (Murray et al., 2015).

Prospective correlational evidence (e.g. Scherzer et al., 2001) and RCTs (e.g. Coppack et al., 2012; Evans & Hardy, 2002) demonstrate that goal setting interventions related to achieving specific rehabilitation criteria, attending a specific number of rehabilitation sessions, profiling improvements and re-adjusting goals all show improvements in self- and physiotherapist-perceived RA. Within the goal setting processes, having goals which relate to individual sessions, progression through stages of return to sport, return to sport goals and lifestyle goals can all benefit athletes. The most likely explanation for associated improvements in RA is likely to be influenced by increases in patient self-efficacy and perceived treatment efficacy (e.g. Coppack et al., 2012; Evans & Hardy, 2002) or simply that the patient becomes more focussed on achieving a specific outcome (e.g. Scherzer et al., 2001).

Case study

Ellen is a 25-year-old professional basketball player who is currently injured with a grade three ankle ligament sprain. She has a history of persistent ankle injuries, including requiring surgical repair 3 years ago. Neither Ellen nor the medical team can give you an indication as to why her ankle keeps getting injured, beyond her history of previous injuries, but everyone is getting very frustrated at the problem. Ellen keeps asking lots of questions about why her ankle keeps getting injured and has asked more advice about what she can do to stop the recurrent injuries. She proudly talks to you about how she is already doing more than she should be, as her coach said they need her back as soon as possible. She also discusses how she has been 'researching different rehab' on the internet, in an attempt to expedite her return to sport.

Due to her injury history, Ellen has always played with a certain degree of pain because 'that's what athletes do'. She frequently talks about basketball being 'a tough game' and that 'real athletes don't quit'. Ellen has come to see you and said that people keep giving her lots of information, but she doesn't understand half of what people say. She finds herself pretty confused with different parts of the advice but is scared to ask questions because she doesn't want people to think she lacks intelligence. During the conversation with you, Ellen repeatedly tells you that being an athlete is 'who she is' and she doesn't know what to do without it. She's fed up with feeling like she is doing everything that she can, but 'nothing works' to make her better.

Questions

1. What are the important psychosocial factors in the case study that are influencing RA and what influence are they having?
2. What are the key health and sport-related risks for the client, based on the rehabilitation behaviours they are displaying?
3. Plan and justify a multimodal approach to enhancing rehabilitation adherence for this athlete, making specific links between the needs of the athlete and the proposed benefits of the interventions.

References

Ardern, C. L., Glasgow, P., Schneiders, A., Witvrouw, E., Clarsen, B., Cools, A., Gojanovic, B., Griffin, S., Khan K. M., Moksnes, H., Mutch, S. A., Phillips, N., Reurink, G., Sadler, R., Silbernagel, K. G., Thorborg, K., Wangensteen, A., Wilk, K. E., & Bizzini, M. (2016). 2016 Consensus statement on return to sport from the First World Congress in Sports Physical Therapy, Bern. *British Journal of Sports Medicine, 50*, 853–864.

Bahr, R., Clarsen, B., & Ekstrand, J. (2018). Why we should focus on the burden of injury and illnesses, not just their incidence. *British Journal of Sports Medicine, 52*, 1018–1021.

Bollen, J. C., Dean, S. G., Siegert, R. J., Howe, T. E., & Goodwin, V. A. (2014). A systematic review of measures of self-reported adherence to unsupervised home-based rehabilitation exercise programmes, and their psychometric properties. *BMJ Open, 4*, e005044. DOI: 10.1136/bmjopen-2014-005044.

Braddock, C. H., Edwards, K. A., Hasenberg, N. M., Laidley, T. L., & Levinson, W. (1999). Informed decision making in outpatient practice: Time to get back to basics. *JAMA, 282*, 2313–2320.

Brewer, B. W., Andersen, M. B. and Van Raalte, J. L. (2002). Psychological aspects of sport injury rehabilitation: Toward a biopsychosocial approach. In D. L. Mostofsky and L. D. Zaichkowsky (Eds.), *Medical and psychological aspects of sport and exercise* (pp. 41–54). Fitness Information Technology.

Brewer, B. W., Cornelius, A. E., Van Raalte, J. L., Petitpas, A. J., Sklar, J. H., Pohlman, M. H., Krushell, R. J., & Ditmar, T. D. (2003). Age-related differences in predictors of adherence to rehabilitation after anterior cruciate ligament reconstruction. *Journal of Athletic Training, 38*, 158–162.

Brewer, B. W., Van Raalte, J. L., & Linder, D. E. (1993). Athletic identity: Hercules' muscles or Achilles heel? *International Journal of Sport Psychology, 24*(2), 237–254.

Brewer, B. W., Van Raalte, J. L., Petitpas, A. J., Sklar, J. H., Pohlman, M. H., Krushell, R. J., Ditmar, T. D., Daly, J. M., & Weinstock, J. (2000). Preliminary psychometric evaluation of a measure of adherence to clinic-based sport injury rehabilitation. *Physical Therapy in Sport, 1*, 68–74.

Carson, F., & Polman, R. (2017). Self-determined motivation in rehabilitating professional rugby union players. *BMC Sports Science, Medicine and Rehabilitation, 9*(2). DOI: 10.1186/s13102-016-0065-6.

Chan, D. K., & Hagger, M. S. (2012). Self-determined forms of motivation predict sport injury prevention and rehabilitation intentions. *Journal of Science and Medicine in Sport, 15*, 398–406.

Chan, D. K., Lonsdale, C., Ho, P. Y., Yung, P. S., & Chan, K. M. (2009). Patient motivation and adherence to postsurgery rehabilitation rehabilitation exercise recommendations: The influence of physiotherapists' autonomy support behaviours. *Archives of Physical Medicine & Rehabilitation, 90*, 1977–1982.

Coppack, R. J., Kristensen, J., Karageorghis, C. I. (2012). Use of a goal setting intervention to increase adherence to low back pain rehabilitation: A randomised controlled trial. *Clinical Rehabilitation, 26*, 1032–1042.

Daly, J. M., Brewer, B. W., Van Raalte, J. L., Petitpas, A. J., & Sklar, J. H. (1995). Cognitive appraisal, emotional adjustment, and adherence to rehabilitation following knee surgery. *Journal of Sport Rehabilitation, 4*, 23–30.

Deci, E. L., & Ryan, R. M. (2000). The "what" and "why" of goal pursuits: Human needs and the self-determination of behavior. *Psychological Inquiry: An International Journal for the Advancement of Psychological Theory, 11*, 227–268.

Dishman, R. K. & Ickles, W. (1981). Self-motivation and adherence to therapeutic exercise. *Journal of Behavioural Medicine, 4*, 421–438.

Ekstrand, J. (2013). Keeping your top players on the pitch: The key to football medicine at a professional level. *British Journal of Sports Medicine, 47*, 723–724.

Eliakim, E., Morgulev, E., Lidor, R., & Meckel, Y. (2020). Estimation of injury costs: Financial damage of English Premier League teams' underachievement due to injuries. *BMJ Open Sport & Exercise Medicine*. DOI: 10.1136/bmjsem-2019-000675.

Evans, L., & Hardy, L. (2002). Injury rehabilitation: A goal-setting intervention study. *Res Quart Ex Sport, 3*, 310–319.

Forsdyke, D., Smith, A., Jones, M., & Gledhill, A. (2016). Psychosocial factors associated with outcomes of sports injury rehabilitation in competitive athletes: A mixed studies systematic review. *British Journal of Sports Medicine, 50*, 537–544.

Gledhill, A. (2020). Biopsychosocial factors in sports injury rehabilitation. In A. Ivarsson, & U. Johnson (Eds.), *Psychological bases of sports injury* (4th ed., pp. 79–100). Fitness Information Technology.

Gledhill, A., & Forsdyke, D. (2018a). An ounce of prevention is better than a pound of cure: Shouldn't we be doing EVERYTHING to reduce sports injury incidence and burden. *British Journal of Sports Medicine, 52*, 1292–1293.

Gledhill, A., & Forsdyke, D. (2018b). Return to Sport: On the way off the pitch, my first thought was "How fast can I be back?" *BASEM Today, 45*, 36–37.

Gledhill, A., Forsdyke, D., & Goom, T. (2020). "I'm asking you to believe – not in my ability to create change, but in yours." Four strategies to enhance patients' rehabilitation adherence. *British Journal of Sports Medicine*. Published Online First: 03 November 2020. DOI: 10.1136/bjsports-2020-102245.

Gledhill, A., Forsdyke, D., & Murray, E. (2018). Psychological interventions used to reduce sports injuries: A systematic review of real-world effectiveness. *British Journal of Sports Medicine, 52*, 967–971.

Gledhill, A., & Ivarsson, I. (2020). Reducing sports injury risk: Making a case for psychological intervention. *The Sport and Exercise Scientist*, 65, 26–27.

Goddard, K., Roberts, C-M., Byron-Daniel, J., & Woodford, L. (2020). Psychological factors involved in adherence to sport injury rehabilitation: A systematic review. *International Review of Sport and Exercise Psychology*. DOI: 10.1080/1750984X.2020.1744179.

Gourlan, M., Bernard, P., Bortolon, C., Romain, A. J., Lareyre, O., Carayol, M., Ninot, G., & Boiché, J. (2016). Efficacy of theory-based interventions to promote physical activity: A meta-analysis of randomised controlled trials. *Health Psychology Review, 10*(1), 50–66.

Granquist, M. D., Gill, D. L., & Appaneal, R. N. (2010). Development of a measure of rehabilitation adherence for athletic training. *Journal of Sport Rehabilitation, 19*, 249–267.

Granquist, M. D., Podlog, L., Engel, J. R., & Newland, A. (2014). Certified athletic trainers' perspectives on rehabilitation adherence in collegiate athletic training settings. *Journal of Sport Rehabilitation, 23*, 123–133.

Hägglund, M., Waldén, M., Magnusson, H., Kristenson, K., Bengtsson, H., & Ekstrand, J. (2013). Injuries affect team performance negatively in professional football: An 11-year follow-up of the UEFA Champions League injury study. *British Journal of Sports Medicine, 47*, 738–742.

Hildingsson, M., Tranaeus-Fitzgerals, U., & Alricsson, M. (2018). Perceived motivational factors for female football players during rehabilitation after sports injury: A qualitative interview study. *Journal of Exercise Rehabilitation, 14*, 199–206.

Hilliard, R. C., Blom, L., Hankemeier, D., & Bolin, J. (2017). Exploring the relationship between athletic identity and beliefs about rehabilitation overadherence in college athletes. *Journal of Sport Rehabilitation, 26*, 208–220.

Holden, M. A., Nicholls, E. E., Young, J., Hay, E. M., & Foster, N. E. (2009). UK-based physical therapists' attitudes and beliefs regarding exercise and knee osteoarthritis: Findings from a mixed methods study. *Arthritis Care & Research, 61*, 1511–1521.

Ivarsson, A., Tranaeus, U., Johnson, U., & Stenling, A. (2017). Negative psychological responses of injury and rehabilitation adherence effects on return to play in competitive athletes: A systematic review and meta-analysis. *Open Access Journal of Sports Medicine, 8*, 27–32.

Johnson, U., Ivarsson, A., Karlsson, J., Hägglund, M., Waldèn, M., & Börjesson, M. (2016). Rehabilitation after first-time anterior cruciate ligament injury and reconstruction in female football players: A study of resilience factors. *BMC Sports Science, Medicine and Rehabilitation, 8*, 20. DOI: 10.1186/s13102-016-0046-9.

Kolt, G. S., Brewer, B. W., Pizzari, T., Schoo, A. M. M., & Garrett, N. (2007). The sport injury rehabilitation adherence scale: A reliable scale for use in clinical physiotherapy. *Physiotherapy, 93*, 17–22.

Levy, A. R., Polman, R. C. J., & Borkoles, E. (2008a). Examining the relationship between perceived autonomy support and age in the context of rehabilitation adherence in sport. *Rehabilitation Psychology, 53*(2), 224–230. https://doi.org/10.1037/0090-5550.53.2.224

Levy, A. R., Polman, R. C. J., & Clough, P. J. (2008b). Adherence to sport injury rehabilitation programs: An integrated psychosocial approach. *Scandinavian Journal of Medicine and Science in Sports, 18*, 798–809.

Levy, A. R., Polman, R. C. J., Nicholls, A. R., & Marchant, D. C. (2009). Sport injury rehabilitation adherence: Perspectives of recreational athletes. *International Journal of Sport and Exercise Psychology, 7*, 212–229.

Lonsdale, C., Hall, A. M., Murray, A., Williams, G. C., McDonough, S. M., Ntoumanis, N., Owen, K., Schwarzer, R., Parker, P., Kolt, G. S., & Hurley, D. A. (2017). Communication skills training for practitioners to increase patient adherence to home-based rehabilitation for chronic low back pain: Results of a cluster randomized controlled trial. *Archives of Physical Medicine and Rehabilitation*, 98, 1732–1743.

Lonsdale, C., Hall, A. M., Williams, G. C., McDonough, S. M., Ntoumanis, N., Murray, A., & Hurley, D. A. (2012). Communication style and exercise compliance in physiotherapy (CONNECT): A cluster randomized controlled trial to test a theory-based intervention to increase chronic low back pain patients' adherence to physiotherapists' recommendations: study rationale, design, and methods. *BMC Musculoskeletal Disorders, 13*(1), 104.

Meichenbaum, D., & Turk, D. C. (1987). *Facilitating treatment adherence*. Plenum.

Milne, M., Hall, C., & Forwell, L. (2005). Self-efficacy, imagery use and adherence to rehabilitation by injured athletes. *Journal of Sport Rehabilitation, 14*, 150–167.

Murphy, P., & Waddington, I. (2007). Are elite athletes exploited? *Soccer and Society, 10*, 239–255.

Murray, A., Hall, A. M., Williams, G. C., McDonough, S. M., Ntoumanis, N., Taylor, I. M., Jackson, B., Matthews, J., Hurley, D. A., & Lonsdale, C. (2015). Effect of a self-determination theory–based communication skills training program on physiotherapists' psychological support for their patients with chronic low back pain: A randomized controlled trial. *Archives of Physical Medicine and Rehabilitation, 96*(5), 809–816.

Ng, J. Y. Y., Ntoumanis, N., Thøgersen-Ntoumani, C., Deci, E. L., Ryan, R. M., Duda, J. L., & Williams, G. C. (2012). Self-determination theory applied to health contexts: A meta-analysis. *Perspectives on Psychological Science, 7*, 325–340.

Ntoumanis, N. (2012). A self-determination theory perspective on motivation in sport and physical education: Current trends and possible future directions. In G. C. Roberts, & D. C. Treasure (Eds.), *Advances in motivation in sport and exercise* (pp. 91–128). Human Kinetics.

Podlog, L., Gao, Z., Kenow, L., Kleinhert, J., Granquist, M., Newton, M., Hannon, J. (2013). Injury rehabilitation overadherence: Preliminary scale validation and relationships with athletic identity and self-presentation concerns. *Journal of Athletic Training, 48*, 372–381.

Poget, F., Blackburn, T., Descloux, F., & Fiddler, H. (2019). Participating in an exercise group after anterior cruciate ligament reconstruction (ACLR) is perceived to influence psychosocial factors and successful recovery: A focus group qualitative study. *Physiotherapy, 105*, 492–500.

Putukian, M. (2016). The psychological response to injury in student athletes: A narrative review with a focus on mental health. *British Journal of Sports Medicine, 50*, 145 –148.

Ristolainen, L., Kettunen, J. A., Kujala, U. M., & Heinonen, A. (2012). Sport Injuries as the Main Cause of Sport Career Termination among Finnish Top-Level Athletes. *European Journal of Sport Science, 12*, 274–282. https://doi.org/10.1080/17461391.2011.566365.

Ryan, R. M., Patrick, H., Deci, E. L., & Williams, G. C. (2008). Facilitating health behaviour change and its maintenance: Interventions based on self-determination theory. *The European Health Psychologist, 10*(1), 2–5.

Scherzer, C. B., Brewer, B. W., Cornelius, A. E., Van Raalte, J. L., Petitpas, A. J., Sklar, J. H., Pohlman, M. H., Krushell, R. J., & Ditmar, T. D. (2001). Psychological skills and adherence to rehabilitation after reconstruction of the anterior cruciate ligament. *Journal of Sport Rehabilitation, 10*, 165–172.

Slade, S. C., Molloy, E., & Keating, J. L. (2009). Listen to me, tell me: A qualitative study of partnership in care for people with non-specific chronic low back pain. *Clinical Rehabilitation, 23*(3), 270–280.

Stephan, Y., & Brewer, B. W. (2007). Perceived determinants of identification with the athletic role among elite competitors. *Journal of Applied Sport Psychology, 19*, 67–79.

Tasiemski, T., & Brewer, B. (2011). Athletic identity, sport participation, and psychological adjustment in people with spinal cord injury. *Adapted Physical Activity Quarterly, 28*, 233–250.

Truong, L. K., Mosewich, A. D., Holt, C. J., Lee, C. Y., Miciack, M., & Whittaker, J. (2020). Psychological, social and contextual factors across recovery stages following a sport-related knee injury: A scoping review. *British Journal of Sports Medicine, 54*, 1149–1156. DOI: 10.1136/bjsports-2019-101206.

Wiese-Bjornstal, D. M., Smith, A. M., Shaffer, S. M., & Morrey, M. A. (1998). An integrated model of response to sport injury: Psychological and sociological dynamics. *Journal of Applied Sport Psychology, 10*, 46–69. https://doi.org/10.1080/10413209808406377.

Williams, G. C., Niemiec, C. P., Patrick, H., Ryan, R. M., & Deci, E. L. (2016). Outcomes of the Smoker's Health Project: A pragmatic comparative effectiveness trial of tobacco-dependence interventions based on self-determination theory. *Health Education Research, 31*(6), 749–759.

7 ARE YOU A BUFFER OR AN AMPLIFIER?

THE ROLE OF SOCIAL SUPPORT IN THE EFFECTIVE RETURN TO SPORT FOLLOWING INJURY

Dr Dale Forsdyke

In sport the burden of injury is high and return to sport outcomes are frequently less than optimal (e.g. Ekstrand et al., 2020; Webster & Feller, 2019). This may be because numerous physical and psychosocial factors influence the readiness of an athlete to return to sport (Brewer et al., 2002). In comparison to the physical factors influencing return to sport, psychosocial factors are relatively poorly understood (Forsdyke et al., 2016). Consequently, a deeper understanding of the psychosocial factors influencing return to sport may be key to facilitating more optimal return to sport outcomes. Whilst there is some research traction around psychological factors, the role of social factors relating to return to sport outcomes is underdeveloped (Truong et al., 2020). As returning to sport following injury is a social process involving interactions with many different stakeholders, one potentially important psychosocial factor requiring consideration is social support.

This chapter begins with an outline of the conceptual considerations around social support and return to sport following injury. The different types of social support injured athletes may require are discussed, and the key providers of social support to injured athletes are outlined. Additionally, the causal processes of how social support may benefit or hinder injured athletes are discussed with the impact of these processes on return to sport outcomes. Evidence-informed strategies to enhance social support for injured athletes are explained. Last, this chapter concludes with a case study with accompanying questions, which will enable readers to apply the chapter content.

WHAT IS SOCIAL SUPPORT?

Social support is a complex and multidimensional factor made up of actual (e.g. the available social support network) and perceptual features (e.g. appraisals over the quality of social support). It can be considered as interactions between individuals with the intention of augmenting a positive outcome (Bianco & Eklund, 2001). Social support interactions provided to an injured athlete are comprised of social support activities and the social support messages arising from such activities. Generally, social support activities are what individuals actually do to help the injured athlete and tend to be observable and overt, for example a clinician accompanying an injured athlete to appointment or a team-mate offering words of encouragement via a phone call. On the other hand, social support messages are what the injured athletes perceive as to what is being implied or the implicit meaning of such activities. In this sense, social support messages tend to be non-observable and covert. For example, a coach conscientiously asking an athlete about their readiness to return to sport based on some inconsistent training form may be interpreted by the athlete as the coach looking for an excuse not to integrate them back into competition. Social support messages are thought to be more important than social support activities (Bianco & Eklund, 2001). In other words, what appears most important to injured athletes is not the quantity or type of social support activity, it is what this activity says about how the provider regards them and their relationship. After all, inferring from the well-known Theodore Roosevelt quote, injured athletes do not necessarily care about what you do or how much you know until they know how much you care (see King et al., 2019).

The social support activities and messages that an athlete experiences are moderated by several contextual factors (Bianco & Eklund, 2001). This may extend to: (1) the sociocultural context of the sport, (2) the characteristics of the pre-injury relationship between support provider and the athlete and (3) characteristics of the support provider and the athlete. First, the sociocultural context of the support determines the range and availability of potential social support providers. In other words, in high performance sport, there may be routine access to a greater range of social support providers (e.g. coaches, clinicians, sports science practitioners, fans) compared to recreational or semi-professional sport due to increased resourcing. Second, the characteristics of the pre-injury relationship between support provider and athlete may impact on the uptake of support activities and the messages arising from such activities. On one hand, experiencing positive and meaningful interactions with team clinicians prior to injury may augment the impact of social support activities and messages during injury (Maurice et al., 2017; Rees et al., 2010). On the other, with little or no pre-injury relationship, the impact of social support may be diminished. The characteristics of the support provider and athlete refer to each individual's aptitude to offer support, seek out support and adhere to the support when offered. For example, due to an adverse previous injury experience, some athletes may become apathetic towards certain social support activities. Additionally, some stakeholders may find it over-challenging to provide certain types of social support to injured athletes due to a lack of a specific training input (Alexanders et al., 2015; Heaney et al., 2017). Together, the awareness of moderating contextual factors is potentially important as these may provide the basis for thinking and planning around how to optimally support athletes when they are injured.

WHAT TYPES OF SOCIAL SUPPORT DO INJURED ATHLETES NEED?

In the management of injured athletes, it is the more perceptual features of support that are more reliably associated with injury outcomes (Clement & Shannon, 2011). This means effectively providing the correct types of social support, in the right amount, at the right time based on the athletes' particular needs (Corbillon et al., 2008). Consequently, not all athletes will have the same social support needs. The social support needs of injured athletes and support activities provided may come in several types. Broadly, the types of social support provided to an injured athlete are emotional support (i.e. caring and comfort), esteem support (i.e. encouragement and positive feedback), tangible support (i.e. practical assistance and services) and informational support (advice and guidance) (Freeman et al., 2011; Hassell et al., 2015). Several studies have suggested that of the different types of support, it is emotional support that appears most important at affecting return to sport outcomes by enhanced well-being (e.g. Carson & Polman, 2008; Yang et al., 2010), whereas more recently, perceived availability of informational support was the strongest predictor of reduced re-injury risk (Gledhill & Craig, in press). Consequently, during the return to sport process, it is likely that each type of social support will fulfil important functions for injured athletes.

The return to sport process is dynamic (i.e. changes in injury-related stressors, Carson & Polman, 2012) and as such the types of social support an injured athlete requires will likely change. For example, early in the return to sport process, injured athletes may need more tangible, informational and emotional support (e.g. transporting to appointment, explaining the injury diagnosis and treatment options, comfort from negative emotions). However, towards the point of return to training and competition, the athlete may need more informational and esteem support (e.g. understanding return to sport criteria, positive feedback on their readiness to return to sport). This highlights that in order to effectively manage injured athletes, their social support needs should be routinely evaluated throughout the return to sport process (Truong et al., 2020).

WHO ARE THE KEY PROVIDERS OF SOCIAL SUPPORT?

Frequently, sustaining injury provides challenges to athletes that they are ill-equipped to deal with (Carson & Polman, 2012). At this point, athletes are likely to look to their available network of support providers for additional and different types of social support when compared to being injury-free. In other words, injury changes the regular social support patterns of athletes (Yang et al., 2010). Prior to injury, athletes may require social support from coaches, sports science staff, clinicians, family and friends, and teammates in equal parts. However, during injury athletes will likely require greater amounts of social support, and in particular from clinicians and coaches (Corbillon et al., 2008; Yang et al., 2010). The additional support required from clinicians (e.g. doctor, physiotherapist, sports therapist, athletic trainer) is presumably required for injury diagnosis, treatment and rehabilitation, whereas the additional support required from coaches may, in part, reflect the need to still feel professionally and socially valued at a time where they may have little or no impact on team performance. Research suggests that together the social support from clinicians and coaches plays an important role during rehabilitation and upon return to sport (Rees et al., 2010; Yang et al., 2014). Therefore, clinicians and coaches need to be well equipped to provide various types of social support to injured athletes.

It is common for athletes to have a large range of social support providers. However, this does not necessarily mean that high-quality social support is provided. In fact, this may present a sizeable challenge for those working with injured athletes as the social support activities provided should be consistent and coherent. With a large number of providers, it is easy for social support activities to become fragmented and contradictory as each stakeholder may have different return to sport goals (Ardern et al., 2016). For example, a clinician may want the athlete to return to sport when they are physically and psychologically ready with reduced risk of re-injury, whereas a coach may want the athlete back as soon as possible in order to improve team performance. This can give injured athletes mixed messages over return to sport. Together, the providers of social support to injured athletes need to operate as a unified therapeutic alliance in order to better augment return to sport outcomes (Babatunde et al., 2017; Rossettini et al., 2018).

HOW DOES SOCIAL SUPPORT HELP OR HINDER INJURED ATHLETES?

Understanding the processes by which social support influences return to sport outcomes is important in order to effectively manage injured athletes. Social support is thought to influence return to sport outcomes through its relationship with injury-related stress and motivated behaviour. Together these mechanisms should be seen as complimentary as opposing one another (Bianco & Eklund, 2001; Rees et al., 2010).

First, social support is thought to modulate the potential harmful effect of excessive injury-related stress on injured athletes via preventative (i.e. main effects model) and palliative mechanisms (i.e. stress-buffering effects hypothesis, Bianco & Eklund, 2001; Cohen & Wills, 1985). The preventive mechanism implies that in the presence of high-quality social support (i.e. amount, type, coherency, consistency), injured athletes will be inoculated from excessive injury-related stress. In other words, high-quality social support will have an effect on return to sport outcome as excessive levels of injury-related stress are not experienced because of enhanced well-being and coping. The palliative mechanism suggests that high-quality social support acts as a buffer during periods of excessive injury-related stress (e.g. setbacks, integrating back into training and competition). In this sense, high-quality social support will have an effect on return to sport outcomes as a function of injury-related stress (Hartley & Coffee, 2019). If an injured experiences poor-quality social support (i.e. insufficient amounts and types, fragmented, inconsistent), this can then become an additional injury-related stressor. In this regard, social support providers can either be amplifiers or buffers of injury-related stress.

Second, social support shares similarities with the concept of relatedness (i.e. being connected, being cared for, externally validated). According to basic psychology needs theory (Deci & Ryan, 2000), relatedness is one of three core psychological needs that are central in moderating self-determined (i.e. autonomous) forms of motivation. As such, social support may be associated with return to sport through its relationship with motivated behaviour. For example, high-quality social support may lead to greater adherence to injury advice and guidance (Bejar et al., 2019; Bianco, 2001; Pizzari et al., 2002).

Possible other causal mechanisms can be found in domain-specific theoretical frameworks (e.g. biopsychosocial model of sports injury rehabilitation, integrated model of psychological response to sports injury and rehabilitation process). According to the biopsychosocial model (Brewer et al., 2002), social support is identified as a socio-contextual factor that impacts on return to sport outcomes via its relationship with several psychological factors (e.g., personality, cognition, affect, behaviour). In the integrated model (Wiese-Bjornstal et al., 1998), social support is named as a situational factor that by influencing cognitive appraisals will impact on subsequent emotional and behavioural responses of the injured athlete and as such impact return to sport outcomes. When looking to these domain-specific frameworks for causal explanations, it is worthy to note that there is little overall empirical support for these propositions, although there is developing evidence for some of the individual components (Brewer, 2010; Walker et al., 2007).

Taken together, these mechanisms all indicate that high-quality social support will have a positive effect on outcomes, and vice versa. There is a current lack of empirical evidence examining social support and specific return to sport outcomes (e.g. returning to pre-injury sport in the long term, returning to pre-injury levels of performance, remaining injury-free). However, previous research has found several important benefits of high-quality social support for injured athletes such as improved motivation (Carson & Polman, 2012), reduced musculoskeletal pain (Rossettini et al., 2018), reduced experience of negative emotions (Covassin et al., 2014; Mitchell et al., 2014; Yang et al., 2014) and the development of greater psychological readiness to return to sport (Meierbachtol et al., 2018; Podlog et al., 2015). Consequently, this denotes that it is advantageous for stakeholders to optimize the social support that injured athletes experience during the return to sport process.

HOW CAN SOCIAL SUPPORT BE IMPROVED?

If social support is associated with return to sport outcomes, how to enhance the social support experienced by injured athletes is an important consideration for all stakeholders. Research indicates that any strategic planning to improve social support for injured athletes could be applied prior to injury and during injury (e.g. Maurice et al., 2017; Rees et al., 2010).

Prior to an injury occurring, several specific social support strategies should be considered. The pre-injury relationship between provider and athlete is an important moderator of social support (Bianco & Eklund, 2001) and as such clinicians should seek to have meaningful interactions with non-injured athletes in addition to injured athletes. One example is having an 'open door' policy for the medical room where informal day-to-day interactions can take place (e.g. Maurice et al., 2017). Sports teams should also consider the make-up and functioning of the athlete-centred therapeutic alliance prior to injury. In other words, a plan of how stakeholders will work with injured athletes within their context. For example, which stakeholders are included, what role does each stakeholder have, who will take the leadership role, are there any training needs and how this will practically operate? The conditions thought to be required for positive working relationships with injured athletes' include being present, receptive, genuine and committed (Miciak, Mayan, Joyce & Gross, 2018). Details, such as these, are thought to be the foundation of effective shared decision-making around return to sport (Ardern et al., 2016).

During injury, the athlete-centred therapeutic alliance should routinely meet to evaluate social support needs of injured athletes. This is important for two important empirically derived reasons. First, the return to sport process is dynamic and as such injured athletes are likely to encounter challenges of different type and magnitude which are likely to require different types and quantities of social support (Clement et al., 2015; Truong et al., 2020). Second, athletes tend to experience more social support early in the return to sport process and that this diminishes as they approach return to training and competition (Johnston & Carroll, 1998). As such, athletes may be returning to training and competition in an emotionally and motivationally vulnerable state. In other words, this would safeguard that the amount and type of social support relative to the athlete's needs is of consistently high quality throughout the whole return to sport process. This is potentially important given that experiencing excessive stress is associated with several negative return to sport outcomes (e.g. Ivarsson et al., 2017). Additionally, during injury, opportunities for injured athletes to engage with teammates and team activities should be provided, for example injured athletes being given different team-based roles during injury and maintaining involvement in team briefing and de-briefing following competition. This would optimize the opportunity for interactions with teammates and stakeholders leading to injured athletes feeling less isolated, more professionally valued and provide an opportunity for more informal social support activities (Corbillon et al., 2008).

CONCLUSION

In conclusion, as recovering from sports injury is a social process, the quality and quantity of social support an athlete experiences is an important consideration for practitioners in order to enhance return to sport outcomes. In this regard, clinicians and mutlidisciplinary teams working with injured athletes can be amplifiers of injury stress, or more favourably, provide a buffer from injury stress.

Case study: 'Injury is the worst roller-coaster of my life'

Tasha, a 16-year-old international-level female footballer, sustained a non-contact injury to her right knee during a game for her club academy team. Following assessment and diagnosis by her club clinicians, she was referred for diagnostic scanning at a local hospital. The advice given to Tasha and her parents was that she required surgical intervention and that she would not be able to participate in any football activities for 12 months. The injury occurred at a really bad time. Tasha was breaking into the club senior team and next year was a World Cup and was feeling positive about her inclusion in the squad for the tournament. To further compound the situation, she was also completing coursework for her academic exams in which participating in and evaluating fitness tests was required.

Following surgery, Tasha was required to attend various hospital appointments with consultant surgeons and hospital-based clinicians (e.g. physiotherapists) and attend club training for in-house treatment and reconditioning. In addition to this, she mentions her international team coach and clinicians have been in touch giving injury-related advice and guidance and checking on her progress. Her schoolteachers are also being unhelpful about her ability to successfully complete her coursework. As this is Tasha's first severe injury, she is feeling over-whelmed, confused and distressed. She feels like she is getting too much advice, and this is making her anxious about her progress and whether she will ever get back to playing football at the same level.

Questions

1. If you had the responsibility to co-ordinate a therapeutic alliance for Tasha, who might be involved?
2. Based on the context of the athlete, what different types of social support might Tasha require?
3. How would you ensure that Tasha maintained some involvement with team activities and her teammates?
4. Which strategies could you employ to optimize the quality of social support Tasha experiences?

References

Alexanders, J., Anderson, A., & Henderson, S. (2015). Musculoskeletal physiotherapists' use of psychological interventions: A systematic review of therapists' perceptions and practice. *Physiotherapy*, *101*(2), 95–102.

Ardern, C. L., Glasgow, P., Schneiders, A., Witvrouw, E., Clarsen, B., Cools, A., Gojanovic, B., Griffin, S., Khan K. M., Moksnes, H., Mutch, S. A., Phillips, N., Reurink, G., Sadler, R., Silbernagel, K. G., Thorborg, K., Wangensteen, A., Wilk, K. E., & Bizzini, M. (2016). 2016 Consensus statement on return to sport from the First World Congress in Sports Physical Therapy, Bern. *British Journal of Sports Medicine*, *50*, 853–864.

Babatunde, F., MacDermid, J., & MacIntyre, N. (2017). Characteristics of therapeutic alliance in musculoskeletal physiotherapy and occupational therapy practice: A scoping review of the literature. *BMC Health Services Research*, *17*, 375.

Bejar, M., Raabe, J., Zakrajsek, R., Fisher, R., & Clement, D. (2019). Athletic trainers influence on national collegiate athletic association division 1 athletes basic psychological needs during sport injury rehabilitation. *Journal of Athletic Training, 54*(3), 245–254.

Bianco, T. (2001). Social support and recovery from injury: Elite skiers share their experiences. *Research Quarterly for Sport and Exercise, 72*, 376–388.

Bianco, T., & Eklund, R. C. (2001). Conceptual considerations for the social support research in sport and exercise settings: The case of sport injury. *Journal of Sport and Exercise Psychology, 23*, 85–107.

Brewer, B. W. (2010). The role of psychological factors in sport injury rehabilitation outcomes. *International Review of Sport and Exercise Psychology, 3*(1), 40–61.

Brewer, B. W., Anderson, M., & Van Raalte, J. (2002). Psychological aspects of sports injury rehabilitation: Towards a biopsychosocial approach. In D. Mostofsky, & L. Zaichkowky (Eds.), *Medical aspects of sport and exercise* (pp. 41–54). Fitness Information Technology.

Carson, F., & Polman, R. (2008). ACL injury rehabilitation: A psychological case study of a professional rugby union player. *Journal of Clinical Sports Psychology, 2*, 71–90.

Carson, F., & Polman, R. (2012). Experiences of professional rugby union players returning to competition following anterior cruciate ligament reconstruction. *Physical Therapy in Sport, 13*(1), 35–40.

Clement, D., Arvinen-Barrow, M., & Fetty, T. (2015). Psychosocial responses during different phases of sport-injury rehabilitation: A qualitative study. *Journal of Athletic Training, 50*(1), 95–104.

Clement, D., & Shannon, V. R. (2011). Injured athletes' perceptions about social support. *Journal of Sport Rehabilitation, 20*(4), 457–470.

Cohen, S., & Wills, T. A. (1985). Stress, social support, and the buffering hypothesis. *Psychological Bulletin, 98*, 310–357.

Corbillon, F., Crossman, J., Jamieson, J. (2008). Injured athletes' perceptions of the social support provided by their coaches and teammates during rehabilitation. *Journal of Sport Behaviour, 31*(2), 93–107.

Covassin, T., Crutcher, B., Bleecker, A., Heiden, E. O., Dailey, A., & Yang, J. (2014). Postinjury anxiety and social support among collegiate athletes: A comparison between orthopaedic injuries and concussions. *Journal of Athletic Training, 49*(4), 462–468.

Deci, E. L., & Ryan, R. M. (2000). The 'what' and 'why' of goal pursuits: Human needs and the self-determination of behavior. *Psychological Inquiry, 11*, 227–268.

Ekstrand, J., Krutsch, W., Spreco, A., et al. (2019). Time before return to play for the most common injuries in professional football: A 16-year follow-up of the UEFA elite club injury study. *British Journal of Sports Medicine*, Published Online First: 10 June 2019. DOI: 10.1136/bjsports-2019-100666.

Forsdyke, D., Smith, A., Jones, M., & Gledhill, A. (2016). Psychosocial factors associated with outcomes of sports injury rehabilitation in competitive athletes: A mixed studies systematic review. *British Journal of Sports Medicine, 50*, 537–544.

Freeman, P., Coffee, P., & Rees, T. (2011). The PASS-Q: The perceived available support in sport questionnaire. *Journal of Sport & Exercise Psychology, 33*, 54–74.

Gledhill, A., & Craig, R. (in press). Psychosocial factors are associated with lower re-injury risk in competitive athletes. *British Journal of Sports Medicine*, IOC World Conference on the Prevention of Illness and Injury in Sport Supplement.

Hartley, C., & Coffee, P. (2019). Perceived and received dimensional support: Main and stress buffering effects on dimensions of burnout. *Frontiers in Psychology*. DOI: 10.3389/fpsyg.2019.01724.

Hassell, K., Sabiston, C., & Bloom, G. (2005). Exploring the multiple dimensions of social support among elite female adolescent swimmers. *International Journal of Sport Psychology*, *41*(4), 340–359.

Heaney, C. A., Walker, N., Green, A. J., & Rostron, C. L. (2017) The impact of a sport psychology education intervention on physiotherapists. *European Journal of Physiotherapy*, *19*(2), 97–103.

Ivarsson, A., Johnson, U., Andersen, M., Tranaeus, U., Stenling, A., & Lindwall, M. (2017). Psychosocial factors and sport injuries: Meta-analyses for prediction and prevention. *Sports Medicine*, *47*(2), 353–365.

Johnston, L. H., & Carroll, D. (1998). The provision of social support to injured athletes: A qualitative analysis. *Journal of Sport Rehabilitation*, *7*, 267–284.

King, J., Roberts, C., Hard S., et al. (2019). Want to improve return to sport outcomes following injury? Empower, engage, provide feedback and be transparent: 4 habits! *British Journal of Sports Medicine*, *53*, 526–527.

Maurice, S., Kuklick, C., & Anderson, M. (2017). Providing social support to injured athletes: Applications of the international sport coaching framework. *International Journal of Physical Education, Sports and Health*, *4*(5), 166–175.

Meierbachtol, A., Yungtum, W., Paur, E., Bottoms, J., & Chmielewski, T. L. (2018). Psychological and functional readiness for sport following advanced group training in patients with anterior cruciate ligament reconstruction. *Journal of Orthopaedic & Sports Physical Therapy*, *48*(11), 864–872.

Miciak, M., Mayan, M., Brown, C., Joyce, A. S., & Gross, D. P. (2018). The necessary conditions of engagement for the therapeutic relationship in physiotherapy: An interpretive description study. *Archives of physiotherapy*, *8*, 3.

Mitchell, I., Evans, L., Rees, T., & Hardy, L. (2014). Stressors, social support, and tests of the buffering hypothesis: Effects on psychological responses of injured athletes. *British Journal of Health Psychology*, *19*, 486–508.

Pizzari, T., McBurney, H., Taylor, N., & Feller, J. (2002). Adherence to anterior cruciate ligament rehabilitation: A qualitative analysis. *Journal of Sport Rehabilitation*, *11*(2), 90–102.

Podlog, L., Banham, S. M., Wadey, R., & Hannon, J. C. (2015). Psychological readiness to return to competitive sport following injury: A qualitative study. *The Sport Psychologist*, *29*(1), 1–14.

Rees, T., Mitchell, I., Evans, L., & Hardy, L. (2010). Stressors, social support and psychological responses to sport injury in high- and low-performance standard participants. *Psychology of Sport & Exercise*, *11*(6), 505–512.

Rossettini, G., Carlino, E., & Testa, M. (2018). Clinical relevance of contextual factors as triggers of placebo and nocebo effects in musculoskeletal pain. *BMC Musculoskeletal Disorders*, *19*(1), 27.

Truong, L. K., Mosewich, A., Holt, C., et al. (2020). Psychological, social and contextual factors across recovery stages following a sport-related knee injury: A scoping review. *British Journal of Sports Medicine*, published on-line first: 14 February 2020. DOI: 10.1136/bjsports-2019-101206.

Walker, N., Thatcher, J., & Lavallee, D. (2007). Review: Psychological responses to injury in competitive sport: A critical review. *Journal of the Royal Society for the Promotion of Health*, *127*(4), 174–180.

Webster, K. E., & Feller, J. A. (2019). Expectations for return to preinjury sport before and after anterior cruciate ligament reconstruction. *The American Journal of Sports Medicine*, *47*(3), 578–583.

Wiese-Bjornstal, D. M., Smith, A. M., Shaffer, S. M., & Morrey, M. A. (1998). An integrated model of response to sport injury: Psychological and sociological dimensions. *Journal of Applied Sport Psychology*, *10*, 46–69.

Yang, J., Peek-Asa, C., Lowe, J. B., Heiden, E., & Foster, D. T. (2010). Social support patterns of collegiate athletes before and after injury. *Journal of Athletic Training*, *45*(4), 372–379.

Yang, J., Schaefer, J. T., Zhang, N., Covassin, T., Ding, K., & Heiden, E. (2014). Social support from the athletic trainer and symptoms of depression and anxiety at return to play. *Journal of Athletic Training*, *49*(6), 773–779.

8 SEEING IS BELIEVING

THE ROLE OF IMAGERY IN SPORTS INJURY REHABILITATION

Dr Adam Gledhill and Dr Dale Forsdyke

As is well established, injuries, particularly severe or recurrent injuries, can have significant negative consequences for the injured athlete, including changing for the worse the ways that an athlete thinks, feels and acts (Forsdyke et al., 2016; Ruddock-Hudson et al., 2014; Tracey, 2003). It stands to reason, therefore, that there is growing interest and appreciation in the role of psychological interventions within the injury rehabilitation process; arguably chief amongst these has been the role of imagery (e.g. Driediger et al., 2006; Slimani et al., 2016; Zach et al., 2018).

This chapter will (1) define imagery and its potential benefits within sports injury rehabilitation; (2) highlight some of the main theories of imagery use; (3) discuss some of the proposed psychophysiological, neurobiological and neurocognitive underpinnings for the proposed benefits of imagery; (4) discuss suggestions for applied practice whilst also highlighting some of the research limitations and (5) present an applied case study.

IMAGERY IN INJURY REHABILITATION

Imagery is the polysensorial creation of recreation of an experience in the mind (Vealey & Forlenza, 2015) and is part of a series of psychological skills that, whilst still relatively under-utilized by injured athletes (Arvinen-Barrow et al., 2015), are valuable to those who do engage with them as part of injury rehabilitation (Arvinen-Barrow et al., 2015; Clement et al., 2013; Schwab Reese et al., 2012; Zach et al., 2018). There are many proposed benefits of imagery for injured athletes, each of which is linked to some of the negative responses associated with injury. For example, imagery is shown to increase confidence (e.g. Callow et al., 2001), improve self-efficacy (e.g. Cupal & Brewer, 2001; Zach et al., 2018), improved knee laxity (e.g. Maddison et al., 2012), functional mobility (e.g. Zach et al., 2018), perceived pain (Zach et al., 2018), healing-related neurobiological factors (Maddison et al., 2012), manage unfamiliar situations (e.g. Munroe et al., 2000), reduced re-injury anxiety (e.g. Cupal & Brewer, 2001), skill acquisition (Ingram

Table 8.1 Theories and models of imagery (adapted from Hale et al., 2005; Morris et al., 2005)

Theory name	*Summary*
Psychomeuromuscular Theory	Imagery enhances performance by producing low intensity muscle movement commands (innervations) that are identical in pattern to the actual performance of a movement. This provides neuromuscular feedback that allows changes to be made to movement patterns
Symbolic Learning Theory	Imagery provides an opportunity to rehearse the sequence of movements that are performed during an activity, which will help the person learning the action to *symbolically code* the movement patterns in the central nervous system. Imagery can help the athlete to focus on specific aspects of a skill to increase performance and can also help to reduce distractions during performance of the skill
Dual-Code Theory	Information can be stored in the memory as one of two independent codes, either an image or a word. Either of these can result in recall
Bioinformational Theory	This is possibly the most complex explanation. Images are propositional structures, of which there are three main types: (1) stimulus (the scene), (2) response (the response to the scene) and (3) meaning (how you interpret different events). Stimulus propositions provide the scene for imagery (e.g. the shape and colour of your leg after a serious injury); response propositions influence how an athlete will react physiologically, emotionally and kinaesthetically (e.g. feelings of frustration) to the scene; and the meaning proposition makes the imagery significant to the athlete (e.g. the time in the game)
Triple-Code Model	Imagery has three important components: (1) the image (I), (2) the somatic response (S) and (3) the meaning of the image (M). You may sometimes see this theory referred to as ISM to represent the three codes
Gross Framework or Insight Theory	Imagery helps the learner to get a *general idea* or the *whole* of the skill (i.e. the gross framework) rather than concentrating on the fine details of the movement. Skill learning results from an insight into the skill rather than through gradual improvement
Attention-Arousal Set Theory	Imagery works as a preparatory set that helps the athlete to achieve an optimal level of arousal prior to competition
Self-Efficacy/Self Confidence Theories	Imagery increases the athlete's expectations of success and their belief in their ability to produce performances that will result in a successful outcome, which can have a beneficial influence on performance. This is partly because imagery increases the amount of time spent preparing for competition
Motivational Explanations	Imagery plays a motivational and cognitive role in enhancing performance. Imagery increases the amount of time spent in practice and as a result increases motivation
Functional Equivalence/ Neurophysiological Theories	Imagery and perception or imagery and movement use the same parts of the nervous system, but when you are only imaging an activity, the actual physical performance of the movement is blocked

et al., 2016) and has been used for good effect in case studies of athletes with severe injuries (e.g. Gledhill et al., 2020). Table 8.1 (adapted from Hale et al., 2005; Morris et al., 2005) provides an overview of the major theories, which seek to explain *how* imagery can elicit some of these benefits.

Given these wide-ranging and established benefits, it is perhaps surprising to note that imagery still isn't a widely used technique within injury rehabilitation (Arvinen-Barrow et al., 2015). One can only assume that this may be due to either a lack of awareness of benefits, a lack of skill in imagery use or existing stigmas towards adopting sport psychology techniques (e.g. Gledhill et al., 2020).

PSYCHOPHYSIOLOGICAL, NEUROBIOLOGICAL AND NEUROCOGNITIVE UNDERPINNINGS FOR THE PROPOSED BENEFITS OF IMAGERY

Principles of psychophysiology suggest that physiological changes in the body bring about changes in psychological-emotional states, and vice-versa (Green et al., 1979). Thanks in part to the advent of electromyography, electroencephalography and functional magnetic resonance imaging, we are now better placed to understand a lot the potential reasons behind the benefits of imagery. For example, Ang et al. (2014) noted that imagery has the potential to restore motor function by inducing activity-dependent brain plasticity, whilst it has also been noted that imagery influences brain activations during motor imagery of locomotor-related tasks (e.g. Malouin et al., 2003). When creating/recreating a movement via imagery, imagery activates the same neural mechanisms that are associated with actual perception, motor control and emotions of movement (Holmes & Collins, 2001; Jeannerod, 1994; Sharma & Baron, 2013). Imagery can also elicit neuromuscular patterning which innervates targeted muscles in the same way, albeit to a lesser degree, as physically performing movements (Lebon et al., 2012; Suinn, 1972). Finally, imagery use is also shown to influence levels of noradrenaline and dopamine (Maddison et al., 2012), which may be important throughout the healing process. Collectively, these points provide a wealth of evidence to support the notion that imagery 'works' and have informed suggestions that imagery training may well be a helpful adjunct to physical therapy during injury rehabilitation and when aiming to prevent re-injury risk (e.g. Gledhill et al., 2018; Lebon et al., 2012; Zach et al., 2018).

APPLYING IMAGERY IN PRACTICE

Notwithstanding the theories and models outlined in Table 1, the majority of modern thinking regarding imagery application is underpinned by the PETTLEP model (Holmes & Collins, 2001). PETTLEP stands for Physical, Environment, Task, Timing, Learning, Emotion and Perspective. This approach essentially combines the tenets from Functional Equivalence Theory (Jeannerod, 1994) and the Bioinformational Theory (Lang, 1979) and suggests that effective imagery should consider the following (Holmes & Collins, 2001; Slimani et al., 2016; Wakefield & Smith, 2012):

- *Physical:* Refers to imaging the perceived physical sensations that would usually be experienced whilst performing the skill. This can be enhanced by the athlete wearing the same clothes they would compete in, holding any relevant sports implements, adopting particular stances etc.
- *Environment:* Involves the athlete completing the imagery in the performance environment. Where this is not possible, videos or photographs of the environment can be used as a replacement.
- *Task:* Refers to making the imaged task similar to the actual task that the athlete would actually perform and should replicate the expected performance level.
- *Timing:* Refers to the imagery training the same or similar length of time to complete as physically performing the task.
- *Learning:* Refers to the imagery being progressively advanced and remaining consistent with the physical capabilities of the athlete, particularly once the athlete has become autonomous and proficient with the task.
- *Emotion:* Any emotions associated with performance should be incorporated into the imagery training, including any feelings of nervousness, apprehension or worry, or replicating any scenarios of particularly high emotion.
- Perspective: Refers whether the athlete completes their imagery from an internal or external perspective. Internal imagery may be more effective at eliciting physical outcomes than external imagery, and this internal imagery can be aided by videos.

Understanding the PETTLEP approach is important as adopting this approach can increase the vividness of images as well as the ease of use of imagery (Anuar et al., 2016). This in turn is important as the vividness of images is likely to impact on imagery effectiveness (Lebon et al., 2018; Wilson et al., 2010).

As with any other skill, imagery can take time to master and requires deliberate training in order to be most effective (Williams & Cumming, 2012). Imagery training is often conducted using a script (Williams et al., 2013), but this can be aided by action observation and the use of videos (e.g. Gledhill et al., 2020; Wright et al., 2015). Using videos of actions to supplement scripts can benefit the injured athlete in a number of ways. First, imagery, action observation and action execution elicit similar brain activation (Williams & Cumming, 2012; Wright et al., 2015). Furthermore, athletes seeing themselves performing sporting movements that they are otherwise unable to perform can increase their confidence in their ability to complete these activities (e.g. Gledhill et al., 2020). Involving the athlete in the process of producing the imagery script is also considered best practice (Williams et al., 2013) and can have greater benefits for the athlete, including increased neuromuscular activity and imagery ability (Wilson et al., 2010).

PLANNING IMAGERY SCRIPTS

Williams et al. (2013) provide a helpful set of guidelines, an imagery script checklist and an example of an imagery script that adopt these guidelines. We'll summarize and contextualize these guidelines, referred to as the 5Ws (who? where and when? what? and why?), below:

- *Who:* It is important to tailor the script to the individual and have personalised content. If working with children, metaphors (e.g. strong as a lion) can be helpful, whereas older and more experienced athletes can benefit from clearer descriptions/more detail.

  The imagery experience and ability of the individual is also important. If you don't know the athlete's experience or ability level, measuring their imagery ability (e.g. by using the Sport Imagery Ability Questionnaire) could be helpful. Novice imagers will require more basic scripts with fewer details, whereas more experienced imagers may benefit from more complex scenarios. Novice imagers may require shorter, more focused timeframes (e.g. 1–2 min maximum); however, approaches to imagery use in injury settings currently lack consistency (Zach et al., 2018).

  As injury is a time when athletes can feel a sense of loss of control (e.g. Forsdyke et al., 2016), having more self-referenced comparisons that emphasize personal improvements could be helpful. However, knowing the athlete is important here as some may still have a preference for externally referenced scripts (e.g. showing them successfully competing against an opponent, being successful and remaining injury free), especially as they transition through the phases of return to sport.
- *Where and when:* This may vary, dependent on the stage of the rehabilitation journey. For example, an athlete in the early stages of the return to sport process (e.g. just entering return to participation stage) may still be spending time frequently in the injury clinic, which could provide a calm and quiet setting. However, an individual in the later stages (e.g. entering or is currently in the return to performance stage) may want to practice their imagery on the team bus. Giving flexibility in how the script is planned to account for these things can help, but it is becoming increasingly common that athletes prefer a recorded imagery script that they can listen to on their mobile phone or other portable devices and often like it if the script and audio recording can be supplemented with appropriate videos (e.g. Gledhill et al., 2020). If recording an audio script for the athlete, the voice, clarity, tempo, tone, pronunciation, enunciation and any pauses are such that the athlete is able to immerse themselves in the recording.
- *Why:* Broadly speaking, athletes use imagery for reasons that fall broadly into one of five functions (Hall et al., 1998; Paivio, 1985). These functions are (1) cognitive specific, (2) cognitive general functions, (3) motivational specific functions, (4) motivational general-arousal functions and (5) motivational general-mastery functions. Understanding their reasons behind imagery use will help guide the imagery content (i.e. the 'what?').
- *What:* The content should be closely linked to the reasons the athlete is using the imagery and the 'who'-related factors that we described earlier.

The imagery should include familiar feelings, situations and/or environments, so that the athlete can easily recall these details from memory. This is important as it can create a more vivid image, thus enhancing the potential imagery benefits (Anuar et al., 2016; Lebon et al., 2018; Wilson et al., 2010). In the case of sports injury, it is not uncommon that athletes may experience elements of nervousness, apprehension, worry or fear as they approach their return to sport (Forsdyke et al., 2016); hence, it can be important to incorporate these into the imagery script so as to help the athlete accept, control and move past them (e.g. Gledhill et al., 2020). However, it is also important to remain mindful of the potential for re-traumatization of the athlete when recreating these emotions, particularly in the case of athletes rehabilitating from severe injuries. Whilst having the athlete involved in writing the script or producing the content is considered good practice anyway, it can be particularly helpful when considering injury-related imagery scripts so as to reduce the chances of such retraumatization occurring. This is in part because the person designing the script is able to receive concurrent feedback from the athlete regarding the content and any potential negative impact (e.g. Gledhill et al., 2020).

It is also important to gain feedback from the athlete once they begin to use the script and as time progresses, so that any necessary amendments can be made. It is not uncommon that, as time progresses, the athlete will become more skilled in their imagery use and will benefit from more detailed and refined imagery scripts.

CONCLUSION

Regardless of whether they are at a stage of return to participation, returning to sport or returning to performance, imagery is an effective skill for athletes that can aid their injury rehabilitation. Whilst, as is the case with much applied sport psychology intervention research, there remain concerns with sample sizes, the lack of replication research and concerns over statistical power, imagery training has shown to be effective in improving a broad range of injury-related concerns (e.g. self-efficacy, motivation, reduced fear). Given that imagery can elicit the same types of changes caused by physically performing movements (e.g. brain activation, muscle innervation), albeit to a smaller level, imagery training then becomes an attractive option during times when an athlete may experience periods of immobilization or reduced mobility. Based on all of the above, we can be confident that, when it comes to imagery, seeing is believing.

Case study

Below is an example of an imagery script (Gledhill et al., 2020) used with an experienced injured athlete. They had played at the highest level of football for a number of years but had suffered a torn anterior cruciate ligament, which was surgically repaired. The athlete was in the return to performance phase (i.e. they had made the return to full competition) but still had lingering injury-related emotions, cognitions and behaviours (e.g. fear of re-injury, lack of confidence in the previously injured limb, performance concerns, avoidance, sleep disturbance). The script was designed with the athlete, audio-recorded and used alongside appropriate videos. The athlete agreed that they would take part in three imagery training sessions per day, for no longer than 3–5 min at a time.

> I am at the ground and the game is going well. We are in control of the game and we have just started a counter-attack after a midfield regain. I am positioned near the side-line on the right wing, and the ball has come loose. I get a little nervous when this happens. My heart races a little and I feel myself shake. I take a deep breath and tell myself: 'My knee is strong. I've prepared well. I'm a stronger player now'. I force out the deep breath, and sprint towards the ball. It is close between me and the opposing defender. I block their attempt to win the ball, controlling the ball with my left foot and then flicking it away with the back of my right heel. I twist and power off in a strong, determined sprint. I twist back inside, beating the defender once again, before placing a perfectly timed pass through zone 14 to the centre forward, who scores.

Questions

1. Given the athlete's injury and the reported associated emotions, cognitions and behaviours, why do you think imagery would be helpful in this circumstance?
2. Which of Paivio's five functions are evident from the imagery script?
3. Critique the imagery script, using the recommendations for producing effective imagery scripts as a guide. Make any amendments that you think would make viable alternatives for this type of athlete.
4. How would you amend the imagery script, if you were working with a younger athlete, who was playing at a lower level of football, who had less experience of performance environments, but who had suffered the same injury?

References

Ang, K., Chua, K., Phua, K., Wang, C., Chin, Z., Kuah, C., Low, W., & Guan, C. (2014). A randomised controlled trial of EEG-based motor imagery brain-computer interface robotic rehabilitation for stroke. *Clinical EEG and Neuroscience*, *46*, 310–320.

Anuar, N., Cumming, J., & Williams, S. E. (2016). Effects of applying the PETTLEP model on vividness and ease of imaging movement. *Journal of Applied Sport Psychology*, *28*, 185–198.

Arvinen-Barrow, M., Clement, D., Hamson-Utley, J., Zakrajsek, R., Lee, S., Kamphoff, C., Lintunen, T., Hemmings, B., & Martin, S. (2015). Athletes' use of mental skills training during sport injury rehabilitation. *Journal of Sport Rehabilitation*, *24*, 189–197.

Callow, N., Hardy, L., & Hall, C. (2001). The effects of motivational-general imagery intervention on the sport confidence of high-level badminton players. *Research Quarterly for Exercise and Sport*, *72*, 389–400.

Clement, D., Granquist, M. D., & Arvinen-Barrow, M. M. (2013). Psychosocial aspects of athletic injuries as perceived by athletic trainers. *Journal of Athletic Training, 48*, 512–521.

Cupal, D. D., & Brewer, B. W. (2001). Effects of relaxation and guided imagery on knee strength, reinjury anxiety, and pain following anterior cruciate ligament reconstruction. *Rehabilitation Psychology, 46*, 28–43.

Driediger, M., Hall, C., & Callow, N. (2006). Imagery use by injured athletes: A qualitative analysis. *Journal of Sports Sciences, 24*, 261–272.

Forsdyke, D., Smith, A., Jones, M., & Gledhill, A. (2016). Psychosocial factors associated with outcomes of rehabilitation in competitive athletes: A mixed-studies systematic review. *British Journal of Sports Medicine, 50*, 537–544.

Gledhill, A. Ahmed, O. H., & Forsdyke, D. (2020). Effectively managing anterior cruciate ligament injury and return to performance in elite women's soccer. In J. Dixon, J. Barker, R. Thelwell, & I. Mitchell (Eds.). *The Psychology of Soccer*. Routledge.

Green, E. E., Green, A. M., & Waters, E. D. (1979). Biofeedback for mind body self-regulation: Healing and creativity. In E. Peper, S. Ancoli, & M. Quinn (Eds.), *Mind body integration: Essential readings in biofeedback*. Plenum Press.

Hale, B. D., Seiser, L., McGuire, E. J., & Weinrich, E. (2005). Mental imagery. In J. Taylor, & G. Wilson (Eds.), *Applying sport psychology* (pp. 187–206). Human Kinetics.

Hall, C., Mack, D., Paivio, A., & Hausenblas, H. (1998). Imagery use by athletes: Development of the sport imagery questionnaire. *International Journal of Sport Psychology, 29*, 73–89.

Holmes, P., & Collins, D. (2001). The PETTLEP approach to motor imagery: A functional equivalence model for sport psychologists. *Journal of Applied Sport Psychology, 13*, 60–83.

Ingram, T., Kraeutner, S., Soloman, J., Westwood, D., & Boe, S. (2016). Skill acquisition via motor imagery relies on both motor and perceptual learning. *Behavioural Neuroscience, 130*, 252–260.

Jeannerod, M. (1994). The representing brain: Neural correlates of motor intention and imagery. *Behavioural and Brain Sciences, 17*, 187–245.

Lang, P. J. (1979). A bio-informational theory of emotional imagery. *Psychophysiology, 16*, 495–512.

Lebon, F., Guillot, A., & Collet, C. (2012). Increased muscle activation following motor imagery during the rehabilitation of the anterior cruciate ligament. *Applied Psychophysiology and Biofeedback, 37*, 45–51.

Lebon, F., Horn, U., Domin, M., & Lotze, M. (2018). Motor imagery training: Kinaesthetic imagery strategy and inferior parietal fMRI activation. *Human Brain Mapping, 39*, 1805–1813.

Maddison, R., Prapavessis, H., Clatworthy, M., Hall, C., Foley, L., & Brewer, B. (2012). Guided imagery to improve functional outcomes post-anterior cruciate ligament repair: Randomized-controlled pilot trial. *Scandinavian Journal of Medicine and Science in Sports, 22*, 816–821.

Malouin, F., Richards, C. L., Jackson, P. L., Dumas, F., & Doyon, J. (2003). Brain activations during motor imagery of locomotor-related tasks: A PET study. *Human Brain Mapping, 19*, 47–62.

Morris, T., Spittle, M., & Watt, A. P. (2005). *Imagery in sport*. Human Kinetics.

Munroe, K., Giacobbi, P., Hall, C., Weinberg, R. (2000). The 4Ws of imagery use: Where, when, why and what. *The Sport Psychologist, 14*, 119–137.

Paivio, A. (1985). Cognitive and motivational functions of imagery in human performance. *Canadian Journal of Applied Sport Science, 10*, 22S–28S.

Ruddock-Hudson, M., O'Halloran, P., & Murphy, G. (2014). The psychological impact of long-term injury on Australian Football League players. *Journal of Applied Sport Psychology, 26*, 377–394.

Schwab Reese, L. M., Pittsinger, R., & Yang, J. (2012). Effectiveness of psychological intervention following sport injury. *Journal of Sport and Health Science, 1*, 71–79.

Sharma, N., & Baron, J. (2013). Does motor imagery share the same neural networks with executed movements: A multivariate fMRI analysis. *Frontiers in Human Neuroscience, 7*. DOI: 10.3389/fnhum.2013.00564.

Slimani, M., Tod, D., Chaabene, H., Miarka, B., & Chamri, K. (2016). Effects of mental imagery on muscular strength in healthy and patient participants: A systematic review. *Journal of Sport Science and Medicine, 15*, 434–450.

Suinn, R. M. (1972). Behaviour rehearsal training for ski racers. *Behaviour Therapy, 3*, 519–520.

Tracey, J. (2003). The emotional response to the injury and rehabilitation process. *Journal of Applied Sport Psychology, 15*, 279–293.

Vealey, R. S., & Forlenza, S. T. (2015). Understanding and using imagery in sport. In J. Williams (Ed.), *Applied sport psychology: Personal growth to peak performance* (pp. 240–273). McGraw-Hill.

Wakefield, C., & Smith, D. (2012). Perfecting practice: Applying the PETTLEP model of motor imagery. *Journal of Sport Psychology in Action, 3*, 1–11.

Williams, S. E., Cooley, S. J., Newell, E., Weibull, F., & Cumming, J. (2013). Seeing the difference: Designing effective imagery scripts for athletes. *Journal of Sport Psychology in Action, 4*, 109–121.

Williams, S. E., & Cumming, J. (2012). Athletes' ease of imaging predicts their imagery and observational learning use. *Psychology of Sport and Exercise, 13*, 363–370.

Wilson, C., Smith, D., Burden, A., & Holmes, P. (2010). Participant-generated imagery scripts produce greater EMG activity and imagery ability. *European Journal of Sport Science, 10*, 417–425.

Wright, D. J., McCormick, S. A., Birks, S., Loporto, M., & Holmes, P. S. (2015). Action observation and imagery training improve the ease with which athletes can generate imagery. *Journal of Applied Sport Psychology, 27*, 156–170.

Zach, S., Dobersek, U., Filho, E., Inglis, V., & Tenebaum, G. (2018). A meta-analysis of mental imagery effects on post-injury functional mobility, perceived pain, and self-efficacy. *Psychology of Sport and Exercise, 34*, 79–87.

9 DOES IT PAY TO PAY ATTENTION?

MAKING A CASE FOR MINDFULNESS-BASED APPROACHES IN INJURY REHABILITATION

Dr Adam Gledhill

It seems strange starting a chapter like this, but what follows is not a chapter that draws on a significant number of studies on mindfulness in sports injury rehabilitation settings to clearly say: 'mindfulness works'. I can't do that; we don't have that many studies of mindfulness and its role within sports injury rehabilitation. What this chapter does intend to do, however, is make a case as to why we *should* be adopting mindfulness-based approaches into sports injury rehabilitation. This position is based on the burgeoning evidence that we do currently have from sports injury settings, as well as the almost omnipresent perspective that mindfulness-based approaches improve athletes' health and performance (e.g., Bühlmayer et al., 2017; Noetel et al., 2017). As such, this is a little different to some of the other chapters in the book; more exploratory in nature, slightly shorter, and drawing on arguments from different schools of thought in psychology, to form a series of arguments and questions that can be used to guide future research and practice.

Throughout this chapter, I'll look to achieve three key aims: (1) outline the concept of mindfulness and the different mindfulness-based approaches, (2) discuss some of the mindfulness literature that draws relevant conclusions that could underpin mindfulness application within sports injury rehabilitation and (3) share an applied case study for consideration.

INTRODUCTION TO MINDFULNESS

One of the earliest definitions of mindfulness notes that it is 'paying attention in a particular way: on purpose, in the present moment, and non-judgementally' (Kabat-Zinn, 1994, p. 4). Later, Kabat-Zinn (2005) noted the importance of open-heartedness, being non-judgemental and having awareness.

In an alternative perspective, Langer, a social psychologist who considered mindfulness to be more of an interaction between an individual and their environment, defines mindfulness as:

> a general style or mode of functioning through which the individual actively engages in reconstructing the environment through creating new categories or distinctions, thus directing attention to new contextual cues that may be consciously controlled or manipulated as appropriate. (Langer, 1989, p. 4)

More recently, Baltzell and Summers (2016, p. 527) defined mindfulness as 'a quality of awareness that objectifies the contents of experience, internally and externally, promoting greater tolerance, interest and clarity towards the content'. Irrespective of which definition one ascribes to, the consistent element that runs throughout each holds that mindfulness includes an awareness of the present. When considering the definitions above, it stands to reason that mindfulness could help an athlete in the different stages of injury rehabilitation become more aware an accepting of their current injury state. Mindfulness could also facilitate an injured athlete becoming more aware of different rehabilitation options that are available to them. In adopting mindfulness interventions, it is likely that an injured athlete in rehabilitation will be more accepting and less resistant to their injury, meaning that they will be able to better focus their energies on rehabilitation activities. Moreover, instead of becoming bored and frustrated with the same rehabilitation activities, it might be that mindfulness enacts a situation where injured athletes become more interested and engaged in different options for their rehabilitation activities.

There are three main mindfulness approaches used in sport psychology: (1) Mindfulness, Acceptance and Commitment (Gardner & Moore, 2007); (2) Mindfulness Meditation Training in Sport (Baltzell & Summers, 2018) and (3) Mindful Sport Performance Enhancement (Kaufman et al., 2018). Table 9.1 (adapted from Glass et al., 2020) provides an overview of the different mindfulness approaches. Readers are invited to view the original texts for full descriptions and details of each of the different approaches.

Whilst it is important to note that this chapter doesn't advocate any mindfulness-based approach over another, of the different mindfulness-based approaches, the MAC approach (Gardner & Moore, 2007) appears most frequently in sport injury-related literature (Josefsson et al., 2020). In a sports injury context, the application of the MAC approach consistently shows the ability to positively impact on achieving medical/injury priorities (see Gledhill & Ivarsson, 2020 for a summary). However, one real-world challenge with the application of the MAC approach is that athletes can find it quite demanding. This is perhaps due to the volume of sessions, independent activities to be undertaken, unfamiliarity with the subject matter and difficulties with seeing how it relates to their sport (Josefsson et al., 2020). These findings from sport performance-based applications of the MAC approach

Table 9.1 Comparison of mindfulness interventions (adapted from Glass et al., 2020)

	Mindfulness Acceptance Commitment (MAC)	*Mindful Meditation Training in Sport (MMTS)*	*Mindful Sport Performance Enhancement (MSPE)*
Authors	Gardner and Moore (2007)	Baltzell and Summers (2018)	Kaufman et al. (2018)
Formal/Informal meditation practices	Formal and informal	Formal and informal	Formal and informal
Influenced by	Acceptance Commitment Therapy (ACT; Hayes et al., 1999)	Mindful Self-Compassion (MSC; Germer & Neff, 2013, 2019)	Mindfulness-based Stress Reduction (MSBR; Kabat-Zinn, 1994)
Structure	Didactic, interactive, with structured and consistent meditative exercises	Instruction, mindfulness exercises and meditation, group discussion, home practice	Didactic, sedentary and active meditation, group discussion, home practice
Number of components	Seven modules (session number can vary) Module 1: Preparation and psychoeducation Module 2: Mindfulness and cognitive diffusion Module 3: Values and value-driven behaviour Module 4: Acceptance Module 5: Commitment Module 6: Skill consolidation and poise – Mindfulness, acceptance and commitment Module 7: Maintaining and enhancing mindfulness acceptance, commitment	6 or 12 sessions Mindfulness and self-compassion Mindfulness: labelling experience Concentration and performance Self-compassion and performance Values and somatic regulation Adapting, adjusting to the now during performance	6 sessions Mindfulness, flow, non-judgement and autopilot Present-moment attention and performance facilitators Expectations, limits and somatic awareness Attachments and acceptance Non-striving and sport-specific anchors for attentions Program review, building an ongoing practice
Session length	1–1.5 h	30 or 60 min	90 min (Flexible)
Duration of program	7–12 weeks	6 weeks (6 h in total)	6 weeks

may provide helpful insights into how the approach can be adopted during injury rehabilitation (e.g. discussing the injury-related benefits of engaging with the approach at the outset; emphasizing during initial consultations that mindfulness practice over a longer period of time tends to elicit greater improvements for athletes).

MINDFULNESS LITERATURE RELEVANT TO SPORTS INJURY REHABILITATION

Whilst the body of research that examines mindfulness in sports injury rehabilitation is sparse, there exists a body of research that allows us to make realistic recommendations regarding mindfulness practice within sports injury rehabilitation. Therefore, this section of the chapter draws on notions of psychological flexibility and inflexibility, the role of mindfulness in sports injury prevention, and a small body of work that has considered mindfulness in injury rehabilitation.

PSYCHOLOGICAL FLEXIBILITY AND INFLEXIBILITY IN SPORTS INJURY REHABILITATION

Psychological flexibility refers to a willingness to remain in contact with undesirable internal experience in the service of one's values or important goals (Bond et al., 2011). It encompasses several processes that take place over time and is most prominent in an individual's ability to adapt to the fluctuating demands in situations, reconfigure mental resources, shift their perspective and balance desires, needs and life domains (Kashdan & Rottenberg, 2010). The six core processes of psychological flexibility (known as the 'hexaflex'; Hayes et al., 1999) are acceptance, cognitive diffusion, self as context, being present, values and committed action. Conversely, an absence of psychological flexibility is characterized by experiential avoidance, cognitive fusion, attachment to conceptualized self, dominance of conceptualized past and weak self-knowledge, lack of clarity with values and inactivity, impulsivity and avoidance (Harris, 2009). A lack of psychological flexibility could be important in injury rehabilitation as the associated avoidant behaviour can serve to exacerbate the very situation that the avoidance was there to protect against. Consider the example of a sprinter with a troublesome, recurrent hamstring injury not attending a scheduled rehabilitation appointment because they woke feeling some re-injury anxiety or a heightened sense of tension, or pain perception. They didn't attend the session, because they didn't want to make things worse. However, by avoiding the rehabilitation session, inherently they increase the chances of making the situation worse further down the line.

One of the major objectives of ACT is to increase psychological flexibility (Josefsson et al., 2020). This may be relevant within sports injury rehabilitation as there is preliminary evidence from student athletes in the USA that suggests psychological flexibility is positively associated with rehabilitation adherence (DeGaetano et al., 2016). This is noteworthy on at least two levels. First, student athletes in the USA typically report low levels of rehabilitation adherence; hence, understanding ways their adherence can be influenced and improved is an important step. Second, improvements in rehabilitation adherence are associated with improved rehabilitation outcomes (Ivarsson et al., 2017).

Next, the absence of psychological flexibility is also associated with an increased risk of depression (Skinner et al., 2010). We also know that injured athletes, particularly those with severe or recurrent injuries, are at a high risk of depression (Putukian, 2016). Moreover, aside from the obvious human impact created by depression, negative responses to injury are also associated with reduced rehabilitation adherence (Ivarsson et al., 2017).

Drawing on the two lines of thought above, we reach the next of our arguments. If, through the use of mindfulness-based approaches, we might improve the mental health of injured athletes and we might also improve outpatient/home-based rehabilitation adherence as a result of increased psychological flexibility, we should consider adopting mindfulness-based approaches in sports injury rehabilitation. The obsequious amongst us will note that underpinning an argument which suggests the needs for trial-based research to inform practice with correlational research and narrative review evidence is stretching our existing understanding too far, in order to meet a pre-determined aim (or, more simply, being biased towards an argument). However, I contend that this argument formation is in-keeping with principles of best evidence synthesis (e.g. Gledhill et al., 2018) and offer the argument as a suggestion for further research to advance the evidence-base as pertains specifically to sports injury rehabilitation.

MINDFULNESS AND SPORTS INJURY RISK AND REHABILITATION

Consistently, the application of mindfulness (specifically MAC) interventions shows the ability to reduce injury risk (Gledhill & Ivarsson, 2020). Whilst the majority of findings talk to reducing injury risk, there are some emerging findings that hint at an importance during rehabilitation. MAC approach has shown to reduce injury rates in treatment groups over control group (Naderi et al., 2020; Zadeh et al., 2019), have a greater proportion of intervention group players remain injury free (Ivarsson et al., 2015) and have fewer average injuries per team in intervention groups (Naderi et al., 2020). In a hint towards rehabilitative benefits, MAC intervention groups have also demonstrated fewer days lost due to injury Naderi et al., 2020), which suggests a faster recovery time may be possible.

The research examining mindfulness-based intervention in sports injury rehabilitation is even more sparse. However, within the available studies benefits are reported. In their case study of a physically recovered athlete but whom was still demonstrating fear of re-injury and avoidant behaviour, Bennett and Lindsay (2016) reported the following improvements within the athlete: increased adherence to stretching, increased attendance at training, reduction in pain and anxiety, improved confidence and increased amount of training time. In an additional investigation of the impact of MSBR on perceptions of pain, anxiety, stress, mindfulness and mood during injury rehabilitation, Mohammed et al. (2018) noted a statistically significant difference in pain tolerance between the intervention and control groups. There were also improvements in mood and mindfulness and decreases in stress and anxiety, but none of these differences were statistically significant. Consequently, there are pockets of evidence that suggest mindfulness may be beneficial during injury rehabilitation.

HOW MIGHT MINDFULNESS-BASED INTERVENTIONS WORK?

Given these encouraging findings, it is important to consider *how* mindfulness-based interventions might 'work' for an athlete rehabilitating from a sports injury. First, a common explanation for reductions in injury risk is due to enhanced attentional processes (Ivarsson et al., 2015; Naderi et al., 2020), particularly speed and accuracy of information processing (Naderi et al., 2020). Mindfulness practice could lead to functional changes in the brain's different attention systems (Fox et al., 2006), such as causing changes in the anterior cingulate cortex where executive attention is housed (Hölzel et al., 2011), resulting in an athlete's ability to pay attention to the relevant stimulus. For example, a rugby player progressing from return to participation into the return to sport phase of rehabilitation may benefit from these changes by being able to notice earlier when they were about to be tackled, which could put them in a position to take evasive or protective action and reduce the risk of injury.

Second, it is not uncommon, especially in cases of severe or recurrent injuries, that athletes can have maladaptive thoughts (e.g. that they'll never recover from their injury or that they'll just get injured over and again; e.g. Gledhill et al., 2020). Consequently, athletes may then change their rehabilitation behaviours to be more indicative of escape or avoidance (e.g. have poorer rehabilitation adherence; e.g. Ivarsson et al., 2017). Mindfulness-based interventions can help to change the injured athlete's relationships with these thoughts, so that they recognize these thoughts as just thoughts (Baer, 2003) and help the athlete to respond with increased psychological flexibility.

Third, it is also not uncommon that injured athletes – again, especially those with severe or recurrent injuries – can experience other types of generally unhelpful and negative feelings towards their injury (e.g. frustration that they then become pre-occupied with; Forsdyke et al., 2016; Ivarsson et al., 2017). Mindfulness can help injured athletes to accept their current situation (i.e., accept that they are injured) and be less attached to the feelings of frustration. In doing so, the injured athlete is more able to make rational decisions about their rehabilitation behaviours moving forward (e.g. make the decision to engage with rehabilitation activities).

Fourth, during injury rehabilitation, athletes can experience heightened emotional upheaval, signs of increased fatigue and increased pain. Mindfulness might be helpful in this respect as the increased awareness afforded by mindfulness may give the injured athlete advanced warning when these changes start to happen. This early warning system then provides the athlete with the opportunity to adjust their activities, so as to prevent further injury. For example, it could prompt the athlete to seek advice from their sports medicine practitioner about why they are increasing heightened pain; they may seek sport psychology support regarding their emotional challenges, which then aids sleep quality etc. and then uses these to make any appropriate amendments to activities.

Fifth, as athletes transition through the different stages of rehabilitation, whilst they will typically be pleased about progress made, there may also be some lingering stress or doubt about their ability to meet the demands of the next stage. For example, during return to performance, athletes can question their ability to reach a minimum of pre-injury levels of performance (Forsdyke et al., 2016). Athletes can then start to negatively appraise this, and their questions then turn into a stressful situation that negatively impacts on their confidence. Based on recent findings in football, mindfulness may be able to help athletes positively reappraise their circumstances (Naderi et al., 2020).

Finally, away from sport populations, mindfulness-based interventions have shown to have positive impacts on a number of variables that, for varying reasons, may be important during injury rehabilitation. These include changes in diurnal variations in cortisol levels (e.g. Ho et al., 2020), beneficial effects in early stages of wound healing (e.g. Meesters et al., 2018) and immune system recovery (e.g. Sanada et al., 2017). According to different models within the sports injury domain (e.g. Appaneal & Perna, 2014; Brewer et al., 2002), these variables may influence further injury risk and intermediate and eventual rehabilitation outcomes. However, as these findings are not from sporting populations and there are concerns over study designs and risk of bias in places. Well-controlled, sport-based studies are needed to determine the efficacy of mindfulness-based interventions in a context specific manner.

CONCLUSIONS

Mindfulness-based interventions have become more prominent in psychology of sports injury literature over the past 5–10 years, with the MAC approach being the most commonly cited in this domain. Whilst athletes can find mindfulness approaches demanding in the early stages of use, which presents a real-world challenge for those seeking to adopt mindfulness-based interventions, ubiquitous amongst the findings is that mindfulness is beneficial for athletes. These benefits can be both injury and performance related, and, if the athlete is adherent to their mindfulness practice, it is likely that these benefits will be long term. So, does it pay to pay attention and is there a case for mindfulness-based interventions within injury rehabilitation? Arguably, yes.

Case study

Anastasia is an international gymnast who 3 weeks ago underwent surgical repair of a traumatic proximal adductor avulsion injury. The technique was a multiple suture anchor technique, which is viewed as allowing for safe return to pre-injury levels of sport performance. The surgery and the rehabilitation do, however, mean that Anastasia will miss the summer tournament games. Her surgeon has told her how relatively uncommon this type of injury and the associated surgical procedures have been in the past, but that the outcomes are generally good.

Anastasia is getting really stressed about her future in her sport and she can't believe that all of her hard work to be able to compete in the summer tournament games has been 'for nothing': because of a 'freak accident' where she 'doesn't even know how she did it'. She constantly talks about how she is so unlucky and regularly questions 'why her'. Whenever she tries to speak to her support staff about her injury rehabilitation and her future career, Anastasia just tells everyone that she 'can't think straight', that she is 'so stressed', really 'frustrated' and she doesn't know if she is 'ready to do any more rehab'.

Despite being a high-level and elite athlete for a number of years, Anastasia has never really engaged with sport psychology support. The support has been available to her and she has attended sessions as required by her international team, but she does not actively engage with any specific forms of psychological skills training.

Questions

1. Discuss some of the key elements of the case study that leads you to believe a mindfulness-based intervention might be appropriate for this client and any factors that might influence how well it could be adopted.
2. Describe the different, common mindfulness-based interventions, then select the intervention that you think would be most appropriate for Anastasia.
3. What would be the main benefits of mindfulness-based interventions for this client?

References

Appaneal, R., & Perna, F. (2014). Biopsychosocial model of injury. In R. Eklund & G. Tenenbaum (Eds.), *Encyclopedia of sport and exercise psychology* (pp. 74–76). Sage Publications, Inc.

Baer, R. A. (2003). Mindfulness training as a clinical intervention: A conceptual and empirical review. *Clinical Psychology: Science and Practice, 10*, 125–143.

Baltzell, A., & Summers, J. (2016). The future of mindfulness and performance across disciplines. In A. L. Baltzell (Ed.), *Mindfulness and performance: Current perspectives in social and behavioural sciences* (pp. 515–541). Cambridge University Press.

Baltzell, A., & Summers, J. (2018). *The power of mindfulness: Mindfulness meditation training in sport (MMTS)*. Springer.

Bennett, J., & Lindsay, P. (2016). Case Study 3: An acceptance commitment and mindfulness based intervention for a female hockey player experiencing post-injury performance anxiety. *Sport & Exercise Psychology Review, 12*, 36–46.

Bond, F. W., Hayes, S. C., Baer, R. A., et al. (2011). Preliminary psychometric properties of the acceptance and action questionnaire – II: A revised measure of psychological inflexibility and experiential avoidance. *Behavior Therapy, 42*, 676–688. DOI: 10.1016/j.beth.2011.03.007.

Brewer, B., Andersen, M. B., & Van Raalte, J. L. (2002). Psychological aspects of sport injury rehabilitation: Toward a biopsychological approach. In D. I. Mosoftsky and L. D. Zaichowsky (Eds.), *Medical aspects of sport and exercise* (pp. 41–54). Fitness Information Technology.

Bühlmayer, L., Birrer, D., Röthlin, P., Faude, O., & Donath, L. (2017). Effects of mindfulness practice on performance-relevant parameters and performance outcomes in sports: A meta-analytical review. *Sports Medicine, 47*(11), 2309–2321.

DeGaetano, J. J., Wolanin, A. T., Marks, D. R., & Eastin, S. M. (2016). The role of psychological flexibility in injury rehabilitation. *Journal of Clinical Sport Psychology, 10*, 192–205.

Forsdyke, D., Smith, A., Jones, M., & Gledhill, A. (2016). Psychosocial factors associated with outcomes of sports injury rehabilitation in competitive athletes: A mixed studies systematic review. *British Journal of Sports Medicine, 50*, 537–544.

Fox, M. D., Corbetta, M., Snyder, A. Z., Vincent, J. L., & Raichle, M. E. (2006). Spontaneous neuronal activity distinguishes human dorsal and ventral attention systems. *Proceedings of the National Academy of Sciences of the United States of America, 103*, 10046–10051.

Gardner, F. L., & Moore, Z. E. (2007). *The psychology of enhancing human performance: The mindfulness-acceptance-commitment approach*. Springer.

Germer, C., & Neff, K. (2013). Self-compassion and clinical practice. *Journal of Clinical Psychology, 69*, 856–867.

Germer, C., & Neff, K. (2019). *Teaching the mindful self-compassion program: A guide for professionals*. Guilford Press.

Glass, C., Pineau, T., Kaufman, K. A., Gardner, F., Moore, Z., & Baltzell, A. (2020). Clarifying the mindfulness muddle: A response to Wilson and Gearity's book review of three popular mindfulness interventions. *Journal of Sport Psychology in Action, 11*, 138–141.

Gledhill, A., Ahmed, O. H., & Forsdyke, D. (2020). Effectively managing anterior cruciate ligament injury and return to performance in elite women's soccer. In J. Dixon, J. Barker, R. Thelwell, & I. Mitchell (Eds.). *The Psychology of Soccer*. Routledge.

Gledhill, A., Forsdyke, D., & Murray, E. (2018). Psychological interventions used to reduce sports injuries: A systematic review of effectiveness. *British Journal of Sports Medicine, 52*, 967–971.

Gledhill, A., & Ivarsson, A. (2020). Reducing sports injury risk: Making a case for psychological intervention. *The Sport and Exercise Scientist, 65*, 26–27.

Harris, R. (2009). *ACT Made Simple: An easy-to-read primer on acceptance and commitment therapy*. New Harbinger Publications.

Hayes, S. C., Strosahl, K., & Wilson, K. G. (1999). *Acceptance and commitment therapy: An experiential approach to behavior change*. Guilford Press.

Ho, R. T. H., Lo, H. H. M., Fong, T. C. T., & Choi, C. E. (2020). Effects of a mindfulness-based intervention on diurnal cortisol pattern in disadvantaged families: A randomised controlled trial. *Psychoneuroendocrinology, 117*. https://doi.org/10.1016/j.psyneuen.2020.104696.

Hölzel, B. K., Lazar, S. W., Gard, T., Schuman-Olivier, Z., Vago, D. R., & Ott, U. (2011). How does mindfulness meditation work? Proposing mechanisms of action from a conceptual and neural perspective. *Perspectives on Psychological Science, 6*, 537–559.

Ivarsson, A., Johnson, U., Andersen, M. B., Fallby, J., & Altemyr, M. (2015). It pays to pay attention: A mindfulness-based program for injury prevention with soccer players. *Journal of Applied Sport Psychology, 27*, 319–334.

Ivarsson, A., Tranaeus, U., Johnson, U., & Stenling, A. (2017). Negative psychological responses of injury and rehabilitation adherence effects on return to play in competitive athletes: A systematic review and meta-analysis. *Open Access Journal of Sports Medicine, 8*, 27–32.

Josefsson, T., Tornberg, R., Gustafsson, H., & Ivarsson, A. (2020). Practitioners' reflections of working with the Mindfulness-Acceptance-Commitment (MAC) approach in team sport settings. *Journal of Sport Psychology in Action, 11*, 92–102.

Kabat-Zinn, J. (1994). *Full catastrophe living: Using the wisdom of your body and mind to face stress, pain, and illness*. Delta.

Kabat-Zinn, J. (2005). *Coming to our senses: Healing ourselves and the world through mindfulness*. Hyperion.

Kashdan, T. B. & Rottenberg, J. (2010). Psychological flexibility as a fundamental aspect of health. *Clinical Psychology Review, 30*(7), 865–878.

Kaufman, K. A., Glass, C. R., & Pineau, T. R. (2018). *Mindful sport performance enhancement: Mental training for athletes and coaches*. American Psychological Association.

Langer, E. (1989). *Mindfulness*. Da Capo Press.

Meesters, A., den Bosch-Meevissen, Y. M. C. I., Weijzen, C. A. H., et al. (2018). The effect of mindfulness-based stress reduction on wound healing: A preliminary study. *Journal of Behavioural Medicine, 41*, 385–397.

Mohammed, W. A., Pappous, A., & Sharma, D. (2018). Effect of Mindfulness Based Stress Reduction (MSBR) in increasing pain tolerance and improving the mental health of injured athletes. *Frontiers in Psychology, 9*, 722. DOI: 10.3389/fpsyg.2018.00722

Naderi, A., Shaabani, S., Zandi, H. G., Calmeiro, L., & Brewer, B. (2020). The effects of a mindfulness-based program on the incidence of injuries in young male soccer players. *Journal of Sport and Exercise Psychology, 42*, 161–171.

Noetel, M., Ciarrochi, J., Van Zanden, B., & Lonsdale, C. (2017). Mindfulness and acceptance approaches to sporting performance enhancement: A systematic review. *International Review of Sport and Exercise Psychology, 1*, 1.

Putukian, M. (2016). The psychological response to injury in student athletes: A narrative review with a focus on mental health. *British Journal of Sports Medicine, 50*, 145–148.

Sanada, K., Alda Díez, M., Salas Valero, M., et al. (2017). Effects of mindfulness-based interventions on biomarkers in healthy and cancer populations: A systematic review. *BMC Complementary and Alternative Medicine*, 17, 125. DOI: 10.1186/s12906-017-1638-y.

Skinner, T. C., Robertson, T., Allison, G. T., Dunlop, S., & Bucks, R. S. (2010). Experiential avoidance, mindfulness and depression in spinal cord injuries: A preliminary study. *Australian Journal of Rehabilitation Counselling, 16*, 27–35.

Zadeh, M. M., Ajilchi, B., Salman, Z., & Kisely, S. (2019). Effect of a mindfulness programme training to prevent the sport injury and improve the performance of semi-professional soccer players. *Australasian Psychiatry, 27*, 589–595.

Part IV

THE PSYCHOLOGY OF RETURN TO SPORT DECISIONS

In the previous parts of the book, you've progressed through the earlier stages of the sports injury journey, from being susceptible to injury, through to ways in which we might be able to enhance athletes' injury experiences and rehabilitation adherence in the last part. Arguably, the goal of enhancing an athlete's injury experience and helping them to improve their rehabilitation adherence is with a view to providing them the best chance of making a return to pre-injury levels of sport without an elevated risk of re-injury. However, for some athletes returning to their pre-injury sport is not an option and they will retire.

In the first chapter of Part 4, Dale Forsdyke discusses the key psychological factors that are important during being reintegrated back to sport following injury. We know that return to sport decision-making has become an increasingly hot topic within both sport psychology and sports medicine (e.g. Forsdyke et al., 2017). We commonly accept now that physical and psychological recovery from an injury frequently do not occur at the same time, and a common dilemma for sports injury practitioners is how they will know when an athlete is really ready to return to their pre-injury sport.

In seeking to address that question, Dale will consider the different factors that are reported by athletes, coaches and injury practitioners as being indicative of psychological readiness to return to sport. He will then offer a critical perspective on the different psychometric measures that can be used to support return to sport decisions. Lastly, Dale provides a heuristic framework that can be used to inform return to sport decisions. This chapter will be framed within the Bern Consensus Statement on Return to Sport (Ardern et al., 2016) and will be an advocate for athlete-centred, multidisciplinary return to sport decision-making.

For the majority of athletes, the undoubtedly preferred sports injury outcome is a successful return to pre-injury levels of sport. However, for some, the decision to retire is either enforced on them or their preferable option. Adam Gledhill will use the next chapter in Part 4 of this book to discuss the different psychological considerations within retirement decisions from sports injury. In recent years, there has been increased attention given to reasons behind athletes making the decision to retire from sport, even in circumstances when the injury didn't necessitate retirement (voluntary retirement), as well as other instances whereby the severity of the injury has necessitated retirement (involuntary retirement). Understanding both sets of circumstances is important for sports injury practitioners, so that they can best support athletes through these types of injury transitions.

References

Ardern, C. L., Glasgow, P., Schneiders, A., Witvrouw, E., Clarsen, B., Cools, A., Gojanovic, B., Griffin, S., Khan K. M., Moksnes, H., Mutch, S. A., Phillips, N., Reurink, G., Sadler, R., Silbernage, K. G., Thorborg, K., Wangensteen, A., Wilk, K. E., & Bizzini, M. (2016). Consensus statement on return to sport from the First World Congress in Sports Physical Therapy, Bern. *British Journal of Sports Medicine, 50*, 853–864.

Forsdyke, D., Gledhill, A., & Ardern, C. (2017). Psychological readiness to return to sport: Three key elements to help the practitioner decide whether the athlete is REALLY ready? *British Journal of Sports Medicine, 51*(7), 555–556.

10

IS MY ATHLETE REALLY READY TO RETURN TO SPORT?

PSYCHOLOGICAL FACTORS AND RETURNING TO SPORT FOLLOWING INJURY

Dr Dale Forsdyke and Dr Adam Gledhill

Sports injury represents a significant challenge for both athletes and practitioners. The burden of injury in sport tends to be high, while the prognosis in the form of return to sport outcomes is frequently poor (e.g. Drew et al., 2017; Harris et al., 2013). Following injury, many athletes will make the decision to cease involvement in their pre-injury sport (Ardern et al., 2014). For those athletes who do return to their pre-injury sport, they do so against a background of high rates of re-injury and a reduced capability to return to their pre-injury levels of performance and status (e.g. Ekstrand et al., 2020; Ishøi et al., 2018; Kyritsis et al., 2016). As such the return to sport landscape is daunting. In an attempt to optimize outcomes, research and consensus guidelines advocate that athletes should only return to sport when they are physically, psychologically, technically and tactically ready to do so (see Ardern et al., 2016; Forsdyke et al., 2016). Frequently, return to sport decisions are made from a reduced perspective with psychological factors seldom evaluated (Barber-Westin & Noyes, 2011; Burgi et al., 2019). Therefore, enhancing the decision-making process around determining whether an athlete is really ready to return to sport following injury is important.

This chapter begins with a contextual outline of the return to sport process. Next, the concept of readiness to return to sport is discussed. Following this, the construct of psychological readiness to return to sport is explored. Additionally, how psychological factors can be integrated in the decision-making process to inform impressions of psychological readiness is outlined. Last, this chapter concludes with a case study with accompanying questions, which will enable readers to apply the content of the chapter.

WHAT IS RETURN TO SPORT?

Returning an athlete back to sport following injury is a contextually minded, athlete-centred process, incorporating injury assessment, diagnosis and treatment to fully engaging in training and competition. The contextual aspect of returning to sport relates to what the athlete is intending to be returned back to (e.g. nature of the sport, nature of the performance level, nature of the athlete). Generally, for an athlete this is an expected return to a complex and dynamic environment that is influenced by many physical, psychological, technical and tactical factors (Forsdyke et al., 2016; Webster & Feller, 2019a).

According to consensus guidelines, return to sport should be viewed as a continuum that is paralleled with tissue healing processes and rehabilitation (see Ardern et al., 2016). There are three elements of the return to sport continuum: (1) return to participation, (2) return to sport and (3) return to performance. Return to participation describes taking part in modified sport activities (i.e. reconditioning, training, competition). Return to sport refers to the athlete returning to their pre-injury sport but are performing below their pre-injury level. Finally, return to performance describes having returned to the pre-injury sport but at a performance level comparable or above pre-injury levels and with their full status restored. Evidence suggests that while a majority of athletes will return back to their pre-injury sport at some point, returning to pre-injury levels of performance represents more of a challenge (e.g. Ishøi et al., 2018; Lai et al., 2018). Increasingly, in addition to physical factors, psychological factors have been put forward to explain the predictive variance in returning to sport and returning to performance outcomes following injury (e.g. Ardern et al., 2013; Forsdyke et al., 2016; Nwachukwu et al., 2019). It then makes sense that physical and psychological factors are considered at each stage of the return to sport continuum in order to better safeguard an athlete's overall readiness to return to their pre-injury sport.

WHAT IS READINESS TO RETURN TO SPORT?

Despite featuring in theoretical frameworks as a desirable and potentially important return to sport outcome, what the term 'readiness' means is relatively understudied (e.g. the Biopsychosocial Model of Sport Injury Rehabilitation; Brewer et al., 2002). It is likely that an athlete's overall readiness to return to sport following injury can be subdivided into physical and psychological components. These components should be viewed as interacting with one another as opposed to separate dichotomous classifications. As such, the extent that an athlete is physically and psychologically ready to return to sport can be placed into quadrants situated on high-to-low axes (see Figure 10.1).

From Figure 10.1, it can be inferred that an athlete returning to sport following injury when they are anything other than high in physical readiness and high in psychological readiness is not desirable. For example, an athlete that possesses high physical readiness and low psychological readiness will be physically robust but may experience anxieties over their performance and re-injury risk. Likewise, an athlete that possesses low physical readiness and

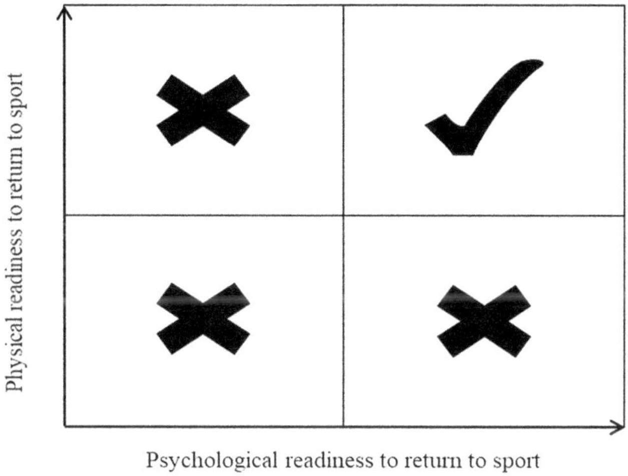

Figure 10.1 Quadrants of readiness to return to sport following injury

high psychological readiness may feel confident and motivated but would likely be unable to withstand the loading demands of the sport (e.g. repeated bouts of high-speed running, single-leg landing). There is evidence to support this perspective. This is because players who do not meet physical and psychological readiness discharge criteria are less likely to return to pre-injury competitive sport (e.g. Ardern et al., 2014; Christino et al., 2016), more likely to sustain re-injury (e.g. Paterno et al., 2017; Webster & Hewett, 2019) and more likely to underperform on return to sport (e.g. Ishøi et al., 2018; Zarzycki et al., 2018). Unfortunately, many athletes will return to sport when they are physically and/or psychologically under prepared (e.g. Phelan et al., 2019; Schmitt et al., 2015). In regard to psychological readiness, this may prove problematic as only a modest number of athletes will experience meaningful improvements in their psychological readiness when they return to training and sport (Zarzycki et al., 2017).

A holistic approach to readiness to return to sport such as this raises several considerations. First, a key challenge for athletes and practitioners is that often physical and psychological readiness may be restored in different timeframes (Podlog & Eklund, 2007). Without clear and shared expectations, this increases the chance of athletes returning to sport when they are physically and not psychologically ready to do so, and vice versa. Second, evidence suggests that despite clear guidance on evaluating physical readiness, many athletes return to sport not fulfilling the stated criteria (Webster & Hewett, 2019). As such, this then impacts on the overall physical and psychological readiness status of the athlete. Achieving physical markers appears important to safeguard physical readiness and also develops psychological readiness in the form of increased confidence and motivation and reduced anxiety (Carson & Polman, 2012; Podlog et al., 2015). Finally, developing and evaluating physical readiness is far more established in research and practice compared to psychological readiness (Forsdyke et al., 2016). As such, what psychological readiness is, how it is developed or diminished and how it can be best evaluated are areas requiring some development (Podlog et al., 2015; Webster et al., 2018).

WHAT IS PSYCHOLOGICAL READINESS TO RETURN TO SPORT?

Even though psychological readiness has appeared in the return to sport literature for many years, working definitions of what psychological readiness is are rare (e.g. Podlog et al., 2015). According to research, psychological readiness is a multifaceted and multidimensional construct (Forsdyke et al., 2017; Webster et al., 2008). In other words, it may be the sum of several psychological factors spanning re-injury and performance dimensions (Forsdyke et al., 2016; Podlog et al., 2015). Athletes tend to present with many concerns over returning to sport with anxiety (including fear), confidence (including self-efficacy), perceived pressure and self-presentational issues predominating (e.g. Meierbachtol et al., 2020; Podlog et al., 2011; Papadopoulos et al., 2018). As such, in the context of performance and re-injury, a psychologically ready athlete can be characterized as having clear return to sport expectations together with high level of confidence and low levels of anxiety (Forsdyke et al., 2017). Psychological readiness can be viewed as an adaptive return to sport outcome that has several behavioural, emotional and performance-related consequences for athletes prior to, upon and after returning to sport (Forsdyke et al., 2016; Phelan et al., 2019).

There is a growing evidence base indicating the important prognostic value of psychological readiness to return to sport (e.g. Webster & Feller, 2019b). One point worthy of consideration is that majority of this research is grounded in the anterior cruciate ligament (ACL) injury literature, although the findings may also have some transferability to other sports injuries (e.g. muscle strain, ligament sprains, overuse injuries). Psychological readiness has been found to be associated with (1) the decision to return to pre-injury sport following injury (e.g. Ardern et al., 2014), (2) the ability to return to pre-injury levels of performance (e.g. Kitaguchi et al., 2019), (3) the risk of sustaining re-injury (e.g. McPherson et al., 2019) and (4) quality of functional performance (e.g. Nagelli et al., 2019; Zarzycki et al., 2018). In other words, an athlete who possesses a high level of psychological readiness will be more likely to return to their pre-injury sport and pre-injury levels of performance when compared with an athlete with low levels of psychological readiness. The goal for many injured athletes is a return to pre-injury levels of sport performance for a prolonged injury-free period of time (Shanley et al., 2019; Webster & Feller, 2019a). As such, psychological readiness appears to be a central consideration in enabling athletes to meet this expectation. Against this background, an awareness of the various factors that may contribute to the development of psychological readiness in athletes is potentially important.

As psychological readiness appears to be a multifaceted construct, several factors will likely contribute to its development (Forsdyke et al., 2017; Webster & Feller, 2018). Measurement instruments infer that improving confidence in performance and remaining injury-free, experiencing fewer negative emotions and having accurate risk appraisals of re-injury will develop psychological readiness (Glazer, 2009; Webster et al., 2008). Research suggests that high-quality social support, achieving clinical outcomes (e.g. physical testing), positive athlete perceptions of symptoms and function, effective goal setting, feeling valued by significant others and expectation management are precursors that may facilitate the development of psychological readiness (Geromatta et al., 2018; Podlog et al., 2015; Webster et al., 2018). Additionally, there are several additional situational factors that may also be associated with psychological readiness, such as sex (i.e. male), age (i.e. younger), interval between injury and surgical intervention (i.e. shorter interval) and pre-injury investment in sport (i.e. higher frequency of participation; Webster et al., 2018). Taken together, there may be many modifiable and non-modifiable factors that may develop psychological readiness. Whereas, an awareness of the non-modifiable factors may serve to stratify the risk of an athlete, the modifiable factors are those that may be of most interest for practitioners working with injured athletes.

HOW TO MAKE DECISIONS OVER PSYCHOLOGICAL READINESS?

Robust decisions should be made at each stage of the return to sport process (Burgi et al., 2019). As such, the combined physical and psychological readiness of athletes should be routinely evaluated to inform progressions (e.g. from the return to participation to the return to sport elements; Ardern et al., 2016). How to make effective decisions over psychological readiness is far less developed in comparison to evaluating physical readiness (e.g. through six established discharge criteria; Kyritsis et al., 2016). For example, in a scoping review of 209 studies focusing on the conditions that athletes are returned to sport following injury, only 1 study reported using a robust of measure of psychological readiness (Burgi et al., 2019).

One framework aimed at supporting practitioners to make decisions over psychological readiness is proposed by Forsdyke et al. (2017). This framework provides three elements to making effective decisions over psychological readiness to return to sport. These elements are as follows: (1) that practitioners should use reliable, valid and responsive psychological measurement instruments to routinely screen and monitor injured players; (2) combine the data obtained from psychological instruments with their working knowledge of the athlete and (3) make all clinical decisions from a player-centred interdisciplinary perspective (i.e. not only use physical criteria). Of particular importance is this framework advocates using all three elements together to inform their impressions on an athlete's psychological readiness as opposed to relying on one element of the framework (i.e. the elements complement each other).

There are several valid and reliable measurement instruments that can be used to inform decisions over psychological readiness to return to sport (see Table 10.1). The general purpose of these instruments would be to screen for psychological factors in order to inform impressions of psychological readiness in preparation for shared decision making (Forsdyke et al., 2017; Shrier, 2015; Slagers et al., 2019). In other words, these instruments should not be seen as diagnostic clinical tools, and if a clinically meaningful psychological disturbance (e.g. depression) is suspected, then practitioners should use the appropriate referral pathways. Of the measures in Table 10.1, the injury-psychological readiness to return to sport scale (I-PRRS) is currently the only direct measure

Table 10.1 Commonly used measurement instruments to screen and monitor psychological factors

Authors and date	*Instrument name (abbreviation)*	*Construct(s) measured*	*Number of items*
Glazer (2009)	I-PRRS	Psychological readiness in the form of confidence	6
Gerometta et al. (2018)	SIRSI	Emotions Confidence Risk appraisal	12
Webster et al. (2008)	ACL-RSI	Emotions Confidence Risk appraisal	12
Webster & Feller (2018)	ACL-RSI short version	Emotions Confidence Risk appraisal	6
Walker et al. (2010)	RIAI	Re-injury anxiety during rehabilitation and re-entry into competition	28
Miller et al. (1991)	TSK	Fear of movement	17
Woby et al. (2005)	TSK-11	Fear of movement	11
Thomeé et al. (2006)	K-SES	Self-efficacy	22
Smith et al. (1990)	ERAIQ	Emotional response Perceived recovery Fear of re-injury Optimism Knowledge of rehabilitation	24
Evans et al. (2008)	PRSII	Restlessness Dispirited Re-organization Isolation Devastation Feeling cheated	19

I-PRRS, Injury-psychological readiness to return to sport scale; SIRSI, Shoulder instability – return to sport after injury scale; ACL-RSI, Anterior cruciate ligament return to sport after injury scale; RIAI, Re-injury anxiety inventory; TSK, Tampa Scale of Kinesiophobia; TSK-11, Tampa Scale of Kinesiophobia short version; K-SES, Knee self-efficacy scale; ERAIQ, Emotional Response of Athletes in Injury Questionnaire; PRSII, Psychological Responses to Sport Injury Inventory.

of psychological readiness. This is because the other instruments are seen as proxy or indirect measures of psychological factors that are associated with, but are distinct from, the construct of psychological readiness (Podlog et al., 2015). The I-PRRS is an injury generic measure that is focussed on performance and injury-related confidence (Conti et al., 2019). However, by doing so a major limitation of the I-PRRS is that it takes a reduced perspective of psychological readiness. As psychological readiness to return to sport appears to be a multifaceted construct, using a combination of measures, together with routine wellness monitoring (e.g. sleep quality, stress, energy, appetite), may provide a more reliable and rounded impressions of psychological readiness (Forsdyke et al. 2017), for example using the I-PRRS together with the RIAI. Several of the other available measures are injury specific (e.g. ACL-RSI, SIRSI, K-SES). Although these measures have been shown to have some predictive ability for athletes returning to sport from that specific injury type, their utility to other injuries that may have similar burden is currently less well known (Kitaguchi et al., 2019; Webster & Feller, 2018).

Users of these measurement instruments should do so in light of two important questions. First, *what are the threshold values of the measure?* Several of the measurement instruments suggest threshold values that may have some clinical relevance to inform decision-making (e.g. ACL-RSI, TSK). In other words, the score that would mean the athlete is in the high or low category. Research has found that such thresholds do have some predictive ability. For example, scoring high on the ACL-RSI (e.g. 60+) appears predictive of a return to pre-injury sport with a reduced risk of re-injury (McPherson et al., 2019; Webster & Feller, 2018). While being aware of threshold values may be of some use to inform overall impressions of athletes, further research is required before decisions can be reliably made on such thresholds. A second related question is *what represents a meaningful change in score?* In other words, the extent a score needs to change to be seen as an important improvement or reduction in the athlete's status. Indicators to interpret this are the minimally important difference (MIC), smallest detectable change (SDC) and standard error of the instrument (SEM; Davidson & Keating, 2014). The MIC, also known as minimally clinically important difference, is the smallest amount of change that would be perceived as important for the athlete. SDC is the smallest change above measurement error of the instrument (usually above 95% CI). SEM is the change in score due to a lack of reliability in the measure. For interpreting a significant change, the MIC should be larger than SDC as it is possible to distinguish change from measurement error with a high degree of certainty (van Kampen et al., 2013). If the SDC is greater than the MIC, the change would be considered important to the athlete but cannot be distinguished from measurement error. A change score greater than both the MIC and SDC is thought to be both significant and important. Such information can be gained from previous studies. For example, the reported MICs of the ACL-RSI and I-PRRS for individual athletes are 2.6 and 0.9, respectively (Slagers et al., 2019). However, the SDCs for these measures are reported as 15.3 and 11.6 (Slagers et al., 2019; Slagers et al., 2017). For practitioners this means that to interpret significant and important changes in psychological status, improvements of 15.3 for the ACL-RSI and 11.6 for the I-PRRS would need to be achieved.

Rather than solely relying on measurement instruments, practitioners should also use their subjective clinical impressions. These impressions are frequently formed from hours and hours of personal interactions with the athlete during the return to sport process. From this exposure, strong collaborative working relationships can be developed from assessment, diagnosis and treatment through to return to sport (King et al., 2019). As such, practitioners will develop a working knowledge and understanding of the athlete. Subjective clinical impressions gleaned from informal conversations and observations have real value in decision-making. Ideally, the working knowledge of the athlete would complement the findings from the measurement instruments and further validate impressions. However, and potentially just as useful, it may also highlight some conflicting messages and facilitate some further questions to resolve the ambiguity. For example, an athlete who may score highly on the I-PRRS may indicate high levels of psychological readiness, but through regular observation they appear to avoid certain injurious movement patterns associated with the pre-injury sport (e.g. tacking, cutting). In turn, this may facilitate further reflection and discussion over the athlete's psychological status.

The third element of the framework is basing all clinical decisions from a player-centred interdisciplinary perspective. An athlete should only return to sport when they are physically, psychologically, technically and tactically ready to do so (Ardern et al., 2016; Forsdyke et al., 2016). As such, clinical decisions to progress through the return to sport process require interdisciplinary 'joined-up' thinking. These decisions are thought to be best made in a collaborative way using the expertise and impressions from members of the multidisciplinary team (Ardern et al., 2016; Shrier, 2015). For example, psychologists, coaches, sports injury practitioners and performance analysis staff may all offer additional insight into the psychological readiness of the athlete to progress. The athlete should always be at the centre of the decision-making process in order to augment empowerment, education and manage everyone's expectations (King et al., 2019). Decisions to progress the athlete during the return to sport process should therefore be a shared and collective responsibility (Dijkstra et al., 2017).

CONCLUSION

So, how do you know whether your athlete is really ready to return to sport? Certainly, your overall impressions of the athlete's psychological readiness which has been informed by diverse evidence is one key consideration. Psychological readiness appears to be an important prognostic and clinically relevant outcome that may help optimise return to sport following injury.

Case study: 'I can't trust my body anymore'

Ravi, a 32-year-old professional Rugby League player, sustained a right shoulder dislocation injury while making a tackle with his outstretched arm. Ravi was immediately removed from the field of players for his protection and for further assessment and diagnosis. Diagnostic imaging revealed a glenohumeral joint dislocation with a Bankart labral tear. This was Ravi's second shoulder dislocation in 2 years. He feels he rushed back to sport from the previous shoulder injury and was not really ready. Following a surgical intervention (i.e. Bankart repair), Ravi was immediately placed into a sling to immobilize his arm and told to avoid contact training for 6 months. The injury occurred at a really bad time for Ravi. He has only 1 year left on his professional contract and has concerns whether anyone will want to employ a 'broken' player who can longer be 'trusted' to do his job in the team.

Following five and half months of rehabilitation and reconditioning, you have been asked to be part of the decision-making process over Ravi's transition back into training and competition. While Ravi appears to be physically robust and athletic, there are no specific data to validate this impression. He mentions to you that he is worried about going through rehabilitation again as it almost certainly would finish his career off. When asked about his return to sport goal, he is uncertain and says he is currently waiting on the decision of others to determine when and if he can get back into training. He mentions he feels weaker on his right side and has been avoiding putting 100% into some overhead exercises. As a consequence of injury, he has lost his place in the senior team to someone much younger and currently doubts his ability to restore his playing status anytime soon. When asked about what people will expect of him and how he will feel about the first collision following returning to sport, he says it has been 'keeping him awake at night'.

Questions

1. What are your impressions about the psychological readiness of Ravi to return to participation and sport following injury?
2. What would be your concerns about Ravi returning to participation and sport based on his current state?
3. What specific data would you want to collect on Ravi to best inform your impressions over his eventual psychological readiness to return to sport?
4. How could you create a return to sport environment that facilitates psychological readiness?

References

Ardern, C. L., Glasgow, P., Schneiders, A., Witvrouw, E., Clarsen, B., Cools, A., Gojanovic, B., Griffin, S., Khan K. M., Moksnes, H., Mutch, S. A., Phillips, N., Reurink, G., Sadler, R., Silbernagel, K. G., Thorborg, K., Wangensteen, A., Wilk, K. E., & Bizzini, M. (2016). 2016 Consensus statement on return to sport from the First World Congress in Sports Physical Therapy, Bern. *British Journal of Sports Medicine, 50*, 853–864.

Ardern, C. L, Österberg, A., Tagesson, S., Gauffin, H., Webster, K. E., & Kvist, J. (2014). The impact of psychological readiness to return to sport and recreational activities after anterior cruciate ligament reconstruction. *British Journal of Sports Medicine, 48*(22), 1613–1619.

Ardern, C. L., Taylor, N. F., Feller, J. A., & Webster, K. E. (2013). A systematic review of the psychological factors associated with returning to sport following injury. *British Journal of Sports Medicine, 47*(17), 1120–1126.

Ardern, C. L., Taylor, N. F., Feller, J. A., & Webster, K. E. (2014). Fifty-five per cent return to competitive sport following anterior cruciate ligament reconstruction surgery: An updated systematic review and meta-analysis including aspects of physical functioning and contextual factors. *British Journal of Sports Medicine, 48*, 1543–1552.

Barber-Westin, S., & Noyes, F. (2011). Objective criteria for return to athletics after anterior cruciate ligament reconstruction and subsequent reinjury rates: A systematic review. *The Physician and Sports Medicine, 39*(3), 100–110.

Brewer, B. W., Andersen, M. B., & Van Raalte, J. L. (2002). Psychological aspects of sport injury rehabilitation: Toward a biopsychological approach. In D. I. Mostofsky, & L. D. Zaichkowsky (Eds.), *Medical Aspects of Sport and Exercise* (pp. 41–54). Fitness Information Technology.

Burgi, C. R., Peters, S., Ardern, C. L., et al. (2019). Which criteria are used to clear patients to return to sport after primary ACL reconstruction? A scoping review. *British Journal of Sports Medicine, 53*, 1154–1161.

Carson, F., & Polman, R. (2012). Experiences of professional rugby union players returning to competition following anterior cruciate ligament reconstruction. *Physical Therapy in Sport, 13*(1), 35–40.

Christino, M. A., Fleming, B. C., Machan, J. T., & Shalvoy, R. M. (2016). Psychological factors associated with anterior cruciate ligament reconstruction recovery. *Orthopaedic Journal of Sports Medicine, 4*(3), 2325967116638341.

Conti, C., di Fronso, S., Robazza, C., & Bertollo, M. (2019). The injury-psychological readiness to return to sport (I-PRRS) scale and the sport confidence inventory (SCI): A cross-cultural validation. *Physical Therapy in Sport, 40*, 218–224.

Davidson, M., & Keating, J. (2014). Patient-reported outcome measures (PROMs): How should I interpret reports of measurement properties? A practical guide for clinicians and researchers who are not biostatisticians. *British Journal of Sports Medicine, 48*, 792–796.

Dijkstra, H. P, Pollock, N., Chakraverty, R., & Ardern, C. L., (2017). Return to play in elite sport: A shared decision-making process. *British Journal of Sports Medicine, 51*, 419–420.

Drew, M. K., Raysmith, B. P., & Charlton, P. C. (2017). Injuries impair the chance of successful performance by sportspeople: A systematic review. *British Journal of Sports Medicine, 51*, 1209–1214.

Ekstrand, J., Krutsch, W., Spreco, A., van Zoest, W., Roberts, C., Meyer, T., & Bengtsson, H. (2020). Time before return to play for the most common injuries in professional football: A 16-year follow-up of the UEFA Elite Club Injury Study. *British Journal of Sports Medicine, 54*, 421–426.

Evans, L., Hardy, L., Mitchell, I., & Rees, T. (2008). The development of a measure to psychological responses to injury, *Journal of Sport Rehabilitation, 1*(16), 21–37.

Forsdyke, D., Gledhill, A., & Ardern, C. (2017). Psychological readiness to return to sport: Three key elements to help the practitioner decide whether the athlete is REALLY ready? *British Journal of Sports Medicine, 51*(7), 555–556.

Forsdyke, D., Smith, A., Jones, M., & Gledhill, A. (2016). Psychosocial factors associated with outcomes of sports injury rehabilitation in competitive athletes: A mixed studies systematic review. *British Journal of Sports Medicine, 50*, 537–544.

Gerometta, A., Klouche, S., Herman, S., Herman, S., Lefevre, N., & Bohu, Y. (2018). The shoulder instability-return to sport after Injury (SIRSI): A valid and reproducible scale to quantify psychological readiness to return to sport after traumatic shoulder instability. *Knee Surgery, Sports Traumatology, Arthroscopy, 26*, 203–211.

Glazer, D. (2009). Development and preliminary validation of the injury-psychological readiness to return to sport (I-PRRS) scale. *Journal of Athletic Training, 44*(2), 185–189.

Harris, J. D., Frank, J. M., Jordan, M. A., Bush-Joseph, C. A., Romeo, A. A., Gupta, A. K., Abrams, G., McCormick, F., & Bach, B. R. (2013). Return to sport following shoulder surgery in the elite pitcher: A systematic review. *Sports Health, 5*(4), 367–376.

Ishøi, L., Thorborg, K., Kraemer, O., & Hölmich, P. (2018). Return to sport and performance after hip arthroscopy for femoroacetabular impingement in 18- to 30-year-old athletes: A cross-sectional cohort study of 189 Athletes. *The American Journal of Sports Medicine*, *46*(11), 2578–2587.

King, J., Roberts, C., Hard S., & Ardern, C. (2019). Want to improve return to sport outcomes following injury? Empower, engage, provide feedback and be transparent: 4 habits! *British Journal of Sports Medicine*, *53*, 526–527.

Kitaguchi, T., Tanaka, Y., Takeshita, S. et al. (2019). Importance of functional performance and psychological readiness for return to preinjury level of sports 1 year after ACL reconstruction in competitive athletes. *Knee Surgery, Sports Traumatology, Arthroscopy*. https://doi.org/10.1007/s00167-019-05774-y.

Kyritsis, P., Bahr, R., Landreau, P., Miladi, R., & Witvrouw, E. (2016). Likelihood of ACL graft rupture: Not meeting six clinical discharge criteria before return to sport is associated with a four times greater risk of rupture. *British Journal of Sports Medicine*, *50*, 946–951.

Lai, C. C., Ardern, C. L., Feller, J. A., & Webster, K. (2018). Eighty-three per cent of elite athletes return to preinjury sport after anterior cruciate ligament reconstruction: A systematic review with meta-analysis of return to sport rates, graft rupture rates and performance outcomes. *British Journal of Sports Medicine*, *52*, 128–138.

McPherson, A. L., Feller, J. A., Hewett, T. E., & Webster, K. E. (2019). Psychological readiness to return to sport is associated with second anterior cruciate ligament injuries. *The American Journal of Sports Medicine*, *47*(4), 857–862.

Meierbachtol, A., Obermeier, M., Yungtum, W., Bottoms, J., Paur, E., Nelson, B., Tompkins, M., Russell, H., & Chmielewski, T. (2020). Injury-related fears during the return-to-sport phase of ACL reconstruction rehabilitation. *Orthopaedic Journal of Sports Medicine*, *8*(3), 2325967120909385.

Miller, R., Kori, S., & Todd, D. (1991). The Tampa scale: A measure of kinesiophobia. *Clinical Journal of Pain*, *7*(1), 51–52.

Nagelli, C., Webster, K., Di Stasi, S., Wordeman, D. S., & Hewett, T. (2019). The association of psychological readiness to return to sport after anterior cruciate ligament reconstruction and hip and knee landing kinematics. *Clinical Biomechanics*, *68*, 104–108.

Nwachukwu, B. U., Adjei, J., Rauck, R. C., Chahla, J., Okoroha, K. R., Verma, N. N., Allen, A. A., & Williams, R. J., 3rd (2019). How much do psychological factors affect lack of return to play after anterior cruciate ligament reconstruction? A systematic review. *Orthopaedic journal of sports medicine*, *7*(5), 2325967119845313.

Papadopoulos, S., Tishukov, M., Stamou, K., Totlis, T., & Natsis, K. (2018). Fear of re-injury following ACL reconstruction: An overview. *Journal of Research and Practice on the Musculoskeletal System*, *2*(4), 124–130.

Paterno, M. V., Huang, B., Thomas, S., Hewett, T. E., & Schmitt, L. C. (2017). Clinical factors that predict a second ACL injury after ACL reconstruction and return to sport: Preliminary development of a clinical decision algorithm. *Orthopaedic Journal of Sports Medicine*, *5*(12), 2325967117745279.

Phelan, B., King, E., Richter, C., Webster, K., & Falvey, E. (2019). A comparison of anterior cruciate ligament: Return to sports after injury (ACL-RSI) scores of male athletes nine-months post-ACL reconstruction with matched uninjured controls. *Physical Therapy in Sport*, *38*, 179–183.

Podlog, L., Banham, S., Wadey, R., & Hannon, J. (2015). Psychological readiness to return to competitive sport following injury: A qualitative study. *The Sport Psychologist, 29*(1), 1–14.

Podlog, L., Dimmock, J., & Miller, J. (2011). A review of return to sport concerns following injury rehabilitation: Practitioner strategies for enhancing recovery outcomes. *Physical Therapy in Sport*, 12(1), 36–42.

Podlog, L., & Eklund, R. C. (2007). The psychosocial aspects of a return to sport following serious injury: A review of the literature from a self-determination perspective. *Psychology of Sport and Exercise, 8*(4), 535–566.

Schmitt, L. C., Paterno, M. V., Ford, K. R., Myer, G. D., & Hewett, T. E. (2015). Strength asymmetry and landing mechanics at return to sport after anterior cruciate ligament reconstruction. *Medicine and Science in Sports and Exercise, 47*(7), 1426–1434.

Shanley, E., Thigpen, C., Brooks, J., Hawkins, R. J., Momaya, A., Kwapisz, A., Kissenberth, J., & Tokish, J. M. (2019). Return to sport as an outcome measure for shoulder instability: Surprising findings in nonoperative management in a high school athlete population. *The American Journal of Sports Medicine, 47*(5), 1062–1067.

Shrier, I. (2015). Strategic assessment of risk and risk tolerance (StARRT) framework for return-to-play decision-making. *British Journal of Sports Medicine, 49*, 1311–1315.

Slagers, A. J., Reininga, I. H., & van Den Akker-Scheek, I. (2017). The Dutch language anterior cruciate ligament return to sport after injury scale (ACL-RSI): Validity and reliability. *Journal of Sports Sciences, 35*(4), 393–401.

Slagers, A. J, van den Akker-Scheek, I., Geertzen, J., Zwerver, J., & Reininga, I. (2019). Responsiveness of the anterior cruciate ligament: Return to sports after Injury (ACL-RSI) and injury – psychological readiness to return to sport (I-PRRS) scales. *Journal of Sports Sciences, 37*(21), 2499–2505.

Smith, A. M., Scott, S. G., O'Fallon, W. M., & Young, M. L. (1990). Emotional responses of athletes to injury. *Mayo Clinic Proceedings, 65*(1), 38–50.

Thomeé, P., Währborg, P., Börjesson, M., Thomeé, R., Eriksson, B. I., & Karlsson, J. (2006). A new instrument for measuring self-efficacy in patients with an anterior cruciate ligament injury. *Scandinavian Journal of Medicine and Science in Sports, 16*(3), 181–187.

van Kampen, D. A., Willems, W. J., van Beers, L., Castelein, R., Scholtes, V., & Terwee, C. (2013). Determination and comparison of the smallest detectable change (SDC) and the minimal important change (MIC) of four-shoulder patient-reported outcome measures (PROMs). *Journal of Orthopaedic Surgery and Research, 8*, 40.

Walker, N., Thatcher, J., & Lavallee, D. E. (2010). A preliminary development of the re-injury anxiety inventory (RIAI). *Physical Therapy in Sport, 11*(1), 23–29.

Webster, K. E., & Feller, J. A. (2018). Development and validation of a short version of the anterior cruciate ligament return to sport after injury (ACL-RSI) Scale. *Orthopaedic Journal of Sports Medicine, 6*(4), 2325967118763763.

Webster, K. E., & Feller, J. A. (2019a). Expectations for return to preinjury sport before and after anterior cruciate ligament reconstruction. *The American Journal of Sports Medicine, 47*(3), 578–583.

Webster, K. E., & Feller, J. A. (2019b). A research update on the state of play for return to sport after anterior cruciate ligament reconstruction. *Journal of Orthopaedics and Traumatology, 20*, 10.

Webster, K. E., Feller, J., & Lambros, C. (2008). Development and preliminary validation of a scale to measure the psychological impact of returning to sport following anterior cruciate ligament reconstruction surgery. *Physical Therapy in Sport*, *9*(1): 9–15.

Webster, K. E., & Hewett, T. E. (2019). What is the evidence for and validity of return-to-sport testing after anterior cruciate ligament reconstruction surgery? *A Systematic Review and Meta-Analysis. Sports Medicine*, *49*, 917–929.

Webster, K. E., Nagelli, C. V., Hewett, T. E., & Feller, J. (2018). Factors associated with psychological readiness to return to sport after anterior cruciate ligament reconstruction surgery. *The American Journal of Sports Medicine*, *46*, 1545–1550.

Woby, S., Roach, N., Urmston, M., & Watson, P. (2005). Psychometric properties of the TSK-11: A shortened version of the Tampa Scale for kinesiophobia. *Pain*, *117*(1), 137–144.

Zarzycki, R., Failla, M., Arundale, A. J. H., Capin, J. J., & Snyder-Mackler, L. (2017). Athletes with a positive psychological response to return to sport training have better outcomes one and two years after ACL reconstruction. *Orthopaedic Journal of Sports Medicine*. https://doi.org/10.1177/2325967117S00324.

Zarzycki, R., Failla, M., Capin, J., & Snyder-Mackler, L. (2018). Psychological readiness to return to sport is associated with knee kinematic asymmetry during gait following ACL reconstruction. *Journal of Orthopaedic & Sports Physical Therapy*, *27*, 1–21.

11

THEY THINK IT'S ALL OVER

INJURY-RELATED RETIREMENT FROM SPORT

Dr Adam Gledhill and Dr Dale Forsdyke

INTRODUCTION

Whilst undoubtedly the preferred option for athletes who have experienced sports injury is to make an injury-free return to a minimum of pre-injury levels of performance (e.g. Ardern et al., 2016) and we should make every effort to support athletes in doing so (e.g. Forsdyke et al., 2017), an unfortunate consequence of sports injury is that athletes do sometimes retire. Indeed, injury-related retirement is a multi-national and cross-continental problem, with injury cited as a leading cause of retirement from sport across a number of countries including Denmark (Moesch et al., 2012), Finland (Ristolainen et al., 2012), Germany (Alfermann et al., 2004), Lithuania (Alfermann et al., 2004), Poland (Grygorowicz et al., 2019), Russia (Alfermann et al., 2004) and South Africa (Steyn & Slattery, 2013). For example, 30% of players within a recent study into retirement decisions of Polish female football players cited sport injury as the cause of retirement, whilst 54% of athletes from Finland, surveyed about their retirement decisions, reported that injury was a leading cause.

To set the landscape for the following chapter, we contend that injury-related retirement should be positioned as either voluntary or involuntary. Whilst historically, career-ending injury has been viewed as a non-normative career transition (Schlossberg, 1995), it is arguable that the understanding of injury-related retirement is potentially more nuanced than this. First, the term 'career-ending injury' connotes that the injury necessitates retirement (i.e. the athlete has no choice but to retire, as the injury prevents them from competing), thus making this an involuntary process. However, there are also instances whereby injuries that do not necessitate retirement from sport may play a role in an athlete's decision to retire. This suggests a more voluntary process, whereby the athlete has been supported to make a decision regarding their sporting future, which may have been informed by health, career, finance and other factors (e.g. Ardern & Khan, 2016; Gledhill & Forsdyke, 2018). It is likely that the voluntariness of the decision to retire will impact on the overall longer term health and wellbeing of the retired athlete and the distinct nature of the voluntariness should be factored into our understanding (e.g. Arvinen-Barrow et al., 2017; Gledhill & Forsdyke, 2018; Grygorowicz et al., 2019). Whilst the distinction is an important one as it will likely influence the impact of retirement on the athlete as well as how we support the athlete (Gledhill & Forsdyke, 2018), it is important to note that the majority of research to date has focused more on involuntary injury-related retirement where the severity of injury has been career-ending (Park et al., 2013).

Drawing on the above, this chapter has four key aims: (1) to discuss the factors underpinning retirement decisions; (2) to discuss the different psychosocial factors that might underpin an injured athlete's decision to retire; (3) to provide suggestions around how to improve the retirement experiences of athletes post-injury, including ways that might enhance health-related quality of life post-retirement and (4) to provide a case study where readers can apply their learning. In an attempt to achieve these aims, we recognize that injury-related retirement is a subjective experience; however, we will draw on patterns from within the literature to provide information around the most consistent themes.

PSYCHOSOCIAL FACTORS UNDERPINNING RETIREMENT DECISIONS

The first, most obvious and arguably most common factor underpinning retirement decisions is that the severity of the injury means that the athlete can no longer compete (Mannes et al., 2019), or it is ill-advised for them to do so. Typically, this will be informed by medical consultants and is most apparent in severe injuries, such as Anterior Cruciate Ligament injuries that require surgical repair (e.g. Tjong et al., 2014).

Notwithstanding this 'involuntary' retirement, there are also instances whereby an athlete will choose to retire from their chosen sport. These factors will likely vary according to age, gender, sport, level of play, stage of life and many other factors (e.g. Ardern & Khan, 2016; Gledhill & Forsdyke, 2018; Tjong et al., 2014). Whilst being largely based on findings from injured athletes who have suffered anterior cruciate ligament injuries, there are some apparent patterns within the body of research of psychosocial factors, which appear to contribute to voluntary retirement decisions. These are reinjury emotions and cognitions, quality of support network, and career or competing demands.

Reinjury emotions and cognitions: A prominent consideration for retirement is that of reinjury emotions and cognitions. Fear of reinjury is established as an important consideration in the return to sport process more broadly (e.g. Truong et al., 2020); however, this can be particularly influential in making the decision to retire (Grygorowicz et al., 2019). Typically, the fear of reinjury can be seen as influencing quality of life, potential impact on future sport performances, mood state and impacting on the love of the sport (e.g. Gledhill & Forsdyke, 2018; Tjong et al., 2014), all of which can contribute to the decision to retire. However, the fear is not always restricted to impacts of the injury on sport-related considerations. Fear can also manifest itself in other ways, including fear of pain, fear of playing sport again and fear of added financial burden through not being able to work (Tjong et al., 2014), all of which can influence an athlete's decision to retire.

More recently, the notion of a continuum of reinjury emotions and cognitions has been forwarded (Gledhill & Forsdyke, 2018), whereby the most severe end of the continuum contains fear of reinjury, then becomes progressively less severe into an expectation of reinjury, then on to the least severe aspect of anticipation of reinjury. In essence, athletes who anticipate a strong likelihood of reinjury, or have been injured so many times that they expect to get injured again, may simply think that a return to sport is no longer worth it and that a retirement decision is more appropriate for them (Gledhill & Forsdyke, 2018; Grygorowicz et al., 2019). This is especially noteworthy in instances where the severity of the injury or the recurrent nature of the injury may have long-term, negative impacts on athlete health (e.g. Ardern & Khan, 2016; Arvinen-Barrow et al., 2017).

Quality of support network: It is unfortunate that there are instances where injured athletes have retired because they feel unsupported and like they have been left to cope with their injury on their own (e.g. Grygorowicz et al., 2019). There are further examples whereby athletes have perceived insufficient support resource (e.g. sport psychology support, sports medicine support) have been available to them and that has contributed to the decision to retire (e.g. Gledhill & Forsdyke, 2018). Moreover, the quality of support network available can impact on perceptions of sporting (in)competence, especially how athletes perceive themselves in the eyes of teammates and coaching staff (Podlog & Eklund, 2006). The negative impact of this perception can contribute to the decision to retire (Gledhill & Forsdyke, 2018).

Career or competing demands: Prominent within literature that has explored experiences of those who are competitive athletes but in typically very low or low paid sports (e.g. Grygorowicz et al., 2019) is the notion of competing demands or other career priorities. For example, female football players are paid significantly less than male players and this can mean that players will take on a second career alongside playing, creating a dual-career demand on the player (e.g. Gledhill & Harwood, 2015). As their additional career may be their main source of income, it becomes a competing priority for the athlete, whereby they will weigh up the cost benefit of retirement and, if the injury or reinjury risk is likely to impact on their long-term financial health through time-off work, there is an increased chance that an athlete will decide to retire (e.g. Gledhill & Forsdyke, 2018; Tjong et al., 2014).

Irrespective of whether the decision to retire is voluntary or involuntary, the outcome is still the same: the athlete retires. This can present a number of challenges for athletes (Mannes et al., 2019). Throughout the following section, we shall discuss the psychosocial impact of injury-related retirement on athletes.

PSYCHOSOCIAL IMPACT OF INJURY-RELATED RETIREMENT

The psychosocial responses to injury-related retirement can be positive or negative (e.g. Arvinen-Barrow et al., 2017, 2019). For some athletes, injury can be a blessing in disguise (Arvinen-Barrow et al., 2019), whilst others feel like they are not ready to leave their sport (Roberts & Davis, 2018). However, arguably, the most consistent findings within the body of research are that injury-related retirement and the associated transitions out of sport are more negative or have a more negative impact, than positive (e.g. Carapinheira et al., 2018; Filbay et al., 2019; Mannes et al., 2019).

Adapting to life post-retirement seems to be more difficult for athletes when their retirement is involuntary, with enforced retirement creating perceptions of social exclusion, a sense of betrayal, a perceived loss of identity and a range of negative emotions (Park et al., 2013). Involuntary retirement from sport is associated with worse health-related quality of life and life satisfaction (Filbay et al., 2019) and can elicit feelings of frustration, disbelief, shock, a sense of loss of control, decreased sense of self, decreased self-esteem, decreased self-identity and a perceived inability to cope with everyday life stressors (Arvinen-Barrow et al., 2017, 2019; Stoltenburg et al., 2011). Repeated concussions and musculo-skeletal injuries are correlates of psychological distress in retired athletes and, where athletes suffer from long-term, detrimental health conditions post-retirement (e.g. osteoarthritis), there is an increased risk of depressive symptoms and substance misuse (Mannes et al., 2019). Furthermore, athletes who have retired from sport are more likely to develop long-term mental health problems if they have experienced more injuries during their playing career (Prinz et al., 2016). In professional athletes, a major life stressor during the transition out of sport and into retirement is finances and income (e.g. Arvinen-Barrow et al., 2017, 2019; Carapinheira et al., 2018). Furthermore, athletes who do not engage in effective post-career planning prior to retirement are more likely to experience a lower quality transition out of sport (Carapinheira et al., 2018).

Collectively, these problems that are in some way associated with injury-related retirement lead to the need to understand ways in which we can enhance athletes' retirement experiences. In the next section of this chapter, we shall discuss different strategies that can be used to achieve this.

IMPROVING RETIREMENT EXPERIENCES

In the previous section, we outlined a number of negative responses to injury-related retirement. Whilst challenging for athletes and the people around them, each of the factors highlighted above is modifiable. That is to say, with appropriate planning and/or intervention, we can support athletes to make improvements in each of these different challenges. It stands to reason that support from an appropriate psychologist may be required or sought post-injury (e.g. Arvinen-Barrow et al., 2019) and should be matched to the needs of athletes. However, this type of support provision is not always available to athletes and engagement with it can vary across age, sport, gender, playing level, playing experience and financial considerations in place with the sport (e.g. Carapinheira et al., 2018; Gledhill & Forsdyke, 2018).

Within the injury retirement literature, four relatively consistent strategies to improve retirement experiences are present. These are planning for retirement (e.g. Arvinen-Barrow et al., 2019; Carapinheira et al., 2018; Stoltenburg et al., 2011), provision of social support (e.g. Arvinen-Barrow et al., 2017; Brown et al., 2018), involving the athlete in decision-making processes about retirement (e.g. Ardern & Khan, 2016) and being physically active (e.g. Mannes et al., 2019), all can serve to enhance the quality of the retirement experience for athletes.

Planning for post-career: One of the most consistent findings within this body of research is that early retirement planning is an important part of managing the retirement transition. As injury-related retirement can be both sudden and unexpected, early post-career planning (i.e. as early as the start of a professional career) could prove the best option to safeguard against the potential negative impact of life stressors on athletes (Arvinen-Barrow et al., 2019; Carapinheira et al., 2018; Stoltenburg et al., 2011). However, unfortunately, many athletes do not engage in this type of post-career planning either at all or until later in their career (Carapinheira et al., 2018). Whilst aspects such as education and insurance seem to be important aspects of retirement planning (e.g. Arvinen-Barrow et al., 2019), education is less important or effective as part of the retirement planning process if it is not part of a wider programme of career planning (Carapinheira et al., 2018). It has been suggested that a more focused retirement planning may be particularly effective for athletes, as they are used to using strategic planning and goal-directed behaviours to achieve desired outcomes and because they are likely to feel more cared for through the process of engaging with key stakeholders during the planning process (Arvinen-Barrow et al., 2019).

Financial planning and insurance appear to be particularly important for athletes (e.g. Arvinen-Barrow et al., 2019). This stands to reason, given that many professional athletes file for bankruptcy after their sport retirement (e.g. Carlson et al., 2015), financial security upon retirement is a major stressor for athletes (e.g. Arvinen-Barrow et al., 2019), and financial insecurity or instability after retirement is a significant correlate with psychological distress (Mannes et al., 2019). Conversely, being employed during retirement is negatively associated with depressive and anxiety symptoms (Gouttebarge et al., 2016).

Social support: Understanding the support needs of their athletes should be a priority for practitioners from the onset of injury (Arvinen-Barrow et al., 2017) and especially in instances where the injury characteristics might increase the chances of injury related-retirement. Whilst there are examples of athletes actively seeking social support as a result of their injury and with the aim of improving their transition into retirement (e.g. Arvinen-Barrow et al., 2017, 2019; Park et al., 2013), there are also a number of instances whereby athletes feel there is insufficient support available (e.g. Gledhill & Forsdyke, 2018; Grygorowicz et al., 2019), or where there remains perceived stigmas attached to social support seeking (e.g. Brown et al., 2018). However, what is clear is that perceived availability and quality of social support are likely to improve the retirement experience of athletes (e.g. Arvinen-Barrow et al., 2017, 2019; Brown et al., 2018; Filbay et al., 2019; Mannes et al., 2019; Park et al., 2013).

The above points refer predominantly to the athlete being in receipt of appropriate social support. More recently, Brown et al. (2018) noted that being a social support provider can also have benefits for athletes. We know that retirement is a time where athletes can experience a negative impact on aspects such as self-esteem, identify and other elements of the self (e.g. Stoltenburg et al., 2011). Therefore, being a support provider for other athletes can help retired athletes to reappraise and redefine this sense of self and to experience a sense of growth after retirement (Brown et al., 2018). Consequently, whilst the importance of receiving appropriate social support has been long established, we now have a more incremental understanding of the importance of being a provider of social support for injured athletes.

Involving the athlete with retirement decisions: Sports injury, especially those which necessitate retirement, contributes to a perceived loss of control for injured athletes (Forsdyke et al., 2016). However, even in instances where the athlete has little choice over whether they retire, it is possible to facilitate a greater sense of self-determination over the decision. This can be achieved by showing trust in the athlete by asking them for their opinions about their body and their understanding of their injury (Defoe, 2018); educating athletes, in a balanced way, about the injury, how it occurred, any associated long-term health risks, and the options available to them (e.g. Ardern & Khan, 2016; Forsdyke et al., 2017; King et al., 2019); and adopting a multi-disciplinary, athlete-centred, shared decision-making approach (e.g. King et al., 2019) which are all ways in which the athlete can be more involved with the retirement decisions. In adopting such approaches, the athlete is likely to feel a greater sense of control over the decision, can have increased confidence in that they have made the correct decision based on their own circumstances and have experienced a sense of social connectedness throughout the process. It is likely that this will increase the chances of the athlete being more at ease with the retirement decision. Further research is needed so support some of these assumptions.

Staying physically active: Remaining physically active in retirement can benefit the overall health and wellbeing of athletes (Mannes et al., 2019). For example, cricket players have reported using swimming and yoga as ways of remaining active and busy during retirement, in such a way that was within their physical capabilities (Arvinen-Barrow et al., 2019). Retired athletes may require appropriate informational support with their activity choices and how these may be influenced by their injury, especially as many athletes with career ending injuries continue to experience pain associated with the injury or other related conditions and aspects of fear (Tjong et al., 2014). Whilst physical activity after retirement can reduce the risk of depression and act as a protective factor against anxiety onset in retired athletes, it is also important to remember that pain-related concerns can reduce the likelihood of retired athletes remaining physically active (Mannes et al., 2019).

CONCLUSION

In summary, injury-related retirement can be either a largely voluntary or involuntary process, depending on different biopsychosocial considerations. Irrespective of the voluntariness of retirement post-injury, the experience is one that can be largely modifiable and can be shaped to be more positive if appropriate within-career and post-career support is available to the athlete.

Case study

Matthew, the injured basketball player

Matthew is an 18-year-old multi-sport athlete, but who sees himself in the long term as a basketball player. Matthew's preference for basketball is based on his playing level: As a tall young player, he was invited to his local national league side to start training when he was 13 years old. He regularly played 'up' in age groups from that point onwards, as his coaches said that he needed to play against bigger, stronger and more experienced players in order to keep developing. He is the record holder for points scored in a single game at his club and has won the league title every year. Matthew also has an extensive injury history but has been offered an athletic scholarship for attending university.

At the age of 12, Matthew was diagnosed with Osgood–Schlatter's disease and advised to restrict activity by his GP, but his coach advised him against this and intimated that his long-term place in the team may be at risk if he stopped training and playing. At the age of 13, he suffered the first of his four lateral ankle ligament injuries (grade 1–grade 3) all sustained whilst playing various sports and all non-contact; at 15 years, he suffered a hairline vertebral fracture, a torn trapezius and a broken finger in a basketball-related incident; at 16, he injured his medial meniscus, medial collateral ligament, lateral collateral ligament and anterior cruciate ligament in his right knee (but cannot provide any specific details beyond this, other than that the surgeon did not want to operate and he wore a knee brace for a while); and at 17, he suffered a strangulated inguinal hernia which required surgical repair. Most recently, Matthew has been diagnosed with a historical posterior cruciate ligament (PCL) injury, after returning to his consultant complaining of persistent pain in his right knee, which radiated down his calf regularly. Matthew has been referred to his sports therapist for conservative management of the PCL injury.

During the initial meeting with Matthew, the therapist asked him about his treatment goals and the level of sport he would like to return to. Matthew replied: 'I don't know' and disclosed that he has 'had enough of being injured' and that he 'can't be bothered to go through it all again'. He said that he'll 'just get injured again' and that he is doubting whether he should even bother going to university, because even after that, he will have the pressure to play because of his scholarship, which also means he'll get injured again.

Matthew's parents, both of whom retired from their respective sports (netball and football) at a young age, have questioned him on numerous occasions about whether he should even be considering returning to sport. His mother particularly is scared about him returning to sport as she is worried about the long-term damage that he is doing to his body. Matthew has asked the medical practitioner whether he should retire from sport.

Questions

1. Who should be involved in the decision-making process and why?
2. What are the key factors that you think may influence a retirement decision?
3. What strategies could be used to support Matthew, should he decide to retire?

References

Alfermann, D., Stambulova, N., & Zemaitye, A. (2004). Reactions to sport career termination: A cross-national comparison of German, Lithuanian and Russian athletes. *Psychology of Sport & Exercise*, *5*, 61–75.

Ardern, C. L., & Khan, K. M. (2016). The old knee in the young athlete: Knowns and unknowns in the return to play conversation. *British Journal of Sports Medicine*, *50*, 505–506.

Ardern, C. L., Glasgow, P., Schneiders, A., Witvrouw, E., Clarsen, B., Cools, A., Gojanovic, B., Griffin, S., Khan K. M., Moksnes, H., Mutch, S. A., Phillips, N., Reurink, G., Sadler, R., Silbernagel, K. G., Thorborg, K., Wangensteen, A., Wilk, K. E., & Bizzini, M. (2016). 2016 Consensus statement on return to sport from the First World Congress in Sports Physical Therapy, Bern. *British Journal of Sports Medicine, 50*, 853–864.

Arvinen-Barrow, M., DeGrave, K., Pack, S., & Hemmings, B. (2019). Transitioning out of professional sport: The psychosocial impact of career-ending non-musculoskeletal injuries among male cricketers from England and Wales. *Journal of Clinical Sport Psychology*, *13*(4), 629–644.

Arvinen-Barrow, M., Hurley, D., & Ruiz, M. C. (2017). Transitioning out of professional sport: The psychosocial impact of career-ending injuries among elite Irish rugby football union players. *Journal of Clinical Sport Psychology*, *11*, 67–84.

Brown, C., Webb, T., Robinson, M., & Cotgreave, R. (2018). Athletes' experiences of social support during their transition out of elite sport: An interpretive phenomenological analysis. *Psychology of Sport and Exercise*, *36*, 71–80.

Carapinheira, A., Mendes, P., Guedes Carvalho, P., Torregrossa, M., & Travassos, B. (2018). Career termination of Portuguese elite football players: Comparison between the last three decades. *Sports*, *6*, 155. https://doi.org/10.3390/sports6040155

Carlson, K., Kim, J., Lusardi, A., & Camerer, C. F. (2015). Bankruptcy rates among NFL players with short-lived income spikes. *American Economic Review*, *105*(5), 381–384.

Defoe, J. (2018). Trusting the experience of the experienced athlete. *British Journal of Sports Medicine*, *52*, 1554–1555.

Filbay, S., Pandya, T., Thomas, B., McKay, C., Adams, J., & Arden, N. (2019). Quality of life and life satisfaction in former athletes: A systematic review and meta-analysis. *Sports Medicine*, *49*, 1723–1738.

Forsdyke, D., Gledhill, A., & Ardern, C. (2017). Psychological readiness to return to sport: Three key elements to help the practitioner decide whether the athlete is REALLY ready? *British Journal of Sports Medicine*, *51*, 555–556.

Forsdyke, D., Smith, A., Jones, M., & Gledhill, A. (2016). Psychosocial factors associated with outcomes of sports injury rehabilitation in competitive athletes: A mixed studies systematic review. *British Journal of Sports Medicine.*, *50*, 537–544.

Gledhill, A., & Forsdyke, D. (2018, May). Psychosocial factors underpinning return to sport decisions of talented and elite female football players. Presentation to the Isokinetics Football Medical Strategies Conference, Barcelona.

Gledhill, A., & Harwood, C. (2015). A holistic perspective on career development in UK female soccer players: A negative case analysis. *Psychology of Sport and Exercise*, *21*, 65–77.

Gouttebarge, V., Aoki, H., Verhagen, E., & Kerkhoffs, G. (2016). Are level of education and employment related to symptoms of common mental disorders in current and retired professional footballers? *Asian Journal of Sports Medicine*, *7*(2), e28447.

Grygorowicz, M., Michalowska, M., Jurga, P., Piontek, T., Jakubowska, H., & Kotwicki, T. (2019). Thirty percent of female football players terminate their careers due to injury: A retrospective study among Polish former players. *Journal of Sport Rehabilitation, 28*, 109–114.

King, J., Roberts, C., Hard, S., & Ardern, C. L. (2019). Want to improve return to sport outcomes following injury? Empower, engage, provide feedback and be transparent: 4 habits! *British Journal of Sports Medicine, 53*, 526–527.

Mannes, Z. L., Waxenberg, L. B., Cottler, L. B., Perlstein, W. M., Burrell, L. E., Ferguson, E. G., Edwards, M. E., & Ennis, N. (2019). Prevalence and correlates of psychological distress among retired elite athletes. *International Review of Sport and Exercise Psychology, 12*, 265–294.

Moesch, K., Mayer, C., & Elbe, A-M. (2012). Reasons for career termination in Danish elite athletes: Investigating gender differences and time-point as potential correlates. *Sport Science Reviews, 21*, 49–68.

Park, S., Lavallee, D., & Tod, D. (2013) Athletes' career transition out of sport: A systematic review. *International Review of Sport and Exercise Psychology, 6*, 22–53.

Podlog, L., & Eklund, R. C. (2006). A longitudinal investigation of competitive athletes' return to sport following serious injury. *Journal of Applied Sport Psychology, 18*, 44–68.

Prinz, B., Dvorak, J., & Junge, A. (2016). Symptoms and risk factors for depression during and after a football career of elite female players. *BMJ Open Sport and Exercise Medicine, 2*, e000124.

Ristolainen, L., Kettunen, J. A., Kujala, H. M., & Heinonen, A. (2012). Sports injuries as the main cause of career termination among Finnish top-level athletes. *European Journal of Sport Science, 12*, 274–282.

Roberts, C-M., & Davis, M. O. (2018). Career transition. In J. Taylor (Ed.). *Assessment in applied sport psychology* (pp. 213–233). Human Kinetics.

Schlossberg, N. (1995). *Counseling adults in transition: Linking practice with theory*. Springer Publishing Company.

Steyn, B., & Slattery, C. (2013). Termination of sporting careers among South African sportswomen. *African Journal of Physical Health Education, Recreation and Dance, 19*, 1–11.

Stoltenburg, A. L., Kamphoff, C. S., Lindstrom Bremer, K. (2011). Transitioning out of sport: The psychosocial effects of collegiate athletes' career ending injuries. *Athletic Insight, 11*, 1–11.

Tjong, V. K., Murnaghan, M. L., Nyhof-Young, J. M., & Ogilive-Harris, D. J. (2014). A qualitative investigation of the decision to return to play to sport after anterior cruciate ligament reconstruction: To play or not to play. *American Journal of Sports Medicine, 42*, 336–342.

Truong, L. K., Mosewich, A. D., Holt, C. J., Le, C. Y., Miciak, M., & Whittaker, J. L. (2020). Psychological, social and contextual factors across recovery stages following a sport-related knee injury: A scoping review. *British Journal of Sports Medicine, 54*, 1149–1156.

Part V

SPECIAL INTERESTS IN SPORTS INJURY

As our understanding of psychological influences across sports injury contexts has grown and continues to grow, there have emerged a number of hot topics that have gathered significant research and applied attention. Some of these are more established (e.g. anterior cruciate ligament injury, ACL), whereas others are much more emerging (e.g. sport-related concussion, spinal cord injury [SCI]). However, what encouraged us to include this section within the book is that everything within it has one thing in common: their impact, both on individual athletes and teams, or within the sports environment more widely, is hugely significant. Consequently, we chose to invite contributions from world-class authorities in these respective fields, to share their insights. We hope this short series of focussed chapters helps promote reflection on practice and foster critical debate.

In the first contributing chapter, Dr Kate Webster discusses the psychology of ACL injuries. ACL injuries are one of the most feared and severe injuries that athletes experience, typically leading to 9–12 months of time loss from sport. They are also the injury that, due to their significant psychological, emotional, social and financial impacts, has received the greatest amount of research attention within the psychology of sports injury literature (Forsdyke et al., 2016). Particular attention within the chapter is given to the prognostic factors that are associated with successful versus unsuccessful return to sport outcomes, psychosocial experiences of surgical versus non-surgical intervention post-ACL injury, and the psychosocial and emotional impact of some of the lasting health conditions that are associated with ACL reconstruction.

Following Kate's contribution regarding ACL injuries, Drs Osman Hassan Ahmed, Eric Hall and Caroline Ketcham provide a novel insight into sport-related concussion. This is one area where interest in the role sport psychology plays is growing, both in the mainstream media and across various academic and applied communities. Osman, Eric and Caroline use this chapter to critically consider athletes' experiences of concussion and recovering from concussion, as well as providing multidisciplinary recommendations for preventing and monitoring concussion.

With a commitment to improving treatment modalities, rehabilitation, and life-long health and well-being following SCI (e.g. Williams et al., 2014), Dr Toni Williams provides an expert overview of SCI in the third chapter of this section. Within it, Toni provides an overview and background to SCI, the psychosocial impact of traumatic SCI and offers a critical overview of physical activity and physical activity promotion associated with SCI. In doing so, she challenges assumptions and poses critical questions for debate that serve to enhance this interesting and growing body of knowledge.

To close this section of the book, Dr Adam Gledhill takes a look at the role of coaches in achieving athlete and team medical outcomes. Whether injured or not, a coach's influence on athletes is significant. Coaches are frequently recognized as 'villains' in the sports injury story, with literature awash with things that coaches could or should have done differently to help their athletes during the injury journey (i.e. adopted a different leadership style or communicated better). Whilst recognizing this quite negative perspective within the chapter, Adam also takes this opportunity to highlight some of the ways that coaches can positively influence (and have influenced) athletes to become the 'heroes' of the sports injury story.

References

Forsdyke, D., Smith, A., Jones, M., & Gledhill, A. (2016). Psychosocial factors associated with outcomes of sports injury rehabilitation in competitive athletes: A mixed studies systematic review. *British Journal of Sports Medicine, 50*, 537–544.

Williams, T. L., Smith, B., & Papathomas, A. (2014). The barriers, benefits and facilitators of leisure time physical activity among people with spinal cord injury: A meta-synthesis of qualitative findings. *Health Psychology Review, 8*, 404–425.

12 THE PSYCHOLOGICAL ASPECT OF ANTERIOR CRUCIATE LIGAMENT INJURIES

Dr Kate E. Webster

INTRODUCTION

Athletic injuries have substantial psychological consequences, which may continue long after the injury has occurred. The role that psychological factors play for a significant athletic injury, such as an anterior cruciate ligament (ACL) rupture, may be heightened because this injury has a long rehabilitation period and a level of uncertainty about whether the athlete will be able to return to their pre-injury level of sport performance (te Wierike et al., 2013). Indeed, it is an injury dreaded by athletes due to the significant physical, psychological, social, emotional and financial impact that it has.

From a psychological perspective, the return-to-sport phase can be particularly challenging following ACL injury. Negative emotions and fears can be heightened once an athlete is cleared to return to sport, which for some athletes may mean that they never return (Ardern, Taylor, Feller, & Webster, 2013). This chapter will explore the evidence-base surrounding the psychology of ACL injuries, with reference to injury recovery, return to sport and potentially adverse consequences such as re-injury and the impact this has on long-term knee health.

PSYCHOLOGICAL IMPACT OF ACL INJURY

It is well demonstrated that athletic injuries have psychological consequences. Injured athletes often experience mood disturbances such as anger and depression, and decreased self-worth (McLean et al., 2008; Smith, 1996; Smith, Scott, O'Fallon et al., 1990; Smith, Scott, & Wiese, 1990). Heightened negative emotions such as shock, frustration and tension have also been reported shortly after an injury and during recovery (Morrey et al., 1999; Walker et al., 2007). Whilst these responses are not specific to ACL injury, they are frequently reported in ACL-injured populations.

The psychological response and impact of the injury may also be linked with athletic identity. For example, competitive athletes who sustained an ACL injury were found to exhibit greater mood disturbances than recreational athletes

(Morrey et al., 1999). Similarly, professional athletes with potentially career-ending injuries (including ACL injury) had stronger negative psychological responses compared to athletes who viewed their injury as minor (Ruddock-Hudson et al., 2012). Lower life satisfaction has also been reported by college athletes who had their athletic careers terminated due to injury (Kleiber et al., 1987).

Recent work has discussed the concept of 'learned helplessness' after ACL injury where it is speculated that neural impairments of the involved limb interact with psychological function to negatively influence performance (Burland et al., 2019). This either creates an avoidance response or a feeling of distress that certain tasks can no longer be completed, and consequently full recovery is never achieved. It is therefore clear that an ACL injury has the potential to elicit a significant psychological response, which may continue long after the injury has occurred, and the chain of psychological sequelae can influence rehabilitation and return-to-sport outcomes, which will be the focus of this chapter.

A THEORETICAL MODEL OF RETURN TO SPORT AFTER ACL INJURY

Theoretical models of return to sport after injury are not typically constructed to be specific to ACL injury, but it is generally accepted that this injury sits well within a biopsychosocial model. Biopsychosocial models conceptualize the many and complex interactions between a range of physical, psychological and social/contextual factors (Brewer et al., 2002; Wiese-Bjornstal et al., 1988), which have both direct and indirect influences on return to sport after athletic injury (Figure 12.1). In such models, psychological factors play a mediating role on physical (e.g. muscle strength), contextual (e.g. expectations regarding recovery) and functional performance (e.g. motor control) factors, and ultimately on return to sport. Injury characteristics and sociodemographic factors (such as age and sex) have an indirect influence on return to sport via their influence on psychological, physical or social/contextual factors.

In a biopsychosocial model, there are clear pathways between psychological factors and outcome as well as the potential for psychological factors to influence return to sport via different pathways (Brewer, 2010). The central role played by psychological factors highlights the importance of addressing them in the overall management and treatment of ACL injury.

PSYCHOLOGICAL ASPECTS RELATED TO RECOVERY FOLLOWING ACL INJURY AND RECONSTRUCTION SURGERY

The psychological response and emotions associated with an ACL injury have been shown to change over time. Whilst a negative emotional response is typically reported immediately following injury, this tends to subside during rehabilitation but may re-emerge once the athlete is cleared to return to sport. Morrey et al. (1999) initially described a U-shaped emotional response pattern following ACL injury with negative peaks immediately following injury but also at the time of clearance for return to sport which was approximately 6 months

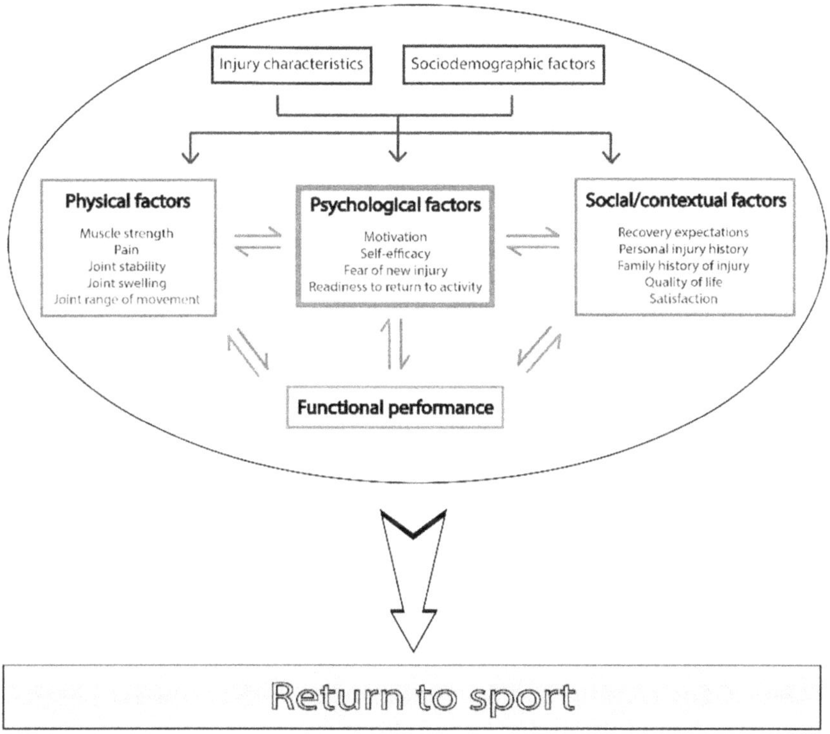

Figure 12.1 Adapted biopsychosocial model for return to sport after injury. Reproduced from Ardern, Kvist, & Webster, 2015

post-ACL reconstruction surgery. This highlighted the return-to-sport phase as a potential challenge for athletes who have ACL injury and subsequent surgery. This phase had not been a focus of previous research, as most of this had been conducted on athletes with injuries that kept them out of sport for a relatively short period of time, days or weeks, rather than the months to years, which is the typical for ACL injuries. Current ACL work is therefore now focussed on the full rehabilitation journey, including return to sport, and as one recent qualitative study states this is 'not always a straight path' (Scott et al., 2018).

There is a lack of information regarding the time course of psychological responses for athletes, who choose a non-operative pathway following ACL injury, but a similar post-injury response would be expected. Whist it may be logical to hypothesize that without experiencing the trauma of surgery the psychological response may be less during rehabilitation and return-to-sport phases, this has not been empirically investigated and it is equally likely that pain, sensations of stability and uncertainty regarding their knee would also cause athletes who choose non-operative pathways to have high level of anxiety and negative emotions throughout recovery.

Two psychological factors which have been highlighted as significant contributors to recovery outcomes following ACL reconstruction are self-efficacy and locus of control (Nyland et al., 2006; Thomeé et al., 2007; Thomeé et al., 2008). Self-efficacy is the belief in one's ability to succeed in a particular situation and has been found to significantly improve as athletes recover from injury. Higher levels of self-efficacy have also been associated with greater patient satisfaction and higher levels of activity following ACL reconstruction (Thomeé et al., 2007). Even preoperative self-efficacy has been found to predict postoperative physical activity and return to sport (Thomeé et al., 2008). Thus, there is convincing evidence that self-efficacy can play a pivotal role in successful rehabilitation and return to sport following ACL injury and subsequent reconstruction surgery.

The second factor is locus of control, which refers to having the belief that there is a relationship between actions and outcomes. There are two types of locus of control, internal or external. An internal locus of control is the belief that you have control of your own life, whereas an external locus of control is the belief that your life is controlled by chance or outside factors, which you cannot influence. Locus of control may thus also contribute to an athlete's sense of self-efficacy. Athletes who have a high internal locus of control score higher on subjective outcomes following ACL reconstruction as well as reporting greater overall knee function (Nyland et al., 2006). Locus of control has also been shown to be a predictor of returning to sport at 12 months after ACL reconstruction surgery (Ardern, Taylor, Feller, & Whitehead et al., 2013).

PSYCHOLOGICAL FACTORS INFLUENCING RETURN TO SPORT AFTER ACL RECONSTRUCTION SURGERY

As noted previously, the return-to-sport phase may be challenging for an athlete who has sustained an ACL injury and undergone reconstruction surgery. Athletes undergoing ACL reconstruction typically expect to be able to return to their pre-injury sport and whilst surgery addresses impairments in knee function, one in every three athletes do not make the transition back to sport after surgery (Ardern, Taylor et al., 2014; Ardern et al., 2011a; Ardern et al., 2011b). Psychological responses have been identified as a potentially modifiable factor associated with returning, or not returning, to the pre-injury level of sport (Ardern et al., 2011a; Czuppon et al., 2014; Everhart et al., 2015; te Wierike et al., 2013).

Athletes, who feel they have a greater level of control over their return to sport, have greater confidence in their body, and who feel more socially connected to their team mates, are more likely to return to their previous sport (Ardern, Kvist et al., 2015; Ardern, Taylor, Feller, & Webster, 2013). Higher levels of motivation prior to surgery and during rehabilitation are also associated with higher rates of return to pre-injury sport following ACL reconstruction (Sonesson et al., 2016). The two most commonly discussed psychological factors in terms of returning to sport are 'fear of re-injury' and 'psychological readiness'.

Fear of re-injury

Using the Tampa Scale of Kinesiophobia, Kvist et al. (2005) identified fear of re-injury as a significant factor for patients who did not return to their previous level of activity after ACL reconstruction. This finding has been supported by numerous subsequent studies and a recent meta-analysis combined the results of 20 studies to show that a staggering 76% of athletes who do not return to sport cite fear of re-injury as the reason (Nwachukwu et al., 2019). Restriction of sporting activity due to fear of re-injury has also been reported (Mann et al., 2007).

Fear is a somewhat broad term and exactly what constitutes fear of re-injury is unclear. For example, it may be fear of the pain of injury itself, fear of the implications for time off work and the related loss of income, fear of not being able to return to the previous level of function or any combination of these. Ross et al. (2017) interviewed patients who reported fear of re-injury as the sole reason for not returning to their pre-injury sport to better understand factors that inform athletes' experience of fear following ACL reconstruction. Undergoing surgery with a long recovery and restricted functional capacity was one of the main factors which informed fear of re-injury. The nature of the pre-injury sport was also important. Specifically, once injured, athletes reported having an increased awareness of how the movement pattern associated with the injury, such as pivoting, was common in their sport. Personality traits and social priorities (i.e. educational commitments) were also found to inform fear of re-injury.

Even if an athlete manages to return to play, fear of re-injury may affect the quality of their performance. Ardern et al. (2012) investigated whether fear of re-injury was still a consideration in athletes who made a successful return to sport after ACL reconstruction surgery. A cohort of 209 athletes answered a series of questions regarding the behavioural manifestations of fear, such as playing with hesitation and being wary of injury provoking situations. Results showed that athletes who had successfully returned to their pre-injury sport generally participated without fear of re-injury. Males who had surgery soon after injury (<3 months between injury and surgery) were found to participate in the pre-injury sport with the least amount of fear.

It has also been shown that athletes who have not been injured are concerned about their chance of being injured in the future. This is most salient for those who participate in high-risk sports, and this concern may be informed by seeing numerous teammates suffer from injury (Phelan et al., 2019). Therefore, some amount of fear associated with returning to sport after ACL injury and reconstruction surgery should be viewed as a normal part of the recovery process. Indeed, a degree of caution may be protective if it means that the athlete does not prematurely or recklessly resume sport without full consideration of the function of their knee (Ardern, Kvist et al., 2015). However, when the level of fear or psychological dysfunction either restricts participation or causes heightened distress targeted psychological intervention may be considered.

Finally, it is interesting to consider the context in which the term fear of re-injury is used and whether it is an appropriate term. In the ACL literature, fear of re-injury is most commonly used in the context of cessation of sport after ACL reconstruction. Walker et al. (Walker et al., 2010) have however suggested that 're-injury anxiety' may be a more appropriate term to describe the emotional response of the athlete. Fear is a biological mechanism which is stimulus-specific and is associated with definite danger, whereas anxiety is associated with anticipation or uncertainly.

Psychological readiness

Psychological readiness to return to sport was suggested to comprise three key aspects: confidence in returning to sport, realistic expectations of sporting capability and motivation to regain pre-injury performance standards (Podlog et al., 2015). Confidence was specifically influenced by the athlete's belief in their rehabilitation program, and their perception that their injury was completely healed and therefore no longer at risk of being reinjured. The belief in being able to perform at the same pre-injury level was also associated with increased psychological readiness to return (Podlog et al., 2015; Webster et al., 2008).

That psychological readiness is important in determining return-to-sport decisions was highlighted by Ardern, Österberg et al. (2014) and Ardern, Taylor, Feller, Whitehead et al. (2013). Although multifactorial, psychological readiness is largely influenced by an athlete's emotions and confidence (Ardern, Kvist, & Webster, 2015). Confidence is thought to be derived from two elements: confidence in the injured body part and confidence in the ability to perform well (Johnston & Carroll, 1998; Quinn & Fallon, 1999). Developing confidence in both these aspects may provide a buffer from injury-related fear and anxiety, resulting in the athlete being in a 'psychologically ready' state to resume sport participation. In line with this, a recent systematic review concluded that an athlete's psychological readiness to return to play is a combination of the lack of fear and anxiety, and confidence in performing well and remaining uninjured (Forsdyke et al., 2016).

There are several measures available to help assess psychological readiness to return to sport (Table 12.1). The Anterior Cruciate Ligament Return to Sport after Injury (ACL-RSI) scale (Webster et al., 2008) was developed as a tool to specifically measure psychological readiness to return to sport after ACL reconstruction and is currently the only scale specific to ACL injury. It is available in multiple languages, having been translated from English to Swedish (Kvist et al., 2013), French (Bohu et al., 2015), German (Müller et al., 2014), Dutch (Slagers et al., 2017), Turkish (Harput et al., 2016), Chinese (Chen et al., 2017; Jia et al., 2018), Brazilian (Silva et al., 2018), Lithuanian (Salatkaite et al., 2019), Korean

Table 12.1 Questionnaires and inventories that can be used to assess psychological readiness to return to sport

Name	*Abbreviation*
Injury Psychological Readiness to Return to Sport Scale (Glazer, 2009)	I-PRRS
Re-injury Anxiety Inventory (Walker et al., 2010)	RIAI
Knee Self Efficacy Scale (Thomeé et al., 2006)	KSES
Tampa Scale of Kinesiophobia (French et al., 2007)	TSK
Anterior Cruciate Ligament Return to Sport after Injury Scale (Webster et al., 2008)	ACL-RSI
Anterior Cruciate Ligament Return to Sport after Injury Scale (Short Form) (Webster, & Feller, 2018)	ACL-RSI (SF)

(Ha et al., 2019) and Spanish (Sala-Barat et al., 2019), with other translations currently underway. Items in this scale are centred on three psychological factors associated with returning to sport: *emotions*, *confidence* and *risk appraisal*. Validation of the scale showed that athletes who had returned to full competition were found to score significantly higher than athletes who had given up sport and athletes who had not recommenced sport but were still planning to return (Webster et al., 2008). A short-form (6 item; ACL-RSI (SF)) version is also available for use in a busy clinical environment where rapid administration may be desirable (Webster, & Feller, 2018). The short-version ACL-RSI is less knee specific and has therefore been modified for use with shoulder, hip and Achilles tendon injuries. Copies of these scales are available from the chapter author.

The factors that contribute to an athlete's psychological readiness have also been investigated (Webster et al., 2018). A cohort of 635 athletes who underwent ACL reconstruction and had been cleared to return to sport completed the ACL-RSI scale 12 months postoperatively. Being male, younger age, a shorter time interval between injury and surgery, a higher frequency of pre-injury sport participation, a higher limb symmetry index on hop tests and a higher self-rating of knee function were all associated with greater psychological readiness. When these factors were included in a multivariate model, subjective knee scores and age accounted for 37% of the variance in psychological readiness. A further comparison between those who had and had not returned to sport showed that female sex was a significant contributor to not returning. Therefore, self-reported knee symptoms and function are most associated with psychological readiness to return to sport after ACL reconstruction. Male and younger patients who participated frequently in sport before ACL injury are more likely to have a positive psychological outlook during the return-to-sport phase after ACL reconstruction surgery. Conversely, females with lower levels of function (both self-reported and on physical testing) may have a more negative outlook and therefore benefit from interventions designed to facilitate a smooth transition back to sport. That females tend to have lower levels of psychological readiness has also been shown in a group of adolescent athletes at multiple time points through recovery and at the return-to-sport phase post-ACL reconstruction surgery (Kostyun et al., 2019).

CAN THE ATHLETE'S PSYCHOLOGICAL RESPONSE TO ACL INJURY BE USED TO PREDICT FUTURE RETURN TO SPORT?

Given the impact of psychological factors on athletes during rehabilitation and return to sport, it is potentially useful to be able to predict which athletes may benefit from psychological counselling or intervention so that psychological recovery can occur in parallel with physical recovery. It is therefore relevant to know whether the psychological responses athletes experience during the rehabilitation period are related to sport resumption.

Two initial large-scale studies were conducted which showed that the ACL-RSI scale could be used to predict return-to-sport outcomes. The first enrolled 100 athletes who completed the ACL-RSI at 3, 6 and 12 months after undergoing ACL reconstruction surgery (Langford et al., 2009). At 12 months, 51% of the athletes had returned to competitive sports. Scores on the ACL-RSI at 6 months were significantly lower in the athletes who did not return to competition sport at 12 months compared to the athletes who did. Therefore, an athlete's readiness to return to sport at 6 months post-ACL reconstruction surgery was related to whether they returned at 12 months, which suggested the possibility of being able to identify athletes at risk of not returning to competitive sport due to psychological reasons.

A second study of 187 patients completed a battery of psychological assessments, before ACL reconstruction surgery, as well as at 4 and 12 months after surgery (Ardern, Taylor, Feller, Whitehead et al., 2013). At 12 months, only 56 athletes (31%) had returned to their previous level of sports participation, despite the majority (91%) having excellent physical recovery. Three variables from the psychological assessments predicted returning to sport by 12 months after surgery: psychological readiness to return to sport, the participant's estimate of the number of months it would take to return to sport and locus of control. Psychological readiness (assessed with the ACL-RSI scale) was the only measure that was predictive of return to sport at both preoperatively and at 4 months postoperatively. The patient cohort was then reviewed at 2 years to specifically see whether those who had not returned by 12 months made a later return (Ardern, Taylor et al., 2015). Once again, greater psychological readiness was associated with participation in the pre-injury sport at 2 years. The clinical relevance of these findings is that they indicate that psychological readiness should be considered throughout all stages of the rehabilitation process. These initial results have been supported by several subsequent research studies (Kostyun et al., 2019; Muller et al., 2015; Rosso et al., 2018; Sadeqi et al., 2018).

There has been much discussion regarding the identification of patients who may benefit from psychological intervention and whether scales such as the ACL-RSI might be useful for categorizing athletes as psychologically ready to return to play or not. This presents a challenge as psychological readiness is essentially a latent trait which, unlike for example body mass, cannot be directly measured and has substantial individual variation. Furthermore, as psychological readiness changes over time any proposed quantitative cut-off score must be interpreted relative to the time, it is measured postoperatively. Nonetheless, there has been work, which is still ongoing, to quantify clinically useful cut-offs to predict return to sport after ACL reconstruction and the suggested values are summarized in Table 12.2. Cut-off values can be calculated for the prediction of athletes who do return to sport, i.e. a score above the cut-off indicates that the athlete is likely to return, and this has been the most common approach. However, some work has also suggested cut-offs that predict non-return, i.e. athletes who score below these cut-offs are likely to not return to their sport.

Taking all data into consideration, it would be reasonable to suggest that athletes who score above 60 points at 4- or 6-month post-surgery are very likely to return to sport by 12 months. Similarly, those who score below 40 points are likely to not have returned. There is less certainty about those who score in between these values. This is not unexpected as there will always be athletes who score low on psychological readiness and yet still return to sport for a variety of

Table 12.2 Cut-off scores for predicting return to sport after ACL reconstruction

Study	*Psychological measure*	*Time of psychological assessment (months)*	*Time of RTS assessment (months)*	*Cut-off score*	*Specificity (%)*	*Sensitivity*
Prediction of return to sport						
Ardern, Taylor, Feller, Whitehead et al. (2013)	ACL-RSI	4	12	56	83	58
Muller et al. (2015)	ACL-RSI	6	7	51.3	63	97
Webster & Feller (2018)	ACL-RSI	6	12	62	81	57
Webster & Feller (2018)	ACL-RSI (SF)	6	12	60	84	50
Kitaguchi et al. (2019)	ACL-RSI	6	12	55	83	69
Prediction of non-return to sport						
Webster & Feller (2018)	ACL-RSI	6	12	42	78	57
Webster & Feller (2018)	ACL-RSI (SF)	6	12	39	74	60

Note: All assessments are post-ACL reconstruction surgery; RTS = return to sport

reasons, including pressure from outside sources. It should be noted that such cut-offs are not suggested to be used for treatment decisions. The clinical utility of a cut-off score is that it provides clinicians with a means to identify which athlete groups may struggle to return to sport from a psychological perspective. This is important given the typically limited resources available for psychological assistance during recovery from injury. This can then initiate a conversation where all available information regarding the athlete's rehabilitation progression and potential re-injury risk are considered.

ASSOCIATIONS BETWEEN THE PSYCHOLOGICAL RESPONSE TO ACL INJURY AND RETURN-TO-SPORT PERFORMANCE

Whilst it has been clearly established that psychological factors can be predictive of return to sport itself, only recently has the association between psychological factors and return-to-sport performance been considered. Webster et al. (2019) studied a large cohort of 222 patients who had undergone primary ACL reconstruction and completed a range of outcome measures at 12 months post-surgery. These included demographic, sport activity level, knee laxity, limb symmetry, subjective function/symptoms (International Knee Documentation Committee subjective knee form) and psychological readiness (ACL-RSI scale). The patient cohort was then followed out to a mean of 3 years (range 2–4 years) post-surgery to determine whether patients had returned to their pre-injury level of performance, which was self-rated. Greater psychological readiness, limb symmetry, subjective knee scores and activity levels were all associated with a return to performance. However, having a greater psychological readiness to return during rehabilitation was the most significant predictor of a subsequent return to comparable performance.

It is perhaps not surprising that psychological readiness contributed most to return-to-sport performance. Recent studies have shown that knee confidence and psychological readiness are related to function (Hart et al., 2019; Paterno et al., 2018) and that lower psychological readiness is associated with greater limb asymmetry (Zarzycki et al., 2018). Psychological factors have also been found to have significant associations with various movement patterns. Trigsted et al. (2018) evaluated 36 females who had undergone ACL reconstruction and found that individuals who reported higher fear of re-injury demonstrated lower peak knee, hip and trunk flexion along with greater motion in the frontal plane during a bilateral drop vertical jump task. Nagelli et al. (2019) also found an association between psychological readiness to return to sport and frontal plane hip and knee joint range of motion during a single-leg landing task in athletes approximately 9 months post-ACL reconstruction surgery. This work is important as it shows clear links between psychological status and physical outcomes and further examination is required to extend this body of research to determine if these movement differences have implications for subsequent performance once the athlete has returned to sport or whether they are also related to future injury risk.

ADVERSE CONSEQUENCE OF THE PSYCHOLOGICAL RESPONSE TO ACL INJURY

Salient consequences of ACL injury as already discussed are the potential for ceasing sports participation and subsequent decrease in activity level, with these factors contributing to a reduced quality of life. For ACL reconstruction surgery to be considered truly successful, it should enable the athlete to return to sport without further injury or damage to the knee (Webster & Feller, 2019). However, rates of further injury are not insignificant, particularly for younger athletes. Cohort studies have shown that between 20% and 30% of younger athletes sustain a second ACL injury (Dekker et al., 2017; Morgan et al., 2016; Paterno et al., 2014; Webster & Feller, 2016). Such statistics are concerning and there has been a recent focus on the development of return-to-sport criteria testing. Most return-to-sport testing is done with the aim of assessing the safety of the patient making a return to sport without suffering a further ACL injury (Feller & Webster, 2019). While there has been much discussion on this topic, the evidence is relatively limited and somewhat conflicting (Webster & Hewett, 2019).

Whilst it has been recommended that psychological factors should be part of return-to-sport test discharge criteria, only recently has there been empirical evidence of their ability to identify those at risk of subsequent injury. Two initial pilot studies showed that fear of re-injury was associated with a second ACL injury. In the first, Tagesson and Kvist (2016) conducted a battery of assessments in a cohort of 19 patients before surgery and at 5 weeks after ACL reconstruction which included fear of re-injury, knee confidence, patient reported function, activity levels, static and dynamic tibial translation and muscle strength. They followed the group for 5 years and found that those who went on to have a second ACL injury had greater fear of re-injury and greater static tibial translation in both knees compared to those who remained uninjured. They suggested these factors may be predictive of subsequent ACL injury. In the second pilot study, Paterno et al. (2018) assessed 40 patients who had been cleared to return to sport and tracked them for 12 months to identify second ACL injuries. Patients with a greater fear of injury (measured using the Tampa Scale of Kinesiophobia) were 13 times more likely to suffer a second ACL injury. These authors suggested that it may be important to measure self-reported fear of movement and incorporate this into return-to-sport discharge criteria to reduce the risk of further ACL injury.

In a subsequent larger study, McPherson et al. (2019) had 429 athletes complete the ACL-RSI both before and at 12 months after ACL reconstruction and then followed the cohort for a minimum 2 years to determine further injury. Given that most ACL injuries occur in the context of sport, only those who had made a return to sport were included in the final analysed cohort of 329 patients. For this group, when measured preoperatively, psychological readiness was not associated with subsequent ACL injury. However, when measured at 12 months, younger injured patients (≤20 years) had significantly lower psychological readiness than younger non-injured patients. A cut-off score of 77 points was calculated which had high sensitivity (90%) but low specificity (47%). From these results, it can be 90% certain that an athlete who has a second ACL injury scores below this cut-off. This may give some guidance, to both patient and clinician, as to what amount of psychological readiness one might be aiming for at this time point of the recovery process to avoid further injury. A follow-up study in the same young cohort showed that those who re-injured had little improvement in ACL-RSI scores from preoperative to 12 months post-surgery, whereas those not injured showed a 20-point increase (out of the 100-point scale). Notably, 15% of those who reinjured had pre- to post-surgery drop in score (McPherson et al., 2019).

While these above-mentioned studies have shown lower levels of fear and greater psychological readiness to be potentially protective of subsequent ACL injury, Paterno et al. (2017) showed that younger female athletes who had high levels of knee-related confidence and high hop symmetry scores were at high risk for second ACL injury. It is therefore possible that having too much confidence may be of concern regarding further injury risk.

Combined, these above studies show an association between psychological factors and further ACL injury. While more work is needed to confirm these findings, they have potential clinical relevance as the long-term consequences of sustaining multiple ACL injuries from a young age will negatively impact on long term knee health and quality of life.

CONCLUSIONS

Psychological factors play a significant and continual role in the sequence of ACL injury and reconstruction, rehabilitation and return to sport. There is also emerging evidence that psychological factors are associated with subsequent

ACL injury. Most of the psychological factors discussed in this chapter are potentially modifiable and should therefore be considered during rehabilitation in order to improve return-to-sport rates and the return-to-sport experience. The use of tools designed to measure psychological factors such as fear of re-injury and psychological readiness may help to identify psychologically at risk athletes and aid clinical decision-making.

Case study

Rhea, a 35-year old Olympic volleyball player, sustained a right knee injury following an awkward single leg landing while blocking an opponent's smash shot. On landing she was unbalanced, her knee buckled, and there was an audible 'pop' followed by intense pain. Having previously torn the ACL on her left knee 18 months ago, Rhea was fairly sure this was a similar injury. She had never really trusted her left knee again and always feared injuring it again. However, she never thought that she would injure her other knee. The thought of going through an arduous and lengthy rehabilitation filled her with dread.

At 35 years, Rhea was coming towards the end of her volleyball career and this would have been her last chance to make another Olympic games. Since returning to sport, she had never performed to the level that she did prior to her first ACL injury, but thought this was just normal. Clinical assessment and diagnostic imaging confirmed that she had a complete rupture of her ACL and the decision was made to have a surgical reconstruction. Following surgery Rhea made slow progress compared with her previous experience of ACL reconstruction. She was doing everything that she was being told to do but was not progressing how she expected and how other people indicated she would. Rhea wondered whether the hard work and heartbreak was worth it, and she often woke in the night questioning 'why me?'. Her return-to-sport expectation was to return to club volleyball as her international career had now been 'destroyed'. At a 6-month evaluation, Rhea mentions that she is concerned that she is getting occasional sharp intermittent pains and her knee just doesn't feel right. Her self-reported knee function and physical test (e.g. muscle strength) scores are low and she doesn't think that her rehabilitation programme is working. Concerned about how the injury is affecting Rhea, you administer the ACL-RSI as a psychological measure. Her score on the ACL-RSI is 39. Against this background, you start to wonder how successful Rhea's return to sport following ACL injury will be.

Questions

1. Do you think that Rhea was ever 'ready' to return to sport following her first ACL injury?
2. Using the biopsychosocial model, what are the specific physical, psychological, social and contextual factors which may influence Rhea's return to sport.
3. How do you think Rhea's psychological response to her ACL injury may consequently influence her functional performance and return to sport?

4. Other than the ACL-RSI, which other questionnaires and inventories might be useful to administer?
5. Which psychological factors would you consider most clinically relevant in order to facilitate Rhea's recovery, and how would you address these?
6. What do you think the likely prognosis is for Rhea at 12-month post-surgery?

References

Ardern, C. L., Kvist, J., & Webster, K. E. (2015). Psychological aspects of anterior cruciate ligament injuries. *Operative Techniques in Sports Medicine, 24*, 77–83.

Ardern, C. L., Österberg, A., Tagesson, S., Gauffin, H., Webster, K. E., & Kvist, J. (2014). The impact of psychological readiness to return to sport and recreational activities after anterior cruciate ligament reconstruction. *The British Journal of Sports Medicine, 48*(22), 1613–1619.

Ardern, C. L., Taylor, N. F., Feller, J. A., & Webster, K. E. (2012). Fear of re-injury in people who have returned to sport following anterior cruciate ligament reconstruction surgery. *The Journal of Science and Medicine in Sport, 15*(6), 488–495.

Ardern, C. L., Taylor, N. F., Feller, J. A., & Webster, K. E. (2013). A systematic review of the psychological factors associated with returning to sport following injury. *The British Journal of Sports Medicine, 47*(17), 1120–1126.

Ardern, C. L., Taylor, N. F., Feller, J. A., & Webster, K. E. (2014). Fifty-five per cent return to competitive sport following anterior cruciate ligament reconstruction surgery: An updated systematic review and meta-analysis including aspects of physical functioning and contextual factors. *The British Journal of Sports Medicine, 48*(21), 1543–1552.

Ardern, C. L., Taylor, N. F., Feller, J. A., Whitehead, T. S., & Webster, K. E. (2013). Psychological responses matter in returning to preinjury level of sport after anterior cruciate ligament reconstruction surgery. *The American Journal of Sports Medicine, 41*(7), 1549–1558.

Ardern, C. L., Taylor, N. F., Feller, J. A., Whitehead, T. S., & Webster, K. E. (2015). Sports participation 2 years after anterior cruciate ligament reconstruction in athletes who had not returned to sport at 1 year: A prospective follow-up of physical function and psychological factors in 122 athletes. *The American Journal of Sports Medicine, 43*(4), 848–856.

Ardern, C. L., Webster, K. E., Taylor, N. F., & Feller, J. A. (2011a). Return to sport following anterior cruciate ligament reconstruction surgery: A systematic review and meta-analysis of the state of play. *The British Journal of Sports Medicine, 45*(7), 596–606.

Ardern, C. L., Webster, K. E., Taylor, N. F., & Feller, J. A. (2011b). Return to the preinjury level of competitive sport after anterior cruciate ligament reconstruction surgery: Two-thirds of patients have not returned by 12 months after surgery. *The American Journal of Sports Medicine, 39*(3), 538–543.

Bohu, Y., Klouche, S., Lefevre, N., Webster, K., & Herman, S. (2015). Translation, cross-cultural adaptation and validation of the French version of the anterior cruciate ligament-return to sport after injury (ACL-RSI) scale. *Knee Surgery, Sports Traumatology, Arthroscopy, 23*(4), 1192–1196.

Brewer, B. (2010). The role of psychological factors in sport injury rehabilitation outcomes. *International Review of Sport and Exercise Psychology, 3*, 40–61.

Brewer, B., Andersen, M. B., & van Raalte, J. L. (2002). Psychological aspects of sport injury rehabilitation: Toward a biopsychosocial approach. In D. Mostofsky, & L. D. Zaichkowsky (Eds.), *Medical and psychological aspects of sport and exercise* (pp. 41–54). Fitness Information Technology.

Burland, J. P., Lepley, A. S., Cormier, M., DiStefano, L. J., Arciero, R., & Lepley, L. K. (2019). Learned helplessness after anterior cruciate ligament reconstruction: An altered neurocognitive state? *Sports Medicine*, *49*(5), 647–657.

Chen, T., Zhang, P., & Li, Y., et al. (2017). Translation, cultural adaptation and validation of simplified Chinese version of the anterior cruciate ligament return to sport after injury (ACL-RSI) scale. *PLoS One*, *12*(8), e0183095.

Czuppon, S., Racette, B. A., Klein, S. E., & Harris-Hayes, M. (2014). Variables associated with return to sport following anterior cruciate ligament reconstruction: A systematic review. *The British Journal of Sports Medicine*, *48*(5), 356–364.

Dekker, T. J., Godin, J. A., Dale, K. M., Garrett, W. E., Taylor, D. C., & Riboh, J. C. (2017). Return to sport after pediatric anterior cruciate ligament reconstruction and its effect on subsequent anterior cruciate ligament injury. *The Journal of Bone and Joint Surgery. American Volume*, *99*(11), 897–904.

Everhart, J. S., Best, T. M., & Flanigan, D. C. (2015). Psychological predictors of anterior cruciate ligament reconstruction outcomes: A systematic review. *Knee Surgery, Sports Traumatology, Arthroscopy*, *23*(3), 752–762.

Feller, J. A., & Webster, K. E. (2019). Where are we with return-to-sport testing following ACL reconstruction? *Orthopaedics & Traumatology: Surgery & Research*, *105*(6), 1037–1038.

Forsdyke, D, Smith, A, Jones, M, & Gledhill, A. (2016). Psychosocial factors associated with outcomes of sports injury rehabilitation in competitive athletes: A mixed studies systematic review. *The British Journal of Sports Medicine*, *50*(9), 537–544.

French, D. J., France, C. R., Vigneau, F., French, J. A., & Evans, R. T. (2007). Fear of movement/(re)injury in chronic pain: A psychometric assessment of the original English version of the Tampa scale for kinesiophobia (TSK). *Pain*, *127*(1–2), 42–51.

Glazer, D. D. (2009). Development and preliminary validation of the injury-psychological readiness to return to sport (I-PRRS) scale. *Journal of Athletic Training*, *44*(2), 185–189.

Ha, J. K., Kim, J. G., & Yoon, K. H., et al. (2019). Korean version of the anterior cruciate ligament-return to sport after injury scale: Translation and cross-cultural adaptation. *Clinics in Orthopedic Surgery*, *11*(2), 164–169.

Harput, G., Tok, D., & Ulusoy, B., et al. (2016). Translation and cross-cultural adaptation of the anterior cruciate ligament-return to sport after injury (ACL-RSI) scale into Turkish. *Knee Surgery, Sports Traumatology, Arthroscopy*. DOI: 10.1007/s00167-016-4288-6.

Hart, H. F., Culvenor, A. G., Guermazi, A., & Crossley, K. M. (2019). Worse knee confidence, fear of movement, psychological readiness to return-to-sport and pain are associated with worse function after ACL reconstruction. *Physical Therapy in Sport*, *41*, 1–8.

Jia, Z. Y., Cui, J., & Wang, W., et al. (2018). Translation and validation of the simplified Chinese version of the anterior cruciate ligament-return to sport after injury (ACL-RSI). *Knee Surgery, Sports Traumatology, Arthroscopy*, *26*(10), 2997–3003.

Johnston, L., & Carroll, D. (1998). The context of emotional responses to athletic injury: A qualitative analysis. *Journal of Sport Rehabilitation*, *7*(3), 206–220.

Kitaguchi, T., Tanaka, Y., & Takeshita, S., et al. (2020). Importance of functional performance and psychological readiness for return to preinjury level of sports 1 year after ACL reconstruction in competitive athletes. *Knee Surgery, Sports Traumatology, Arthroscopy, 28*(7), 2203–2212.

Kleiber, D., Greendorfer, S., Blinde, E., & Samdahl, D. (1987). Quality of exit from university sports and life satisfaction in early adulthood. *Sociology of Sport Journal, 4*, 28–36.

Kostyun, R. O., Burland, J. P., Kostyun, K. J., Milewski, M. D., & Nissen, C. W. (2019). Male and female adolescent athletes' readiness to return to sport after anterior cruciate ligament injuryand reconstruction. *Clinical Journal of Sport Medicine*. Online ahead of print. DOI: 10.1097/JSM.0000000000000751.

Kvist, J., Ek, A., Sporrstedt, K., & Good, L. (2005). Fear of re-injury: A hindrance for returning to sports after anterior cruciate ligament reconstruction. *Knee Surgery, Sports Traumatology, Arthroscopy, 13*(5), 393–397.

Kvist, J., Österberg, A., Gauffin, H., Tagesson, S., Webster, K., & Ardern, C. (2013). Translation and measurement properties of the Swedish version of ACL-return to sports after injury questionnaire. *Scandinavian Journal of Medicine & Science in Sports, 23*(5), 568–575.

Langford, JL, Webster, K, E., & Feller, J. A. (2009). A prospective longitudinal study to assess psychological changes following anterior cruciate ligament reconstruction surgery. *The British Journal of Sports Medicine, 43*(5), 377–381.

Mann, B. J., Grana, W. A., Indelicato, P. A., O'Neill, D. F., & George, S. Z. (2007). A survey of sports medicine physicians regarding psychological issues in patient-athletes. *The American Journal of Sports Medicine, 35*(12), 2140–2147.

McLean, S. G., Huang, X., & van den Bogert, A. J. (2008). Investigating isolated neuromuscular control contributions to non-contact anterior cruciate ligament injury risk via computer simulation methods. *Clinical Biomechanics (Bristol, Avon), 23*(7), 926–936.

McPherson, A. L., Feller, J. A., Hewett, T. E., & Webster, K. E. (2019). Psychological readiness to return to sport is associated with second anterior cruciate ligament injuries. *The American Journal of Sports Medicine, 47*(4), 857–862.

McPherson, A. L., Feller, J. A., Hewett, T. E., & Webster, K. E. (2019). Smaller change in psychological readiness to return to sport is associated with second anterior cruciate ligament injury among younger patients. *The American Journal of Sports Medicine, 47*(5), 1209–1215.

Morgan, M. D., Salmon, L. J., Waller, A., Roe, J. P., & LA, P. (2016). Fifteen-year survival of endoscopic anterior cruciate ligament reconstruction in patients aged 18 years and younger. *The American Journal of Sports Medicine, 44*(2), 384–392.

Morrey, M. A., Stuart, M. J., Smith, A. M., & Wiese-Bjornstal, D. M. (1999). A longitudinal examination of athletes' emotional and cognitive responses to anterior cruciate ligament injury. *Clinical Journal of Sport Medicine, 9*(2), 63–69.

Muller, U., Kruger-Franke, M., Schmidt, M., & Rosemeyer, B. (2015). Predictive parameters for return to pre-injury level of sport 6 months following anterior cruciate ligament reconstruction surgery. *Knee Surgery, Sports Traumatology, Arthroscopy, 23*(12), 3623–3631.

Müller, U., Schmidt, M., Krüger-Franke, M., & Rosemeyer, B. (2014). Die ACL-return to sport after injury skala als wichtiger parameter bei der beurteilung rückkehr zum sport level I und II nach Rekonstruktion des vorderen Kreuzbands. Ihre Übersetzung in die deutsche Sprache (ACL-Return to sport after injury scale as an important predictor for return to sport level I and II after ACL reconstruction. Translation into German language). *Sports Orthopaedics and Traumatology, 30*, 135–144.

Nagelli, C. V., Webster, K. E., Di Stasi, S., Wordeman, S. C., & Hewett, T. E. (2019). The association of psychological readiness to return to sport after anterior cruciate ligament reconstruction and hip and knee landing kinematics. *Clinical biomechanics (Bristol, Avon), 68*, 104–108.

Nwachukwu, B. U., Adjei, J., & Rauck, R. C., et al. (2019). How much do psychological factors affect lack of return to play after anterior cruciate ligament reconstruction? A systematic review. *Orthopaedic Journal of Sports Medicine, 7*(5), 2325967119845313.

Nyland, J., Cottrell, B., Harreld, K., & Caborn, D. N. (2006). Self-reported outcomes after anterior cruciate ligament reconstruction: An internal health locus of control score comparison. *Arthroscopy, 22*(11), 1225–1232.

Paterno, M. V., Flynn, K., Thomas, S., & Schmitt, L. C. (2018). Self-reported fear predicts functional performance and second ACL injury after ACL reconstruction and return to sport: A pilot study. *Sports Health, 10*(3), 228–233.

Paterno, M. V., Huang, B., Thomas, S., Hewett, T. E., & Schmitt, L. C. (2017). Clinical factors that predict a second ACL injury after ACL reconstruction and return to sport: Preliminary development of a clinical decision algorithm. *Orthopaedic Journal of Sports Medicine, 5*(12), 2325967117745279.

Paterno, M. V., Rauh, M. J., Schmitt, L. C., Ford, K. R., & Hewett, T. E. (2014). Incidence of second ACL injuries 2 years after primary ACL reconstruction and return to sport. *American Journal of Sports Medicine, 42*(7), 1567–1573.

Phelan, B., King, E., Richter, C., Webster, K., & Falvey, E. (2019). A comparison of anterior cruciate ligament – Return to sports after injury (ACL-RSI) scores of male athletes nine months post-ACL reconstruction with matched uninjured controls. *Physical Therapy in Sport, 38*, 179–183.

Podlog, L., Banham, S. M., Wadey, R., & Hannon, J. (2015). Psychological readiness to return to competitive sport following injury: A qualitative study. *Sport Psychology, 29*(1), 1–14.

Quinn, A. M., & Fallon, B. J. (1999). The changes in psychological characteristics and reactions of elite athletes from injury onset until full recovery. *Journal of Applied Sport Psychology, 11*(2), 210–229.

Ross, C. A., Clifford, A., & Louw, Q. A. (2017). Factors informing fear of reinjury after anterior cruciate ligament reconstruction. *Physiotherapy Theory and Practice, 33*(2), 103–114.

Rosso, F., Bonasia, D. E., & Cottino, U., Cambursano, S., Dettoni, F., Rossi, R. (2018). Factors affecting subjective and objective outcomes and return to play in anterior cruciate ligament reconstruction: A retrospective cohort study. *Joints, 6*(1), 23–32.

Ruddock-Hudson, M., O'Halloran, P., & Murphy, G. (2012). Exploring psychological reactions to injury in the Australian Football League (AFL). *Journal of Applied Sport Psychology, 24*, 375–390.

Sadeqi, M., Klouche, S., Bohu, Y., Herman, S., Lefevre, N., & Gerometta, A. (2018). Progression of the psychological ACL-RSI Score and return to sport after anterior cruciate ligament reconstruction: A prospective 2-year follow-up study from the French prospective anterior cruciate ligament reconstruction cohort study (FAST). *Orthopaedic Journal of Sports Medicine, 6*(12), 2325967118812819.

Sala-Barat, E., Alvarez-Diaz, P., Alentorn-Geli, E., Webster, K. E., Cugat, R., & Tomas-Sabado, J. (2020). Translation, cross-cultural adaptation, validation, and measurement properties of the Spanish version of the anterior cruciate ligament-return to sport after injury (ACLRSI-Sp) scale. *Knee Surgery, Sports Traumatology, Arthroscopy, 28*(3), 833–839.

Salatkaite, S., Siupsinskas, L., & Gudas, R. (2019). Translation and cultural adaptation of Lithuanian version of the anterior cruciate ligament return to sport after injury (ACL-RSI) scale. *PLoS One, 14*(7), e0219593.

Scott, S. M., Perry, M. A., & Sole, G. (2018). "Not always a straight path": Patients' perspectives following anterior cruciate ligament rupture and reconstruction. *Disability and Rehabilitation, 40*(19), 2311–2317.

Silva, L. O., Mendes, L. M. R., Lima, P. O. P., & Almeida, G. P. L. (2018). Translation, cross-adaptation and measurement properties of the Brazilian version of the ACL-RSI Scale and ACL-QoL Questionnaire in patients with anterior cruciate ligament reconstruction. *Brazilian Journal of Physical Therapy, 22*(2), 127–134.

Slagers, A. J., Reininga, I. H., & van den Akker-Scheek, I. (2017). The Dutch language anterior cruciate ligament return to sport after injury scale (ACL-RSI): Validity and reliability. *Journal of Sports Sciences, 35*(4), 393–401.

Smith, A. M. (1996). Psychological impact of injuries in athletes. *Sports Medicine, 22*(6), 391–405.

Smith, A. M., Scott, S. G., O'Fallon, W. M., & Young, M. L. (1990). Emotional responses of athletes to injury. *Mayo Clinic Proceedings, 65*(1), 38–50.

Smith, A. M., Scott, S. G., & Wiese, D. M. (1990). The psychological effects of sports injuries coping. *Sports Medicine, 9*(6), 352–369.

Sonesson, S., Kvist, J., Ardern, C., Österberg, A., & Grävare Silbernagel, K. (2016). Psychological factors are important to return to pre-injury sport activity after anterior cruciate ligament reconstruction: Expect and motivate to satisfy. *Knee Surgery, Sports Traumatology, Arthroscopy.* DOI: 10.1007/s00167-016-4294-8.

Tagesson, S., & Kvist, J. (2016). Greater fear of re-injury and increased tibial translation in patients who later sustain an ACL graft rupture or a contralateral ACL rupture: A pilot study. *Journal of Sports Sciences, 34*(2), 125–132.

te Wierike, S. C., van der Sluis, A., van den Akker-Scheek, I., Elferink-Gemser, M. T., & Visscher, C. (2013). Psychosocial factors influencing the recovery of athletes with anterior cruciate ligament injury: A systematic review. *Scandinavian Journal of Medicine & Science in Sports, 23*(5), 527–540.

Thomeé, P., Währborg, P., Börjesson, M., Thomeé, R., Eriksson, B. I., & Karlsson, J. (2006). A new instrument for measuring self-efficacy in patients with an anterior cruciate ligament injury. *Scandinavian Journal of Medicine & Science in Sports, 16*(3), 181–187.

Thomeé, P., Währborg, P., Börjesson, M., Thomeé, R., Eriksson, B. I., & Karlsson, J. (2007). Self-efficacy, symptoms and physical activity in patients with an anterior cruciate ligament injury:A prospective study. *Scandinavian Journal of Medicine & Science in Sports, 17*(3), 238–245.

Thomeé P., Währborg P., Börjesson M., Thomeé R., Eriksson B. I., & Karlsson J. (2008). Self-efficacy of knee function as a pre-operative predictor of outcome 1 year after anterior cruciate ligament reconstruction. *Knee Surgery, Sports Traumatology, Arthroscopy, 16*(2), 118–127.

Trigsted, S. M., Cook, D. B., Pickett, K. A., Cadmus-Bertram, L., Dunn, W. R., & Bell, D. R. (2018). Greater fear of reinjury is related to stiffened jump-landing biomechanics and muscle activation in women after ACL reconstruction. *Knee Surgery, Sports Traumatology, Arthroscopy*, *26*(12), 3682–3689.

Walker, N., Thatcher, J., & Lavallee, D. (2007). Psychological responses to injury in competitive sport: A critical review. *Journal of the Royal Society for the Promotion of Health*, *127*(4), 174–180.

Walker, N., Thatcher, J., & Lavallee, D. (2010). A preliminary development of the re-injury anxiety inventory (RIAI). *Physical Therapy in Sport*, *11*(1), 23–29.

Webster, K. E., & Feller, J. A. (2016). Exploring the high reinjury rate in younger patients undergoing anterior cruciate ligament reconstruction. *The American Journal of Sports Medicine*, *44*(11), 2827–2832.

Webster, K. E., & Feller, J. A. (2018). Development and validation of a short version of the anterior cruciate ligament return to sport after injury (ACL-RSI) scale. *Orthopaedic Journal of Sports Medicine*, *6*(4), 2325967118763763.

Webster, K. E., & Feller, J. A. (2019). A research update on the state of play for return to sport after anterior cruciate ligament reconstruction. *Journal of Orthopaedics and Traumatology*, *20*(1), 10.

Webster, K. E., Feller, J. A., & Lambros, C. (2008). Development and preliminary validation of a scale to measure the psychological impact of returning to sport following anterior cruciate ligament reconstruction surgery. *Physical Therapy in Sport*, *9*(1), 9–15.

Webster, K. E., & Hewett, T. E. (2019). What is the evidence for and validity of return-to-sport testing after anterior cruciate ligament reconstruction surgery? A systematic review and meta-analysis. *Sports Medicine*, *49*(6), 917–929.

Webster, K. E., McPherson, A. L., Hewett, T. E., & Feller, J. A. (2019). Factors associated with a return to preinjury level of sport performance after anterior cruciate ligament reconstruction surgery. *The American Journal of Sports Medicine*, *47*(11), 2557–2562.

Webster, K. E., Nagelli, C. V., Hewett, T. E., & Feller, J. A. (2018). Factors associated with psychological readiness to return to sport after anterior cruciate ligament reconstruction surgery. *The American Journal of Sports Medicine*, *46*(7), 1545–1550.

Wiese-Bjornstal, D. M., Smith, A. M., Schaffer, S. M., & Morrey, M. A. (1988). An integrated model of response to sport injury: Psychological and sociological dynamics. *Journal of Applied Sport Psychology*, *10*, 46–69.

Zarzycki, R., Failla, M., Capin, J. J., & Snyder-Mackler, L. (2018). Psychological readiness to return to sport is associated with knee kinematic asymmetry during gait following anterior cruciate ligament reconstruction. *Journal of Orthopaedic & Sports Physical Therapy*, *48*(12), 968–973.

13 'IT'S MY CONCUSSION STORY, AND I WANT IT TO BE HEARD'

UNDERSTANDING THE PSYCHOLOGY OF CONCUSSION EXPERIENCE

Dr Osman Hassan Ahmed, Dr Eric E. Hall and Dr Caroline J. Ketcham

Sports-related concussion (SRC) is arguably one of the most pressing issues in elite and recreational sport at present, and there has been significant attention paid to the frequency and consequences of this injury in both the academic literature (Alla et al., 2011) and mainstream media (Ahmed & Hall, 2017). In terms of the qualitative literature base related to concussion, there is a comparative lack of published research, suggesting that many concussion stories and experiences may not be 'heard' by the wider scientific community.

This chapter begins with an outline of the impact of SRC, and some of the key factors related to this injury. The importance of athlete experiences related to SRC will be discussed, as well as the role of the media in SRC discourse. An exploration of the effect of SRC on athlete well-being is included, along with its association with factors such as depression and loss of identity. The role of the multidisciplinary team (MDT) in the management of this injury will be outlined, including the role of psychology. The chapter concludes with a concussion-related case study and questions associated with this case study, which it is hoped will help the practitioner when dealing with this injury.

BACKGROUND TO CONCUSSION

Unlike many other common sporting injuries, concussion is seen as an 'invisible injury'. This is due in part to the fact that the diagnosis and subsequent management of SRC is dependent upon an individual reporting their symptoms (alongside any observable signs of the injury which may be witnessed). What constitutes a concussion has been a contentious issue historically (McCrory et al., 2017a), with formal definitions being provided by the Concussion in Sport

Group (CISG). Five summary and agreement/consensus statements have been produced through this process, which commenced in 2001 (Aubry et al., 2002). This process has evolved with the inclusion of major sporting organizations, including the International Olympic Committee Medical Commission, the Federation Internationale de Football Association and the International Ice Hockey Federation. The most contemporary definition of concussion from the 2016 CISG meeting states that concussion is a 'traumatic brain injury induced by biomechanical forces' (McCrory et al., 2017b), with this definition giving additional detail relating to the variable, often temporary, and typically functional (rather than structural) nature of this injury.

IMPACT OF CONCUSSION

An oft-quoted statistic is that concussion affects 1.7 million people per year in the USA (Langlois et al., 2006); however, this figure has been suggested as being on the low side with actual figures suggested to be closer to 3 million people per year (Centers for Disease Control and Prevention, 2019). Contact sports such as rugby (Rafferty et al., 2019), ice hockey (Schneider et al., 2018) and soccer (Beaudouin et al., 2019) are all associated with high rates of concussion due to the respective demands of these sports. Other sports, which may not be traditionally viewed as high risk, also have high concussion rates including dancing (Stein et al., 2014) and cheerleading (Shields et al., 2009). In addition, SRC rates have been shown to be high in paralympic sports (Kissick & Webborn, 2018). Recent concussion-related research has identified trends and patterns related to a number of key factors. The importance of sex and gender in relation to SRC has been identified (Mollayeva et al., 2018), with females shown to sustain more concussions than males and have a greater time loss than males (Covassin et al., 2016). Irrespective of gender, the likelihood of having a subsequent SRC having sustained one previously has also been shown by several studies (Daneshvar et al., 2011; O'Brien et al., 2017). In addition, individuals who have experienced a SRC may also be at risk of further musculoskeletal injuries (Herman et al., 2017).

The long-term impact of SRC often focuses on neurodegenerative diseases such as Alzheimer's disease and Chronic Traumatic Encephalography (Sundman et al., 2014). Generally however, the long-lasting effects of a concussion can be seen through changes in both quality of life and sleep (Ahman et al., 2013; Blake et al., 2019; Emanuelson et al., 2003; Kuehl et al., 2010). In the study by Ahman et al. (2013), almost half of the participants still reported fatigue, poor memory, headache, frustration and depression 3 years following a mild traumatic brain injury (mTBI). Some of these participants still reported difficulties 11 years following their mTBI.

Diagnoses of depression and post-traumatic stress disorder are also commonly reported following SRC or mTBI (Cnossen et al., 2017; Levin et al., 2001; Stein et al., 2019). It is also possible that following a concussion with persistent symptoms or with multiple concussions, an athlete may be faced with the decision to retire from sports (Cantu & Register-Mihalik, 2011). The decision to retire from sports can lead to a loss of identity and has been related to retirement difficulties, especially if the retirement is due to injuries (Webb et al., 1998). As such, the role of athletic identity is something that needs to be taken into consideration when retirement occurs (Lavallee et al., 1997).

EMOTIONAL RESPONSES TO CONCUSSION

The integrated model of sport injury and rehabilitation by Wiese-Bjornstal et al. (1998) suggests that personal factors and situational factors will affect any cognitive appraisals following an injury. These cognitive appraisals influence emotional responses to injury, the subsequent behavioural responses and the recovery outcomes from injury. More recently, Wiese-Bjornstal has attempted to adapt this model to include SRC as the injury (Wiese-Bjornstal et al., 2015). The major inclusions in this adaptation came through three main additions: including symptoms in the cognitive, emotional and behavioural responses (because of the intentionality of these along with responses to concussion management); including neurobiological, psychogenic and pathophysiological causes as a mediator between the personal and situational factors to the cognitive symptoms and appraisals; and adding in the importance of post-injury psychological care into the model and how it influences recovery from concussion.

Three recent studies have used qualitative methodology to better examine the lived experiences of athletes who have experienced a concussion (Iadevaia et al., 2015; Moreau et al., 2014; Valovich McLeod et al., 2017). The findings from these studies are fairly consistent, in that they all describe a significant impact in symptoms they experienced. Additionally, these symptoms usually resulted in a significant emotional response, and collectively these experiences caused a change in social relationships. There are a wide variety of signs and symptoms that are often associated with SRC (McCrory et al., 2017b). A recent study by Wasserman et al. (2016) found that the most commonly reported symptoms from SRC include headaches, dizziness and difficulty in concentrating. These primary symptoms may not be labelled as emotional symptoms; however despite the fact that these initial symptoms will typically recover spontaneously in a relatively short period of time, previous studies have suggested that they may lead to a significant emotional response (Iadevaia et al., 2015; Moreau et al., 2014; Valovich McLeod et al., 2017).

Common emotional responses to SRC are frustration and anxiety (Wiese-Bjornstal et al., 2015), which may arise from a number of reasons. One might be that being taken out of sport may have a significant influence on their identity and could lead to feelings of anxiety and depression (Brewer, 1993; Brewer et al., 1993; Sparkes, 1998). The loss of identity for an athlete associated with their injury suggests that there may be some educational implications for those who interact with the injured athlete (Lockhart, 2010). Additionally, Silver (2014) suggests that these feelings of anxiety and frustration are caused by changes in function that occur as a result of SRC and a dysfunctional cognitive feedback loop.

CONCUSSION AND SOCIAL RELATIONSHIPS

Symptoms reported following SRC, as well as the subsequent emotional responses, are made even more difficult by the strained social relationships that these athletes may be experiencing (Iadevaia et al., 2015; Moreau et al., 2014; Valovich McLeod et al., 2017). As predicted by the Wiese-Bjornstal (2015) integrated model, social relationships are included in the situational factors that may influence the cognitive symptoms and appraisals, via psychogenic causes and subsequent emotional responses.

In these studies, athletes often report that social relationships might also influence future behavioural responses, such that they will often report that they 'don't want to let their teammates down' or 'can't contribute to the team' (Valovich McLeod et al., 2017). In addition to the pressure the athletes are placing on themselves, they also experience pressure from coaches, teammates, parents and fans. A recent study found that more than a quarter of participants (college athletes) reported experiencing pressure to continue playing from at least one source (i.e. coaches, teammates, parents and fans) after sustaining an impact to the head (Kroshus et al., 2015). If an athlete reported feeling pressure from all four sources, they were more likely to continue playing. It is not surprising that this pressure placed upon themselves and by others may provoke additional anxiety and frustration and prolong their recovery from concussion.

PSYCHOSOCIAL INTERVENTIONS FOR CONCUSSION

The integrated model of sport injury and rehabilitation adequately captures these experiences of the concussed athlete and provides areas where psychosocial interventions may be relevant (Wiese-Bjornstal et al., 2015). A recent targeted review has suggested that there is an anxiety/mood clinical profile of SRC (Sandel et al., 2017). This clinical profile is one of six that have been suggested as being experienced by an individual who has a concussion, and this review article suggests four forms of targeted treatment that may be useful for this type of concussion (psychoeducation, behavioural regulation, desensitization to environmental stimuli and psychotherapy). Psychoeducation is a common intervention for the management of SRC and provides informational support about the expected signs and symptoms of a concussion to an individual. Common components of such programs include clinicians setting a positive expectation for recovery, descriptions of the pathophysiology of concussion, description of the common signs and symptoms of a concussion and potential strategies to help reduce symptoms (Cooper et al., 2015).

In regard to behavioural regulation, Sandel et al. (2017) suggest that implementing good sleep hygiene and physical activity may be useful behaviours to focus on in order to help mitigate symptoms. Sleep alterations are a common symptom following a concussion; therefore, any intervention to help regulate these symptoms would be beneficial for recovery. Similarly, physical activity has been shown to have an impact on emotions, sleep, cognition and numerous physiological changes (Biddle, 2016) that could be beneficial from concussion recovery. If there are environments that are anxiety provoking for those with a concussion, desensitization through exposure may be a method to help them deal with these anxiety symptoms and aid their recovery. If anxiety and mood are persistent issues following SRC, then psychotherapy is suggested as a possible approach. This may include cognitive behavioural therapy, techniques to improve mindfulness, implementing adaptive coping strategies and potentially pharmacologic interventions.

Based on the social pressures experienced, it may also be important to provide appropriate social support for those suffering from concussion. The work of Covassin et al. (2014) indicated that those who reported having higher levels of social support experienced less anxiety following SRC. The provision of informational and emotional support from parents, coaches and sports medicine staff have been stated as important components in assisting concussion recovery (André-Morin et al., 2017). A recent study found that this emotional support was related to more positive psychosocial reactions and intentions to report future concussion symptoms (Wayment & Huffman, 2019), reinforcing the importance that emotional support can have in the recovery following SRC. Additionally, informational support by physicians and athletic trainers/physiotherapists has been found to be important in the recovery process from concussions (André-Morin et al., 2017).

EFFECT OF THE MEDIA ON SHAPING CONCUSSION EXPERIENCES

Given the impact that concussion has had on sport and those individuals playing it, it is unsurprising that the mainstream media has reported extensively on high-profile concussive injuries. As a consequence, the potential exists for individuals who have experienced SRC to have their attitudes, opinions and potentially their management of concussion shaped by what they encounter online, in print or in other forms of media. This is of concern, as several studies have highlighted inaccuracies and inconsistencies in the reporting of SRC in the mainstream media. Ahmed and Hall (2017) evaluated 153 online news articles and found that almost 10% of all articles contained terminology which could downplay the seriousness of the injury. As a consequence of this, an associated editorial by the same authors made recommendations for journalists in order to help disseminate concussion-related stories in a more accurate manner (Ahmed et al., 2016).

The effect of the media on individuals assessing and managing concussion has also been noted. Martin et al. (2018) explored the effect of television consumption and internet use on the attitudes of Athletic Training students towards SRC. Those Athletic Training students who consumed more internet per day felt that the reporting of concussion accurately educates the public, whereas students who consumed more television per day were more likely to disagree that this positively educates the public about concussion. As Athletic Trainers are often central to the assessment and management of SRC, then the effect of the media on their perceptions of concussion is important to understand.

One of the ways that the media has also impacted upon the public's perception of SRC is in the sharing of emotive stories related to high-profile persons who have experienced an injury. McGannon et al. (2013) used ethnographic content analysis to examine the media discourse regarding the concussion of Sidney Crosby (a star ice hockey player from Canada). From the 68 included articles in the study, the central narrative which emerged was that this concussive injury arose from the culture of risk through sport and the subsequent impact of this risk upon athletes. In an unrelated editorial, Kuhn et al. (2017) also outlined some of the challenges to the media reporting of SRC. These authors highlighted that 'highly publicised and emotionally-charged events' from the media are likely to supersede the public's perception of concussion, over and above any knowledge based on empirical data.

MANAGEMENT OF CONCUSSION

The management of concussion has evolved as researchers know more about the recovery process and the impact on athletes physically, cognitively and emotionally. The most recent recommendations for the management of concussion are to integrate an active rehabilitation model, while monitoring symptom load in an effort to ease athlete and clinician frustration and improve recovery (Leddy et al., 2019; McCrory et al., 2017b; Schneider et al., 2017; Thomas et al., 2015). While this is progress from the previous recommendation of restricted cognitive and physical activity until symptoms subside (McCrory et al., 2013), there is still limited evidence on the specifics to be implemented via this approach. Researchers have therefore shown a keen interest in how much activity to engage in, the specificity of activities and the impact of activity on symptoms, recovery and overall well-being (Leddy et al., 2019; Register-Mihalek et al., 2019). Athletes who sustain an injury are typically recommended rest for 24–48 h and then symptoms are monitored until they subside at which point they engage in a graded exertion protocol. With an active rehabilitation model, during the symptom monitor phase, activity is added at levels that do not increase symptoms and may target symptoms specifically. Engaging athletes in activity and monitoring symptoms has been shown to improve the psychological burden as they are doing something to recover and not increase the typical 7–14-day return to play timeline (Thomas et al., 2015). Researchers are trying to better understand if active rehabilitation changes the overall trajectory of recovery and more importantly improve athletes' psychological well-being.

In addition to the 'what' of concussion management, the 'who' is also important. Athletes work with a MDT and as a concussive injury affects individuals differently, a team of professionals can be instrumental in the recovery process. Typical professionals include the sports medicine staff (physician, athletic trainer, physiotherapists) but may also include other medical professionals (school nurse, family medicine clinicians) and these professionals are usually involved in the standard concussion management team. In addition, many institutions may also include others on the MDT such as mental health professionals (neuropsychologist, sport psychologist) and return to learn or work supports (teacher, speech pathologist, occupational therapist, resource teams, social worker) (Ahmed et al., 2017; Ketcham et al., 2017). While these professionals are usually not incorporated into the MDT unless an athlete has protracted recovery or ongoing symptoms, they may be beneficial earlier in the recovery process even if primarily in an advisory or peripheral support role. There may be value highlighting emotional and cognitive challenges many athletes face in an effort to normalize the complexity of concussion recovery. Athletes who are also students may find that learning is very different in the short term and so providing tips for the classroom may allow them to increase cognitive load (Ketcham et al., 2017). Although every athlete might not need all these resources depending on their recovery, having a MDT in place and accessible to athletes may reduce the frustration of their injury, provide comprehensive and holistic care, and support athlete well-being.

Case study: 'It's my concussion story, and i want it to be heard'

Alexa, a 20-year-old collegiate softball student-athlete, sustained an impact to the head when she dove for a ball in the outfield and hit the wall at her Friday afternoon game. She immediately felt symptoms of dizziness and a headache, and her Athletic Trainer removed her from play. She was advised to 'take it easy' in the following days (both physically and cognitively), and her symptoms were monitored and post-concussion testing scheduled for 48 h later. Alexa's symptoms continued, her neurocognitive performance score was significantly lower than her baseline and the sports medicine physician diagnosed her with a concussion. Instructions to Alexa were to continue to monitor her own cognitive and physical activity, and to limit both of these if her symptoms increased.

Alexa was a high-achieving athlete and student. She was majoring in Public Health and was taking pre-med prerequisites, so missing class and labs gave her great anxiety. She already had to work hard to make up work for missed classes due to travel, but it was even more deflating to her as she now had to miss more classes due to her concussion. It was one of the final few series before her regionals and she hated missing practice and events with her team. She would get dizzy and her head would pound when she would try to attend practice or film sessions. The noise, lights and lots of moving people were too much. Alexa felt more sadness, anxiety and mental fogginess over the next several days. Every time she tried to read books or online material for her courses, her symptoms would increase and she would be unable to remember what she had read.

Her partner Sam was frustrated that she was unable to go out to dinner and hang out with their friends. Alexa had a much shorter temper and would cry much more easily than she would do normally. The arguments between Alexa and Sam seemed constant, and Sam seemed to blame Alexa for this escalation. Everything seemed to be falling apart. After 2 weeks, Alexa's symptoms were improving and she was able to increase physical and cognitive load without her symptoms increasing, but she felt behind in everything. Her teammates were bonding with the 2nd place finish in conference, and with the next games on the horizon, they were working incredibly well together as a team. Alexa was told by her Athletic Trainer and coaches that she could travel, but as part of the return-to-play protocol, she would not be able to play in competition yet.

Although Alexa passed all of her neurocognitive tests and her symptoms had stabilized or were absent, she still did not feel 'like herself' and she struggled to be able to explain this to others or indeed understand this herself. School work was continuing to take longer and she just 'didn't feel sharp'. Sam, her teammates and her friends were clearly annoyed Alexa wasn't as outgoing as usual, and Alexa was frustrated as she did not feel like joining in. As the season ended and summer came, Alexa was cleared to return to full activities and was 'recovered' by all measures and metrics. She felt better, but not completely herself, and she was pretty upset that her course grades were slightly lower than she was used to (or had hoped for). She entered the summer with mixed emotions; both ready for a break, but simultaneously worried about returning in the fall.

1. What are some additional resources or supports that would have benefitted Alexa during this process?
2. Is the Alexa that headed into summer the new baseline for her?
3. Is Alexa's general sadness and anxiety something that should be followed up or typical for a student-athlete who has had a set-back in both?
4. This is Alexa's 3rd diagnosed concussion and she is a rising senior. Should sports medicine staff talk to her about retiring from her sport?

References

Ahman, S., Saveman, B.-I., Styrke, J., Björnstig, U., & Stålnacke, B.-M. (2013). Long-term follow-up of patients with mild traumatic brain injury: A mixed-method study. *Journal of Rehabilitation Medicine*, *45*(8), 758–764. https://doi.org/10.2340/16501977-1182.

Ahmed, O. H., Blake, T., & Hall, E. E. (2016). Educating the masses: Suggestions for improving online concussion information via the mainstream media. *Concussion*, 2(1). https://doi.org/10.2217/cnc-2016-0026.

Ahmed, O. H., & Hall, E. E. (2017). "It was only a mild concussion": Exploring the description of sports concussion in online news articles. *Physical Therapy in Sport*, *23*, 7–13. DOI: 10.1016/j.ptsp.2016.07.003.

Ahmed, O. H., Loosemore, M., Hornby, K., Kumar, B., Sylvester, R., Makalanda, H. L., Rogers, T., Edwards, D., & de Medici, A., (2017). Moving concussion care to the next level: The emergence and role of concussion clinics in the UK. *Progress in Brain Research*, *234*, 205–220. DOI: 10.1016/bs.pbr.2017.06.014.

Alla, S., Sullivan, S. J., McCrory, P., & Hale, L. (2011). Spreading the word on sports concussion: Citation analysis of summary and agreement, position and consensus statements on sports concussion. *British Journal of Sports Medicine*, *45*(2), 132–135. DOI: 10.1136/bjsm.2010.074088.

André-Morin, D., Caron, J. G., & Bloom, G. A. (2017). Exploring the unique challenges faced by female university athletes experiencing prolonged concussion symptoms.

Sport, Exercise, and Performance Psychology, *6*(3), 289–303. https://doi.org/10.1037/spy0000106.

Aubry, M., Cantu, R., Dvorak, J., Graf-Baumann, T., Johnston, K., Kelly, J., Lovell, M., McCrory, P., Meeuwisse, W., & Schamasch, P. (2002). Summary and agreement statement of the first international conference on concussion in sport, Vienna 2001. *British Journal of Sports Medicine*, *36*(1), 6–10.

Beaudouin, F., Aus der Fünten, K., Tröß, T., Reinsberger, C., Meyer, T. (2019) Head injuries in professional male Football (Soccer) over 13 years: 29% Lower incidence rates after a rule change (Red Card). *British Journal of Sports Medicine*, *53*(15), 948–952. DOI: 10.1136/bjsports-2016-097217.

Biddle, S. (2016). Physical activity and mental health: Evidence is growing. *World Psychiatry*, *15*(2), 176–177. DOI: 10.1002/wps.20331.

Blake, A. L., McVicar, C. L., Retino, M., Hall, E. E., & Ketcham, C. J. (2019). Concussion history influences sleep disturbances, symptoms, and quality of life in collegiate student-athletes. *Sleep Health*, *5*(1), 72–77. https://doi.org/10.1016/j.sleh.2018.10.011.

Brewer, B. W. (1993). Self-identity and specific vulnerability to depressed mood. *Journal of Personality*, *61*(3), 343–364. https://doi.org/10.1111/j.1467-6494.1993.tb00284.x.

Brewer, B. W., Van Raalte, J. L., & Linder, D. E. (1993). Athletic identity: Hercules' muscles or Achilles heel? *International Journal of Sport Psychology*, *24*(2), 237–254.

Cantu, R. C., & Register-Mihalik, J. K. (2011). Considerations for return-to-play and retirement decisions after concussion. *PM&R*, *3*(10 Suppl 2), S440–444. https://doi.org/10.1016/j.pmrj.2011.07.013

Centers for Disease Control and Prevention (2019). "TBI: Get the Facts". Accessed 27th July 2019. Available at: https://www.cdc.gov/traumaticbraininjury/get_the_facts.html.

Cnossen, M. C., Scholten, A. C., Lingsma, H. F., Synnot, A., Haagsma, J., Steyerberg, P. E. W., & Polinder, S. (2017). Predictors of major depression and posttraumatic stress disorder following traumatic brain injury: A systematic review and meta-analysis. *The Journal of Neuropsychiatry and Clinical Neurosciences*, *29*(3), 206–224. https://doi.org/10.1176/appi.neuropsych.16090165.

Cooper, D. B., Bunner, A. E., Kennedy, J. E., Balldin, V., Tate, D. F., Eapen, B. C., & Jaramillo, C. A. (2015). Treatment of persistent post-concussive symptoms after mild traumatic brain injury: A systematic review of cognitive rehabilitation and behavioral health interventions in military service members and veterans. *Brain Imaging and Behavior*, *9*(3), 403–420. https://doi.org/10.1007/s11682-015-9440-2.

Covassin, T., Crutcher, B., Bleecker, A., Heiden, E. O., Dailey, A., & Yang, J. (2014). Postinjury anxiety and social support among collegiate athletes: A comparison between orthopaedic injuries and concussions. *Journal of Athletic Training*, *49*(4), 462–468. https://doi.org/10.4085/1062-6059-49.2.03.

Covassin, T., Moran, R., & Elbin, R. J. (2016). Sex differences in reported concussion injury rates and time loss from participation: An update of the national collegiate athletic association injury surveillance program from 2004-2005 through 2008-2009. *Journal of Athletic Training*, *51*(3), 189 194. DOI: 10.4085/1062-6050-51.3.05.

Daneshvar, D. H., Nowinski, C. J., McKee, A. C., & Cantu, R. C. (2011). The epidemiology of sport-related concussion. *Clinics in Sports Medicine*, *30*(1), 1–7. DOI:10.1016/j.csm.2010.08.006.

Emanuelson, I., Andersson Holmkvist, E., Björklund, R., & Stålhammar, D. (2003). Quality of life and post-concussion symptoms in adults after mild traumatic brain injury: A population-based study in Western Sweden. *Acta Neurologica Scandinavica, 108*(5), 332–338.

Herman, D., C., Jones, D., Harrison, A., Moser, M., Tillman, S., Farmer, K., Pass, A., Clugston, J. R., Hernandez, J., & Chmielewski, T. L. (2017). Concussion may increase the risk of subsequent lower extremity musculoskeletal injury in collegiate athletes. *Sports Medicine, 47*(5), 1003–1010. DOI: 10.1007/s40279-016-0607-9.

Iadevaia, C., Roiger, T., & Zwart, M. B. (2015). Qualitative examination of adolescent health-related quality of life at 1 year postconcussion. *Journal of Athletic Training, 50*(11), 1182–1189. https://doi.org/10.4085/1062-6050-50.11.02.

Ketcham, C. J., Bowie, M., Buckley, T. A., Baker, M., Patel, K., Hall, EE. (2017). The value of speech-language pathologists in concussion management. *Current Research: Concussion, 4*, e8–e13. DOI: 10.1055/s-0037-1603645.

Kissick, J., & Webborn, N. (2018). Concussion in para sport. *Physical Medicine and Rehabilitation Clinics of North America, 29*(2), 299–311. DOI: 10.1016/j.pmr.2018.01.002.

Kroshus, E., Garnett, B., Hawrilenko, M., Baugh, C. M., & Calzo, J. P. (2015). Concussion under-reporting and pressure from coaches, teammates, fans, and parents. *Social Science & Medicine*, 134, 66–75. https://doi.org/10.1016/j.socscimed.2015.04.011.

Kuehl, M. D., Snyder, A. R., Erickson, S. E., & Valovich McLeod, T. C. (2010). Impact of prior concussions on health-related quality of life in collegiate athletes. *Clinical Journal of Sport Medicine, 20*(2), 86. https://doi.org/10.1097/JSM.0b013e3181cf4534.

Kuhn, A. W., Yengo-Kahn, A. M., Kerr, Z. Y., & Zuckerman, S. L. (2017). Sports concussion research, chronic traumatic encephalopathy and the media: Repairing the disconnect. *British Journal of Sports Medicine, 51*(24), 1732–1733. DOI: 10.1136/bjsports-2016-096508.

Langlois, J. A., Rutland-Brown, W., & Wald, M.,M. (2006). The epidemiology and impact of traumatic brain injury: A brief overview. *The Journal of Head Trauma Rehabilitation, 21*(5):375–378.

Lavallee, D., Gordon, S., & Grove, J. R. (1997). Retirement from sport and the loss of athletic identity. *Journal of Personal and Interpersonal Loss, 2*(2), 129–147. https://doi.org/10.1080/10811449708414411.

Leddy, J. J., Haider, M. N., Ellis, M. J., Mannix, R., Darling, S. R., Freitas, M. S., Suffoletto, H. N., Leiter, J., Cordingley, D. M., & Willer, B. (2019). Early subthreshold aerobic exercise for sport-related concussion: A randomized clinical trial. *JAMA Pediatrics, 173*(4):319–325. DOI: 10.1001/jamapediatrics.2018.4397.

Levin, H. S., Brown, S. A., Song, J. X., McCauley, S. R., Boake, C., Contant, C. F., Goodman, H., & Kotrla, K. J. (2001). Depression and posttraumatic stress disorder at three months after mild to moderate traumatic brain injury. *Journal of Clinical and Experimental Neuropsychology, 23*(6), 754–769. https://doi.org/10.1076/jcen.23.6.754.1021.

Lockhart, B. D. (2010). Injured athletes' perceived loss of identity: Educational implications for athletic trainers. *Athletic Training Education Journal, 5*(1), 26–31.

Martin, T. G., Wallace, J., Suh, Y. I., Harriell, K., & Tatman, J. (2018). Sport-related concussions pilot study: Athletic training students' media use and perceptions of media coverage. *International Journal of Sport Communication, 11*(1), 75–94.

McCrory, P., Feddermann-Demont, N., Dvořák, J., Cassidy, J. D., McIntosh, A., Vos, P. E., Echemendia, R. J., Meeuwisse, W., & Tarnutzer, A. A. (2017a). What is the definition of sports-related concussion: A systematic review. *British Journal of Sports Medicine, 51*(11), 877–887. DOI: 10.1136/bjsports-2016-097393.

McCrory, P., Meeuwisse, W., Dvorak, J., Aubry, M., Bailes, J., Broglio, S., Cantu, R. C., Cassidy, D., Echemendia, R. J., Castellani, R. J., Davis, G. A., Ellenbogen, R., Emery, C., Engebretsen, L., Feddermann-Demont, N., Giza, C. C., Guskiewicz, K. M., Herring, S.,... Vos, P. E. (2017b). Consensus statement on concussion in sport—The 5th international conference on concussion in sport held in Berlin, October 2016. *British Journal of Sports Medicine, 51*(11), 838–847. https://doi.org/10.1136/bjsports-2017-097699.

McCrory, P., Meeuwisse, W. H., Aubry, M., Cantu, R. C., Dvořák, J., Echemendia, R. J., Engebretsen, L., Johnston, K., Kutcher, J. S., Raftery, M., Sills, A., Benson, B. W., Davis, G. A., Ellenbogen, R., Guskiewicz, K. M., Herring, S. A., Iverson, G. L., Jordan, B. d., Kissick, J.,... Turner, M. (2013). Consensus statement on concussion in sport: The 4th international conference on concussion in sport, Zurich, November 2012. *Journal of Athletic Training, 48*(4), 554–575. DOI: 10.4085/1062-6050-48.4.05.

McGannon, K. R., Cunningham, S. M., & Schinke, R. J. (2013). Understanding concussion in socio-cultural context: A media analysis of a national hockey league star's concussion. *Psychology of Sport and Exercise, 14*(6), 891–899. https://doi.org/10.1016/j.psychsport.2013.08.003.

Mollayeva, T., El-Khechen-Richandi, G., & Colantonio, A. (2018). Sex & gender considerations in concussion research. *Concussion, 3*(1). DOI: 10.2217/cnc-2017-0015.

Moreau, M. S., Langdon, J. L., & Buckley, T. A. (2014). The lived experience of an in-season concussion amongst NCAA division I student-athletes. *International Journal of Exercise Science, 7*(1), 62–74.

O'Brien, M. J., Howell, D. R., Pepin, M. J., & Meehan, W. P., 3rd (2017). Sport-related concussions: Symptom recurrence after return to exercise. *Orthopaedic Journal of Sports Medicine, 5*(10), 2325967117732516. DOI: 10.1177/2325967117732516.

Rafferty, J., Ranson, C., Oatley, G.,Mostafa, M., Mathema, P., Crick, T., & Moore, I. S. (2019). On average, a professional rugby union player is more likely than not to sustain a concussion after 25 matches. *British Journal of Sports Medicine, 53*(15), 969–973.

Register-Mihalik, J. K., Guskiewicz, K. M., Marshall, S. W., McCulloch, K. L., Mihalik, J. P., Mrazik, M., Murphy, I., Naidu, D., Ranapurwala, S. I., Schneider, K., Gildner, P., McCrea, M., & Active Rehab Study Consortium Investigators. (2019). Methodology and implementation of a randomized controlled trial (RCT) for early post-concussion rehabilitation: The Active Rehab Study. *Frontiers in Neurology, 10*, 1176.

Sandel, N., Reynolds, E., Cohen, P. E., Gillie, B. L., & Kontos, A. P. (2017). Anxiety and mood clinical profile following sport-related concussion: From risk factors to treatment. *Sport, Exercise, and Performance Psychology, 6*(3), 304–323. https://doi.org/10.1037/spy0000098.

Schneider, K. J., Leddy, J. J., Guskiewicz, K. M., & Makdissi, M. (2017). Rest and treatment/rehabilitation following sport-related concussion: A systematic review. *British Journal of Sports Medicine, 51*(12), 930–934. DOI: 10.1136/bjsports-2016-097475.

Schneider, K. J., Nettel-Aguirre, A., Palacios-Derflingher, L., Mrazik, M., Brooks, B. L., Woollings, K., Blake, T., McKay, C., Lebrun, C., Barlow, K., Taylor, K., Lemke, N., Meeuwisse, W. H., & Emery, C. A. (2018). Concussion burden, recovery, and risk factors in elite youth ice hockey players. *Clinical Journal of Sport Medicine, 8*. DOI: 10.1097/JSM.0000000000000673.

Shields, B. J., Fernandez, S. A., & Smith, B. A. (2009). Epidemiology of cheerleading stunt-related injuries in the United States. *Journal of Athletic Training, 44*(6), 586–594.

Silver, J. M. (2014). Neuropsychiatry of persistent symptoms after concussion. *Psychiatric Clinics of North America*, *37*(1), 91–102. https://doi.org/10.1016/j.psc.2013.11.001.

Sparkes, A. C. (1998). Athletic identity: An Achilles' heel to the survival of self. *Qualitative Health Research*, *8*(5), 644–664. https://doi.org/10.1177/104973239800800506.

Stein, M. B., Jain, S., Giacino, J. T., Levin, H., Dikmen, S., Nelson, L. D., & Zafonte, R. (2019). Risk of posttraumatic stress disorder and major depression in civilian patients after mild traumatic brain injury: A TRACK-TBI study. *JAMA Psychiatry*. https://doi.org/10.1001/jamapsychiatry.2018.4288.

Stein, C. J., Kinney, S. A., McCrystal, T., Carew, E. A., Bottino, N. M., Meehan III, W. P., & Micheli, L. J. (2014). Dance-related concussion: A case series. *Journal of Dance Medicine & Science*, *18*(2), 53–61. DOI: 10.12678/1089-313X.18.2.53.

Sundman, M. H., Hall, E. E., & Chen, N. (2014). Examining the relationship between head trauma and neurodegenerative disease: A review of epidemiology, pathology and neuroimaging techniques. *Journal of Alzheimer's Disease & Parkinsonism*, *04*(01). https://doi.org/10.4172/2161-0460.1000137.

Thomas, D. G., Apps, J. N., Hoffmann, R. G., McCrea, M., & Hammeke, T. (2005). benefits of strict rest after acute concussion: A randomized controlled trial. *Pediatrics*, *135*(2), 213–223. DOI: 10.1542/peds.2014-0966.

Valovich McLeod, T. C., Wagner, A. J., & Bacon, C. E. W. (2017). Lived experiences of adolescent athletes following sport-related concussion. *Orthopaedic Journal of Sports Medicine*, *5*(12), 2325967117745033. https://doi.org/10.1177/2325967117745033.

Wasserman, E. B., Kerr, Z. Y., Zuckerman, S. L., & Covassin, T. (2016). Epidemiology of sports-related concussions in national collegiate athletic association athletes from 2009–2010 to 2013–2014: Symptom prevalence, symptom resolution time, and return-to-play time. *The American Journal of Sports Medicine*, *44*(1), 226–233. https://doi.org/10.1177/0363546515610537

Wayment, H. A., & Huffman, A. H. (2019). Psychosocial experiences of concussed collegiate athletes: The role of emotional support in the recovery process. *Journal of American College Health*, *0*(0), 1–6. https://doi.org/10.1080/07448481.2019.1577863.

Webb, W. M., Nasco, S. A., Riley, S., & Headrick, B. (1998). Athlete identity and reactions to retirement from sports. *Journal of Sport Behavior*, *21*(3), 338–362.

Wiese-Bjornstal, D. M., Smith, A. M., Shaffer, S. M., & Morrey, M. A. (1998). An integrated model of response to sport injury: Psychological and sociological dynamics. *Journal of Applied Sport Psychology*, *10*(1), 46–69. https://doi.org/10.1080/10413209808406377.

Wiese-Bjornstal, D. M., White, A. C., Russell, H. C., & Smith, A. M. (2015). Psychology of sport concussions. *Kinesiology Review*, *4*(2), 169–189. https://doi.org/10.1123/kr.2015-0012.

14 SPINAL CORD INJURY AND SPORT

Dr Toni Louise Williams

INTRODUCTION

Spinal cord injury (SCI) is a catastrophic injury resulting in often permanent changes in function and sensation below the level of injury. These changes following SCI present individuals with significant challenges to improving and maintaining their health and well-being. A significant proportion of traumatic SCIs are caused by sports-related injury. Therefore, it is important to explore the impact of sports-related SCI to improve treatment modalities, rehabilitation and life-long health and well-being. Accordingly, this chapter begins with a brief overview of how injury to the spinal cord occurs and the prevalence and causes of SCI within sport. The impact of traumatic SCI to health and well-being is then considered along with the role of physical activity in SCI rehabilitation. Next, a critical approach to physical activity promotion to this population is offered. To close, a case study of SCI acquired through sport is presented with associated questions to help explore experiences of SCI.

BACKGROUND TO SCI

SCI is a serious neurological condition where damage to the spinal cord results in temporary or permanent changes in sensory, motor or autonomic function (Singh et al., 2014). The degree of impairment depends upon the location of the injury and whether the spinal cord is partially ruptured (incomplete injury) or completely severed (complete injury) (Ahuja et al., 2017). A complete injury to the cervical vertebrae can result in loss of sensory and motor function in all four limbs, the trunk and pelvic organs (known as quadriplegia or tetraplegia), whereas a complete injury to the thoracic vertebrae and below can result in loss of sensory and motor function in the legs, trunk and pelvic organs (known as paraplegia) (Ahuja et al., 2017). In incomplete injuries, only part of the spinal cord is damaged leaving the individual with some functional and/or sensory impairment and partial paralysis. The causes of SCI can be classified as traumatic or non-traumatic. Traumatic SCI occurs through external physical impact damaging the spinal cord, whereas non-traumatic SCI occurs through disease injuring the spinal cord (Ahuja et al., 2017). According to the World Health Organization (2020), the leading causes of traumatic SCI include road traffic accidents, falls and violence, with a significant number of SCIs attributed to work and sports-related injuries.

SPORT AND SCI

Sport plays a significant role in causing traumatic SCI. Given the serious nature of SCI, much of the literature seeks to understand the prevalence, causes and impact of SCI. This information is important for designing effective injury prevention interventions in sport, and improving treatment modalities, rehabilitation and life-long health and well-being following SCI (Patel et al., 2013; Williams et al., 2014). For example, a review conducted by Nadarajah et al. (2017) examined trends and demographics of sports-related paediatric SCIs in the United States. This study revealed that sports-related injury was the most common cause of SCI in children aged 14–17 and most frequently involved the cervical spine. Boys were identified as four times more likely to suffer a sport-related SCI in comparison to girls, likely explained by the predominance of boys participating in high-impact sports compared to girls. The authors proposed that the high incidence of SCI in this population was likely due to the psychological and behavioural characteristics of this population such as their engagement in risky gameplay within sport.

Another review by Chan et al. (2016) sought to determine patterns and occurrence rates of sport-related SCIs across 25 countries. The authors noted that in six countries, 13–32% of all traumatic SCIs were caused by sports-related injuries (Russia [32.9%], Fiji [32%], New Zealand [20%], Iceland [18.8%], France [15.8%] and Canada [13.1%]). The sports causing the greatest number of SCIs included diving, skiing, rugby and horseback riding. In terms of level of injury, within hockey, skiing, diving, American football and horseback riding, SCIs commonly occurred in the cervical spine. Horseback riding and snowboarding also carried a higher risk for thoracic and lumbo-sacral injuries. For all sports-related SCI, the most frequent neurological outcome at discharge was incomplete tetraplegia (46.9%) and complete tetraplegia (37.4%) with less than 1% of patients experiencing complete neurological recovery. Considering these catastrophic outcomes, the authors recommended improvements regarding regulations, equipment and attitudes towards safety and risk within sport.

Professional sports organisations have faced increased social and political pressure to improve their player safety protocols and understand the impact of serious injuries including SCI. As such, there have been a variety of risk prevention strategies which have successfully reduced the incidence of sports-related SCIs (Patel et al., 2013). Many of these strategies include the design of better protective equipment and regulation changes. For example, rule changes within rugby to decrease collision forces in the scrum, the prohibition of charging and checking from behind in hockey, and the banning of head-first tackling and blocking in American football have all been shown to reduce the prevalence of SCI in these sports (see Chan et al., 2016).

IMPACT OF TRAUMATIC SCI

Spinal cord injured individuals are faced with immediate loss of function, reduced mobility and are at risk of serious future health complications. Secondary health conditions following SCI include pressure ulcers, urinary tract infections, chronic pain, obesity, respiratory dysfunction and cardiovascular disorders (Canning & Hicks, 2014; Hitzig et al., 2008). These secondary health conditions can present as risk factors for poor mental health, increased disability and a decrease in life expectancy (Canning & Hicks, 2014; Krause & Saunders, 2011). Such sudden and significant changes can present spinal cord injured individuals with significant challenges to improving and maintaining their well-being.

In terms of subjective well-being (i.e. perceived happiness and satisfaction with life [Keyes et al., 2002; Ryan & Deci, 2001]), SCI can lead to elevated levels of depression and anxiety and decreased self-esteem (Krause & Saunders, 2011; Post & Van Leeuwen, 2012). Notably, depression has been reported as the most common psychological trauma following SCI (Williams & Murray, 2015). In relation to depressive symptoms and subjective well-being, those with SCI face higher comparative risks for feeling helpless, poor quality of life and reduced life satisfaction (Craig et al., 2009; Williams & Murray, 2015). Furthermore, in association with psychological well-being (i.e. psychological growth and development [Keyes et al., 2002; Ryan & Deci, 2001]), people with SCI report a loss of purpose in life and increased social isolation and exclusion (Geyh et al., 2012).

Formal rehabilitation plays an important role in restoring the health and well-being of a person following SCI (Williams et al., 2018a). The aim of rehabilitation is to go beyond functional independence and return individuals to 'the life they want as far as their disability will allow' (Nunnerley et al., 2013, pp. 1164–1165). To achieve this aim, people need to be educated to take care of their dramatically altered body and learn essential skills of daily living. Yet to continue to improve and maintain health and well-being beyond rehabilitation, it is vital that people with SCI lead a physically active lifestyle.

PHYSICAL ACTIVITY FOLLOWING SCI

Being physically active – general wheeling, exercising in the gym, playing sport – can alleviate or prevent many of the health and well-being complications following SCI (Williams et al., 2014). For example, physical activity participation can decrease the levels of perceived musculoskeletal pain, reduce the risk factors of cardiovascular disease and type 2 diabetes and lead to greater cardiorespiratory fitness, power output and muscle strength (Buchholz et al., 2009; Martin Ginis et al., 2012; Norrbrink et al., 2012; van der Scheer et al., 2017). As such, specific scientific guidelines have been developed which outline the type and minimum dose of exercise needed to improve fitness and cardiometabolic health for people with SCI (Martin Ginis et al., 2018). In addition to health benefits, physical activity can positively impact subjective well-being through enjoyment, reducing depression, enhancing physical self-concept and increasing life satisfaction (Hicks et al., 2003; Williams et al., 2014). Furthermore, psychological well-being can be improved through facilitating sporting experiences, which promote post-traumatic growth (Day, 2013).

Sport and exercise participation can also aid people in developing and embodying a physically active or athletic identity following SCI (Williams et al., 2014). Sport, competition and athletic performance can become central to people's lives when other roles and identities may have been lost (Chun & Lee, 2010;

Stephens et al., 2012). Maintaining a physically active identity is especially important to those who were heavily involved in sport and exercise before their injury (Levins et al., 2004; O'Brien et al., 2008). Athletic identity has also been identified as a key factor in the process of psychological adjustment following SCI (Hawkins et al., 2014; Tasiemski & Brewer, 2011). This relationship between sport and positive psychological adjustment may be explained by a myriad of factors. These include sporting opportunities providing a sense purpose and positive social network for people with SCI (Hawkins et al., 2014; Tasiemski & Brewer, 2011).

A CRITICAL APPROACH TO PHYSICAL ACTIVITY PROMOTION

Despite the health and well-being benefits gained from regular physical activity, people with SCI are among the most inactive in society (Martin Ginis et al., 2010). This lack of activity is the result of multiple barriers constraining a physically active lifestyle (Williams et al., 2014). To address these barriers, physical activity participation and promotion is a key consideration within SCI research and practice (Martin Ginis et al., 2018; Williams et al., 2018a). This focus is in line with the ongoing and expanding global health initiative known as 'Exercise is Medicine' (EiM). The EiM movement is committed to the belief that promoting physical activity is integral for the prevention, management and treatment of a variety of clinical health issues and diseases (Lobelo et al., 2014; Sallis, 2015). In SCI populations, the EiM movement has been conceptualized as a cultural narrative telling a story of improved health and well-being through engagement in SCI (Papathomas et al., 2015), and the preferred narrative within rehabilitation and community contexts (Williams et al., 2018a). Yet within physical activity research, a more critical approach to physical activity promotion by health and exercise professionals and practitioners has been called for (Williams et al., 2014; Williams et al., 2018b).

One concern is that the EiM movement promotes a neoliberal health role whereby individuals are expected to take responsibility for their health and well-being by exercising regularly for their own good (Berryman, 2010). The issue with this personal accountability is that it ignores the social, environmental and cultural barriers preventing people with SCI from leading a physically active lifestyle (Williams et al., 2014). Thus, the neoliberal health role ignores disablism – a form of social oppression – that arises from disabling and discriminatory conditions which impede activities such as sport and exercise participation (Smith & Perrier, 2014). When people with SCI are motivated to be physically active, but cannot access any sport and exercise opportunities, their health and well-being will be negatively impacted (Williams et al., 2014).

Another issue with EiM is when exercise is *perceived as medicine* and people are motivated to be physically active in pursuit of cure from SCI (Williams et al., 2018b). These stories align with the dominant narrative of restitution, which projects hope of recovery following illness and injury (Frank, 2013). For example, restitution has been identified as the dominant narrative structure in stories of SCI acquired through rugby (Smith & Sparkes, 2005), and in stories of exercise following SCI (Papathomas et al., 2015). The restitution narrative aligns with concrete hopes of recovery from SCI whereby people are seeking to return to their pre-injured and pre-disabled identity. The exercise in restitution narrative provides a subtle modification to the restitution narrative where exercise – rather than technological or medical breakthroughs – is the primary means by which a person can return to their former self (Papathomas et al., 2015).

Although restitution can be useful in facilitating a commitment to exercise, the danger is what happens when recovery is not possible? When restitution is not forthcoming, individuals need other stories to live by; otherwise, they can be plunged into a chaotic existence where all hopes of a future worth living are lost (Frank, 2013). Indeed, health and exercise professionals and practitioners face a delicate situation of fostering hopefulness of the future, without promoting false hope of recovery from SCI (Williams et al., 2018a). If exercise is indeed medicine for people with SCI, then we might need to begin promoting and prescribing it in an ethical way (Williams et al., 2018b). This may include being aware of individual's circumstances, passions and priorities to avoid feelings of guilt and self-blame when exercise adherence becomes difficult, or unexpected disappointment when desired outcomes from exercise are not achieved. Furthermore, sharing stories can expand people's narrative resources by highlighting multiple and alternative possibilities following SCI.

CONCLUSION

This chapter explores the catastrophic nature of SCI and the accompanying challenges individuals face in improving and maintaining their health and well-being. Such challenges are brought about by a loss of function and mobility, which predisposes people with SCI to secondary health conditions and a decreased quality of life. The benefits of leading a physically active lifestyle following SCI in alleviating or preventing these health and well-being complications have been highlighted. For example, exercising can improve health and fitness, and playing sport can foster an athletic identity and positive psychological adjustment. That said, this chapter warns against an EiM approach, which promotes physical activity as a cure for all ills and calls upon individuals to take responsibility to be active for their own good. Health and exercise professionals and practitioners are therefore encouraged to take an ethical approach to physical activity promotion and prescription. This includes recognizing the social, cultural and environmental barriers preventing participation, and sharing stories which highlight alternative narratives following SCI.

Case study

The following case study is based upon life-history interviews with individuals with SCI adapted from multiple research projects (see Soundy et al., 2010; Williams et al., 2018b). Please read the case study carefully and consider the questions below.

Mark was 19 years old studying Sport and Exercise Science at university alongside playing for a premiership rugby academy. His dream was to be selected for the first team and play professionally once he had finished his degree course this year. Mark was playing a competitive academy match against a local rival team towards the end of the season. The match was important to Mark as he knew his performance on the pitch could influence his chances of having his contract renewed with the club. In the first half of the rugby match, Mark was feeling sluggish and stiff. He had taken a bad hit to the thigh in training a few days before and hadn't quite recovered. He didn't let on to any of the athlete support personnel or his teammates that he was struggling and managed to avoid any heavy contact in this part of the game.

At half time, the captain called for the team to turn up the pressure on the other side. They were losing the match, but only by one try. They could still win. In the second half, Mark saw an opening and managed to score a try. His teammate Derek converted. They were now in the lead. Determined to keep the win, Mark's gameplay became more aggressive. The other team were coming at them hard, and Mark decided to lead the charge in response. Their centre player had the ball and Mark decided to take him high. Then as the centre got closer, Mark changed his position at the last minute and went low. At the same time, the centre dipped his shoulder to change direction, and his shoulder hit Mark squarely in the top of the head. BANG! It sounded like a gunshot going off. Mark was left lying on the ground feeling weightless. He was not in any pain, but unable to feel or move his arms and legs. This was the moment when Mark became paralyzed.

After the incident, Mark was devastated. The first few months in hospital were particularly challenging. But this is where Mark made the decision to fight for his life. He was determined to get back to his old self and identity as a rugby player. Being able to play rugby involved beating his paralysis and learning to walk again. He was willing to do everything in his power to make this possible. Following discharge from hospital 6 months later, Mark started an activity-based rehabilitation (ABR) programme. ABR is characterized by individual intensive exercise programmes aiming to improve physiological, functional and neurological outcomes. Mark stayed near the ABR centre for a week so that he could participate in the programme as much as possible. He then made the 5-h journey back home with his parents every weekend to watch the rugby matches he can no longer play in. So far, Mark has not regained any function or had any sensation returned below the level of injury. But he is not giving up. He will walk again.

1. What psychosocial factors may have increased Mark's risk of injury?
2. What narrative type do you think best fits Mark's story?
3. What are the possible benefits and pitfalls for Mark when telling this type of story?

References

Ahuja, C. S., Wilson, J. R., Nori, S., Kotter, M. R. N., Druschel, C., Curt, A., & Fehlings, M. G. (2017). Traumatic spinal cord injury. *Nature Reviews Disease Primers*, 3, 17018. DOI: 10.1038/nrdp.2017.18.

Berryman, J. W. (2010). Exercise is medicine: A historical perspective. *Current Sports Medicine Reports, 9*(4), 195–201. DOI: 10.1249/JSR.0b013e3181e7d86d.

Buchholz, A. C., Martin Ginis, K. A., Bray, S. R., Craven, B. C., Hicks, A. L., Hayes, K. C., Latimer, A. E., McColl M. A., Potter, P. J., & Wolfe, D. L. (2009). Greater daily leisure time physical activity is associated with lower chronic disease risk in adults with spinal cord injury. *Applied Physiology, Nutrition and Metabolism, 34*, 640–647. DOI: 10.1139/H09-050.

Canning, K. L., & Hicks, A. L. (2014). Secondary health conditions associated with spinal cord injury. *Critical Reviews in Physical and Rehabilitation Medicine, 26*, 181–191. DOI: 10.1615/CritRevPhysRehabilMed.2014011067.

Chan, C. W. L., Eng, C. J. J., Tator, C. H., Krassioukov, A., & the Spinal Cord Injury Research Evidence Team. (2016). Epidemiology of sport-related spinal cord injuries: A systematic review. *The Journal of Spinal Cord Medicine, 39*, 255–264. DOI: 10.1080/10790268.2016.1138601.

Chun, S., & Lee, Y. (2010). The role of leisure in the experience of posttraumatic growth for people with spinal cord injury. *Journal of Leisure Research, 42*, 393–415. DOI: 10.1080/00222216.2010.11950211.

Craig, A., Tran, Y., & Middleton, J. (2009). Psychological morbidity and spinal cord injury: A systematic review. *Spinal Cord, 47*, 108–114. DOI: 10.1038/sc.2008.115.

Day, M. C. (2013). The role of initial physical activity experiences in promoting posttraumatic growth in Paralympic athletes with an acquired disability. *Disability and Rehabilitation, 35*, 2064–2072. DOI: 10.3109/09638288.2013.805822.

Frank, A. W. (2013). *The wounded storyteller* (2nd ed.). University of Chicago Press.

Geyh, S., Nick, E., Stirnimann, D., Ehrat, S., Müller, R., & Michel, F. (2012). Biopsychosocial outcomes in individuals with and without spinal cord injury: A Swiss comparative study. *Spinal Cord, 50*, 614–622. DOI: 10.1038/sc.2012.21.

Hawkins, C., Coffee, P., & Soundy, A. (2014). Considering how athletic identity assists adjustment to spinal cord injury: A qualitative study. *Physiotherapy, 100*, 268–274, DOI: 10.1016/j.physio.2013.09.006.

Hicks, A. L., Martin, K. A., Ditor, D. S., Latimer, A. E., Craven, C., Bugaresti, J., & McCartney N. (2003). Long-term exercise training in persons with spinal cord injury: Effects on strength, arm ergometry performance and psychological well-being. *Spinal Cord, 41*, 34–43. DOI: 10.1038/sj.sc.3101389.

Hitzig, S. L., Tonack, M., Campbell, K., McGillivray, C. F., Boschen, K., Richards, K., & Craven, C. B. (2008). Secondary health complications in an aging Canadian spinal cord injury sample. *American Journal of Physical Medicine and Rehabilitation, 87*, 545–555. DOI: 10.1097/PHM.0b013e31817c16d6.

Keyes, C. L., Shmotkin, D., & Ryff, C. D. (2002). Optimizing well-being: The empirical encounter of two traditions. *Journal of Personality and Social Psychology, 82*, 1007–1022. DOI: 10.1037/0022-3514.82.6.1007.

Krause, K. S., & Saunders, L. L. (2011). Health, secondary conditions, and life expectancy after spinal cord injury. *Archives of Physical Medicine and Rehabilitation, 92*, 1770–1775. DOI: 10.1016/j.apmr.2011.05.024.

Levins, S. M., Redenbach, D. M., & Dyck, I. (2004). Individual and societal influences on participation in physical activity following spinal cord injury: A qualitative study. *Physical Therapy, 84*, 496–509. DOI: 10.1093/ptj/84.6.496.

Lobelo, F., Stoutenberg, M., & Hutber, A. (2014). The exercise is medicine global health initiative: A 2014 update. *British Journal of Sports Medicine, 48,* 1627–1633. DOI: 10.1136/bjsports-2013-093080.

Martin Ginis, K. A., Jörgensen, S., & Stapleton, J. (2012). Exercise and sport for persons with spinal cord injury. *PM&R, 4,* 894–900. DOI: 10.1016/j.pmrj.2012.08.006.

Martin Ginis, K. A., Latimer, A. E., Arbour-Nicitopoulos, K. P., Buchholz, A. C., Bray, S., Craven, B. C., Hayes, K. C., Hicks, A. L., McColl, M. A., Potter, P. J., Smith, K., & Wolfe, D. L. (2010). Leisure time physical activity in a population-based sample of people with spinal cord injury. Part I: Demographic and injury-related correlates. *Archives of Physical Medicine and Rehabilitation, 91,* 722–728. DOI: 10.1016/j.apmr.2009.12.027.

Martin Ginis, K. A., van der Scheer, J. W., Latimer-Cheung, A. E., Barrow, A. Bourne, C, & Goosey-Tolfrey, V. L. (2018). Evidence-based scientific exercise guidelines for adults with spinal cord injury: An update and a new guideline. *Spinal Cord, 56,* 308–321. DOI: 10.1038/s41393-017-0017-3.

Nadarajah, V., Jauregui, J. J., Perfetti, D., Shasti, M., Koh, E. Y., & Henn III, R. F. (2017). What are the trends and demographics in sports-related pediatric spinal cord injuries? *The Physician and Sportsmedicine, 46,* 8–13. DOI: 10.1080/00913847.2018.1408384.

Norrbrink, C., Lindberg, T., Wahman, K., & Bjerkefors, A. (2012). Effects of an exercise programme on musculoskeletal and neuropathic pain after spinal cord injury—Results from a seated double-poling ergometer study. *Spinal Cord, 50,* 457–461. DOI: 10.1038/sc.2011.160.

Nunnerley, J., Hay-Smith, E., & Dean, S. (2013). Leaving a spinal unit and returning to the wider community: An interpretative phenomenological analysis. *Disability and Rehabilitation, 35,* 1165–1173. DOI: 10.3109/09638288.2012.723789.

O'Brien, A., Renwick, R., & Yoshida, K. (2008). Leisure participation for individuals living with acquired spinal cord injury. *International Journal of Rehabilitation Research, 31,* 225–230. DOI: 0.1097/MRR.0b013e3282fb7d13.

Papathomas, A., Williams, T. L., & Smith, B. (2015). Understanding physical activity participation in spinal cord injured populations: Three narrative types for consideration. *International Journal of Qualitative Studies on Health and Well-being, 14*(10), 27295. DOI: 10.3402/qhw.v10.27295.

Patel, S. A., Vaccaro, A. R., & Rihn, J. A. (2013). Epidemiology of spinal injuries in sports. *Operative Techniques in Sports Medicine, 21,* 146–151. DOI: 10.1053/j.otsm.2013.10.003.

Post, M. W. M., & Van Leeuwen, C. M. C. (2012). Psychosocial issues in spinal cord injury: A review. *Spinal Cord, 50,* 382–389. DOI: 10.1038/sc.2011.182.

Ryan, R. M., & Deci, E. L. (2001). On happiness and human potentials: A review of research on hedonic and eudaimonic well-being. *Annual Review of Psychology, 52,* 141–166. DOI: 10.1146/annurev.psych.52.1.141.

Sallis, R. (2015). Exercise is medicine: A call to action for physicians to assess and prescribe exercise. *The Physician and Sportsmedicine, 43,* 22–26. DOI: 10.1080/00913847.2015.1001938.

Singh, A., Tetreault, L., Kalsi-Ryan, S., Nouri, A., & Fehlings, M.G. (2014). Global prevalence and incidence of traumatic spinal cord injury. *Clinical Epidemiology, 6,* 309–311. DOI: 10.2147/CLEP.S68889.

Smith, B., & Perrier, M-J. (2014) Disability, sport, and impaired bodies: A critical approach. In R. J. Schinke &K. R. McGannon (Eds.), *The psychology of sub-culture in sport and physical activity: A critical approach* (pp. 95–106). Routledge.

Smith, B., & Sparkes, A. C. (2005). Men, sport, spinal cord injury and narratives of hope. *Social Science & Medicine*, *61*, 1095–1105. DOI: 10.1016/j.socscimed.2005.01.011.

Soundy, A., Smith, B., Cressy, F., & Webb, L. (2010). The experience of spinal cord injury: Using Frank's narrative types to enhance physiotherapy undergraduates' understanding. *Physiotherapy*, *96*, 52–58. DOI: 10.1016/j.physio.2009.06.001.

Stephens, C., Neil, R., & Smith, P. (2012). The perceived benefits and barriers of sport in spinal cord injured individuals: A qualitative study. *Disability and Rehabilitation*, *34*, 2061–2070. DOI: 10.3109/09638288.2012.669020.

Tasiemski, T. &Brewer, B. W. (2011). Athletic identity, sport participation, and psychological adjustment in people with spinal cord injury. *Adapted Physical Activity Quarterly*, *28*, 233–250. DOI: 10.1123/apaq.28.3.233.

van der Scheer, J. W., Martin Ginis, K. A., Ditor, D. S., Goosey-Tolfrey, V. L., Hicks, A. L., West, C. R., & Wolfe, D. L. (2017). Effects of exercise on fitness and health of adults with spinal cord injury: A systematic review. *Neurology*, *89*. DOI: 10.1212/WNL.0000000000004224.

Williams, R., & Murray, A. (2015). Prevalence of depression after spinal cord injury: A meta-analysis. *Archives of Physical Medicine and Rehabilitation*, *96*, 133–140. DOI: 10.1016/j.apmr.2014.08.016.

Williams, T. L., Hunt, E. R., Papathomas, A., & Smith, B. (2018b). Exercise is medicine? Most of the time for most: But not always for all. *Qualitative Research in Sport, Exercise and Health*, *10*, 441–456. DOI: 10.1080/2159676X.2017.1405363.

Williams, T. L., Smith, B., & Papathomas, A. (2014). The barriers, benefits and facilitators of leisure time physical activity among people with spinal cord injury: A meta-synthesis of qualitative findings. *Health Psychology Review*, *8*, 404–425. DOI: 10.1080/17437199.2014.898406.

Williams, T. L., Smith, B., & Papathomas, A. (2018a). Physical activity promotion for people with spinal cord injury: Physiotherapists' beliefs and actions. *Disability and Rehabilitation*, *40*, 52–61, DOI: 10.1080/09638288.2016.1242176.

World Health Organization. (2020). *Spinal Cord Injury*. https://www.who.int/newsroom/fact-sheets/detail/spinal-cord-injury [accessed 10 January 2020].

15 'BUT I NEED YOU TO PLAY'

COACH INFLUENCES ON ATHLETE AND TEAM MEDICAL OUTCOMES

Dr Adam Gledhill

'But I need you to play': a statement that many of us will have heard at some point during our careers as either athletes or practitioners. The connotations from this statement are wide ranging: 'Does my coach value me that much that I should play?'; 'Does this mean we'll likely lose if I don't play?'; 'What does it say about everyone else if I'm expected to play when I'm not really ready?'; for many athletes faced with this statement, though, the response would simply be something akin to 'sure, boss, no problem', wherever possible. A simple statement can have many meanings and implications for athletes, all of which are generally related to the power and influence that a coach has within their team environment. We assert that how coaches choose to use that power and influence will be a significant contributory factor to athlete and team medical outcomes, specifically injury risk and the success of rehabilitation outcomes.

For the purposes of this chapter, the 'coach' is someone who has influence over the team in terms of team selection/de-selection, tactical decisions, recruitment etc. This person might be the head coach, or one of the members of the coaching staff; ultimately, the influence that they have is an instrumental factor in the power dynamic of their relationship with athletes. Often, the coach is viewed within the psychology of sports injury literature as either the harbinger of doom who puts unrealistic expectations on athletes and causes injuries or is the hero of the story whereby they've created a psychologically safe environment and meet athletes' support needs during the return-to-sport journey (Gledhill & Forsdyke, 2018a). As such, our aim through this chapter is threefold: (1) to discuss the coach's role in injury risk, (2) to discuss the coach's role in injury rehabilitation and return to sport and (3) to present an applied case study for consideration.

THE COACH'S ROLE IN INJURY RISK

There is opinion that, in elite sport at least, the head coach is the most important person when it comes to injury risk (Ekstrand, 2019). When considering the coach's role in injury risk, there is an emergent pattern that indicates coaches, their influences and their behaviours can either increase or decrease an athlete's re-injury risk (e.g. Ekstrand et al., 2018; Pensgaard et al., 2018; Steffen et al., 2013). Some of the reported patterns also provide some level of understanding regarding the differences in risk of acute versus overuse injuries (Gledhill & Forsdyke, 2018a).

Coach-athlete interactions and injury risk

When considering coach-player interactions, coach behaviours have been associated with injury risk in athletes. For example, athletes experiencing different indices of transformational leadership (e.g. coach vision, supportive leadership, encouragement of development) appear to be at a reduced risk of injury (Ekstrand et al., 2018). An athlete's relationship with their coach might also be a risk factor for sports injury. Athletes who find it difficult to communicate with their coach may under-report pain and injury, particularly under-reporting the onset of injuries (Roderick et al., 2000). Further, poor communication between athletes and coaches is recognized by both athletes and coaches as a risk factor for overuse injuries in sport (van Wilgen & Verhagen, 2012), whereas open communication between athletes and coaches is viewed as an important element of injury prevention (Bolling et al., 2020). Moreover, where the coach is a source of stress, athletes are at a higher risk of overuse injuries (Pensgaard et al., 2018). Furthermore, in parasport athletes, there is a reported view that coaches do not fully understand athletes' needs or the needs of specific impairments and may not be able to effectively structure training, which leads to a sense of inequality and lacking important pre-requisites (Fagher et al., 2016). Athletes perceive these factors to increase their sports injury risk and report them as a source of stress.

These findings related to coach-athlete interactions and their impact on injury risk can largely be explained through the Biopsychosocial Model of Athletic Injury and Health (Appaneal & Perna, 2014). This model suggests that negative life event stress (such as the coach as a life event stressor) elicits stress responses that contribute to physiological mechanisms such as impaired skeletal muscle repair and immunosuppression, as well as behavioural mechanisms such as impaired self-care and poor sleep quality. Collectively, these physiological and behavioural mechanisms can create overtraining-like symptoms in athletes and lead to outcomes including increased injury risk or longer injury recovery times.

Coach-support team interactions and injury risk

In the highest levels of sport, specifically Olympic sports and elite football, interactions between the coach and other stakeholders (e.g. medical personnel) are also suggested to influence injury risk and prevention in sport (e.g. Bolling et al., 2020; Ekstrand, 2019; Ekstrand et al., 2019). Communication between the head coach/manager is vital for keeping football players in the pitch in elite football (Ekstrand, 2019). Clubs with good quality internal communication suffer fewer injuries and experience greater player availability in elite football, when compared to clubs with poor communication. Internal communication between the head coach and the medical team is of great importance, with low or poor communication quality between the head coach and the medical team significantly associated with the injury rate (Ekstrand et al., 2019). Consequently, the notion of 'communicate and co-operate' appears to be an important one for increasing player availability in elite football (Ekstrand, 2019) and is perceived to be important in reducing injury risk in Olympic sports (Bolling et al., 2020).

Coach education and injury risk

The final element of the coach's roles in injury risk is the notion of coach development (e.g. Ageberg et al., 2019; Ekstrand 2019; Fagher et al., 2016; Soligard et al., 2010). Coach development in the form of education is likely to impact on a coach's willingness to implement injury prevention programmes in sport (Ageberg et al., 2019; Ekstrand 2019; Fagher et al., 2016; Soligard et al., 2010). This education may be in the form of understanding how injury prevention correlates to team success (Ekstrand, 2019), learning about and experiencing injury prevention programmes to increase a coach's belief in their ability to implement the programme (Ageberg et al., 2019; Soligard et al., 2010) or learning about the specific needs of athletes (Fagher et al., 2016).

Irrespective of the type of education, there is a view that educating coaches can improve their attitude towards adopting injury prevention programmes (Soligard et al., 2010). This improved attitude and understanding, however, does not necessarily guarantee implementation of injury prevention programmes (Frank et al., 2015; Lindblom et al., 2018). However, in instances where it is appropriate to do so (e.g. amateur sport; youth sport), coach education can lead to a coach's efficacy beliefs in their ability to lead or deliver injury prevention programmes, which is important as coach-led or coach-facilitated delivery of injury prevention programmes can significantly reduce injury risk (Hägglund et al., 2007; Steffen et al., 2013). The likely explanation for this is that coach-led or coach-facilitated injury prevention programmes tend to result in higher athlete compliance and higher compliance is associated with reduced injury risk (Steffen et al., 2013). Ergo, it is apparent that coach education around injury prevention empowers coaches to make informed decisions about adopting behaviours that will ultimately reduce injury risks for their athletes.

THE COACH'S ROLE IN INJURY REHABILITATION AND RETURN TO SPORT

As well as influencing injury risk, the coach is also an important factor during return to sport. Of course, the points above regarding the coach's role in injury risk are also important when it comes to re-injury risk. Anything that is an injury *risk* factor is also a *reinjury* risk factor. Consequently, the points made above, especially those relating to the coach's roles in facilitating athletes' completion of re-injury prevention programmes, effective communication and the coach as a life stressor, are important during the rehabilitation period as well (e.g. Forsdyke et al., 2016; Podlog & Dionigi, 2010). In framing the next part of this chapter, we consider 'rehabilitation' as the process of returning to at least pre-injury levels of performance, transitioning through the stages of return to participation, return to sport and return to performance (Ardern et al., 2016).

THE COACH, SOCIAL SUPPORT AND INJURY REHABILITATION

During injury rehabilitation, coaches can either be a stressor or a stress buffer for athletes (Forsdyke & Gledhill, 2014) and this can influence how the athlete thinks, feels and acts (Forsdyke et al., 2016). Developing strong coach-athlete relationships is fundamental to supporting athletes through their injury (Bianco, 2020). Not least of which is because coaches recognize that they have an important role as a key social support provider or facilitator during injury rehabilitation and they need to understand athletes' needs to fulfil this role (e.g. Gledhill et al., 2020; Gledhill & Forsdyke, 2018a; Podlog & Dionigi, 2010; Podlog & Eklund, 2007; Podlog et al., 2013). This supports and includes directly providing informational, emotional and tangible support at different times throughout rehabilitation (Bianco, 2020). In youth sport, the coach can also impact on the social support relationships away from sport, such as player-parent dyads (Gledhill et al., 2015).

As well as directly providing social support, coaches can have important role in facilitating access to other athletes who have experienced similar injuries (Podlog & Dionigi, 2010), which can have benefits for both the provider and receiver of social support (e.g. Brown et al., 2018). Given the range of rehabilitation, cognitive, social and even financial stressors experienced by athletes (Bianco, 2020), and combined with the perceived importance of the coach on influencing athletes' careers (e.g. Mitchell et al., 2020), it is perhaps unsurprising that social support provision by coaches is chief amongst the coach-focused recommendations for facilitating return to sport (Forsdyke et al., 2016). It is also important, however, that coaches recognize the limitations of the extent of social support that they can provide and that they have an appropriate referral network in place.

THE COACH AND THE INJURY REHABILITATION ENVIRONMENT

A thread throughout this chapter is that the coach is a strong cultural architect during sports injury (e.g. Ekstrand et al., 2019) and this can extend to informing the rehabilitation environment (Podlog & Dionigi, 2010; Podlog & Eklund, 2007). For example, coaches facilitating injured players' access to the team environment is interpreted as supporting rehabilitation activities (Gledhill et al., 2015) as it can help athletes maintain a sense of identity with their team and their sport (Forsdyke et al., 2016). However, coaches do recognize the importance of striking the right balance in this respect, between facilitating access to the team environment and in ensuring that they aren't throwing the injury in the athlete's face, by constantly having them in an environment where they can't be an athlete in the way they would like (Podlog & Dionigi, 2010). Open, honest and regular communication between coaches, athletes and the medical team (e.g. 'checking in' once per week) and communicating with the athlete about this outside of sport as well as in sport will likely give a good indicator of the athlete's progress generally but will also help with decision-making about their involvement with the sporting environment.

More broadly, the coach can be an architect in creating a more positive environment that supports appropriate goal-directed behaviours (Gledhill et al., 2020; Podlog & Dionigi, 2010; Podlog & Eklund, 2007). By helping athletes to focus on what they can do, as opposed to focusing on what they can't do, the coach can have an important impact on how the injured athlete views their injury experience and the degree to which they engage with it (Podlog & Dionigi, 2010; Podlog et al., 2013). Creating a culture and environment whereby the athlete retains a sense of value to the team despite not being able to compete, as opposed to simply discarding the injured athlete until they can play again, is also an important part of facilitating athletes' progress through rehabilitation (Gledhill et al., 2015; Podlog et al., 2013). It is likely that this will impact on an athlete's mood state (Forsdyke et al., 2016) and support their rehabilitation adherence (Goddard et al., 2020).

THE COACH AND RETURN-TO-SPORT DECISION-MAKING

The coach also has an important role to play as part of an athlete-centred, shared decision-making approach regarding return to sport post-injury (Gledhill & Forsdyke, 2018b; King et al., 2019). Within this, the coach may be able to provide feedback regarding re-integration into the sport environment, inform appropriate return-to-sport goals from a technical and tactical perspective and generally work collaboratively with the athlete and support team (Gledhill et al., 2020).

There is also a widely held view that coaches can increase or decrease perceptions of pressure to return to sport (e.g. Dyer & Holt, 2018; Owen, 2019; Philips & Niyonsenga, 2013; Podlog & Dionigi, 2010), which can impact on the return-to-sport decisions. It is not uncommon that sport belies a hyper-masculine culture, which normalizes pain and increases the likelihood of risk-taking behaviours following injury (Truong et al., 2020). In this, the coach can become an important instrument in setting the return-to-sport culture, whereby if there is increased pressure for premature return to sport, this is likely to increase re-injury risk and worsen rehabilitation outcomes (Forsdyke et al., 2016).

However, this pressure to return to sport is not a one-way street. The coach may also experience pressure from players, parents and other key stakeholders to allow players to return to sport earlier than expected. This pressure has multiple foundations, not least of which might be that injury is a perceived barrier to successful athletic career transitions (e.g. Mitchell et al., 2020). Consequently, whilst it is important that coaches provide and facilitate social support for injured athletes, it is also important to recognize that coaches have their own social support needs and can even vicariously experience some of the player-level stressors during injury. Hence, it is important that the social support needs of coaches are also met.

CONCLUSION

Ultimately, every coach's ideal situation is to have as many healthy athletes available for selection as possible (Ekstrand, 2019); therefore, coaches understanding their role in injury prevention is imperative. Adopting transformational leadership principles, creating a threat-free environment that fosters open communication, and educating themselves around injury prevention and strategies for player availability, and, where appropriate, facilitating athletes' injury prevention programme completion, are all likely to go some way towards supporting coaches in achieving their aims of player availability. However, athletes get injured. That's just a fact of sporting life. Therefore, once an athlete has become injured, every coach wants their athlete to make as timely a return to sport as possible, whilst achieving at least pre-injury levels of performance, and remaining injury-free upon return (e.g. Ardern et al., 2016; Forsdyke et al., 2016). This is a 'perfect storm' of challenges for athletes and injury practitioners, one in which coaches play a central role in achieving. Being an effective social support provider and facilitator, facilitating athletes' balanced involvement in the sporting environment, fostering open and effective communication, adopting an athlete-centred, shared decision-making approach and avoiding the pressure for premature return to sport post-injury are all strategies that will help athletes, medical personnel and coaches to navigate this perfect storm.

Case study

Ravinder is a 19-year-old Rugby league player, who is 7 months into his first 1-year professional contract with his boyhood club. He progressed through the youth ranks at the club and is well known to the coaching and support staff as a result. Currently, the clubs have not offered him a contract extension but have spoken to him about the possibility of a new deal. Ravinder and his coaches speak regularly about his development as a player as he has not regularly represented the first team as yet, but they rarely show any interest in him or his life outside of Rugby. The staff say they prefer to keep their personal and professional lives separate. Ravinder has recently got engaged to his long-term partner and they have a child on the way, but this is from an unplanned pregnancy.

For the past 5 weeks or so, Ravinder has noticed that something 'doesn't feel right' in his shoulder. He has some stiffness in his shoulder and it sometimes feels like it is grinding and about to lock in place. He can't move it as far or as easily as usual and he has noticed that the affected shoulder feels a little weaker than the other. Because of these things, Ravinder has started to guard his shoulder a little more during training and doesn't perform his sporting movements to the fullest extent or with his normal intent. His coaches have noticed that his training levels haven't been up to the required standard and have mentioned this to Ravinder, but he doesn't want to say anything to them about his injury because of the uncertainty over his contractual situation. Ravinder confided to his best friend in the team about the situation with his shoulder, who told him not to worry about it because 'shoulder pain is just part of rugby' and that he should 'just carry on because coaches don't give contracts to injured players who don't play'. Ravinder also spoke to one of the more senior players on the team for some advice, who told Ravinder that 'he's in a man's world now' and needs to 'man up'.

A more senior player in the team is now out for the rest of the season with an injury and the coach has told Ravinder that he needs him to play in an upcoming game. Ravinder doesn't know whether he should play.

Questions

1. What are the key injury risk factors within the case study?
2. If you are a part of the support staff in this scenario, what ideas could you discuss with Ravinder to support his decision-making about whether he should play?
3. What are the key recommendations you would make about the sporting environment, to reduce the level of risk for athlete like Ravinder?

References

Ageberg, E., Bunke, S., Lucander, K., Nilsen, P., & Donaldson, A. (2019). Facilitators to support the implementation of injury prevention training in youth handball: A concept mapping approach. *Scandinavian Journal of Medicine and Science in Sports, 29*, 275–285.

Appaneal, R. N., & Perna, F. M. (2014). Biopsychosocial model of injury. In R. Eklund, & G. Tenenbaum (Eds.), *Encyclopedia of sport and exercise psychology* (pp. 73–77). SAGE.

Ardern, C. L., Glasgow, P., Schneiders, A., Witvrouw, E., Clarsen, B., Cools, A., Gojanovic, B., Griffin, S., Khan K. M., Moksnes, H., Mutch, S. A., Phillips, N., Reurink, G., Sadler, R., Silbernagel, K. G., Thorborg, K., Wangensteen, A., Wilk, K. E., & Bizzini, M. (2016). 2016 Consensus statement on return to sport from the First World Congress in Sports Physical Therapy, Bern. *British Journal of Sports Medicine, 50*, 853–864.

Bianco, T. (2020). Sport injury and the need for coach support. In A. Ivarsson, U. Johnson (Eds.), *Psychological bases of sports injuries* (4th ed.; pp. 223–242). Fitness Information Technology.

Bolling, C., Barboza, S. D., van Mechelen, W., & Pasman, H. R. (2020). Letting the cat out of the bag: Athletes, coaches and physiotherapists share their perspectives on injury prevention in elite sports. *British Journal of Sports Medicine, 54*, 871–877.

Brown, C., Webb, T., Robinson, M., & Cotgreave, R. (2018). Athletes' experiences of social support during their transition out of elite sport: An interpretive phenomenological analysis. *Psychology of Sport and Exercise, 36*, 71–80.

Dyer, K., & Holt, O. (2018). *Old too soon, smart too late*. London: Headline Publishing Group.

Ekstrand, J. (2019). Lessons learned from two decades of injury surveillance in elite football. *Aspetar Sports Medicine Journal, 8*, 12–16.

Ekstrand, J., Lundqvist, D., Davison, M., D'Hooghe, M., & Pensgaard, A-M. (2019). Communication quality between the medical team and the head coach/manager is associated with injury burden and player availability in elite football clubs. *British Journal of Sports Medicine, 53*, 304–308.

Ekstrand, J., Lundqvist, D., & Lagerbäck, L. (2018). Is there a correlation between coaches' leadership styles and injuries in elite football teams? A study of 36 teams across 17 countries. *British Journal of Sports Medicine, 52*, 527–531.

Fagher, K., Forsberg, A., Jacobsson, J., Timpka, T., Dahlström, Ö., & Lexell, J. (2016). Paralympic athletes' perceptions of their experiences of sports-related injuries, risk factors and preventative possibilities. *European Journal of Sport Science, 16*, 1240–1249.

Forsdyke, D., & Gledhill, A. (2014). Reaching out for a helping hand: The role of social support in sports injury rehabilitation. *SportEx Medicine, 61*, 8–12.

Forsdyke, D., Smith, A., Jones, M., & Gledhill, A. (2016). Psychosocial factors associated with outcomes of sports injury rehabilitation in competitive athletes: A mixed studies systematic review. *British Journal of Sports Medicine.*, *50*, 537–544.

Frank, B. S., Register-Mihalik, J., & Padua, D. A. (2015). High levels of coach intent to integrate an ACL injury prevention program into training does not translate to effective implementation. *Journal of Science and Medicine in Sport*, *18*, 400–406.

Gledhill, A. Ahmed, O. H., & Forsdyke, D. (2020). Effectively managing anterior cruciate ligament injury and return to performance in elite women's soccer. In J. Dixon, J. Barker, R. Thelwell, & I. Mitchell (Eds.), *The Psychology of Soccer*. Routledge.

Gledhill, A., & Forsdyke, D. (2018a). Football coaches' roles in achieving player and team medical outcomes of (re)injury prevention and successful return to performance: A realist synthesis. *Journal of Sports Sciences*, *36*(S1), 13.

Gledhill, A., & Forsdyke, D. (2018b). Return to sport: On the way off the pitch, my first thought was: "How fast can I be back?". *BASEM Today*, *45*, 36–37.

Gledhill, A., & Forsdyke, D., & Sutton, G. (2015). The role of player–parent dyads in sports injury rehabilitation and the return to competition of elite female youth soccer players. *Journal of Sports Sciences*, *33*(S1), S72–S74.

Goddard, K., Roberts, C-M., Byron-Daniel, J., & Woodford, L. (2020). Psychological factors involved in adherence to sport injury rehabilitation: A systematic review. *International Review of Sport and Exercise Psychology*. DOI: 10.1080/1750984X.2020.1744179

Hägglund, M., Waldén, M., & Ekstrand, J. (2007). Lower re-injury rate with a coach-controlled rehabilitation programme in amateur male soccer. *American Journal of Sports Medicine*, *35*, 1433–1442.

King, J., Roberts, C., Hard, S., & Ardern, C. L. (2019). Want to improve return to sport outcomes following injury? Empower, engage, provide feedback and be transparent: 4 habits! *British Journal of Sports Medicine*, *53*, 526–527.

Lindblom, H., Carlfjord, S., & Hägglund, M. (2018). Adoption and use of an injury prevention exercise program in female football: A qualitative study among coaches. *Scandinavian Journal of Medicine and Science in Sports*, *28*, 1295–1303.

Mitchell, T., Gledhill, A., Nesti, M., Richardson, D., & Littlewood, M. (2020). Practitioner perspectives on the barriers associated with youth to senior transition in elite youth soccer academy players. *International Sport Coaching Journal*, 1–10. https://doi.org/10.1123/iscj.2019-0015.

Owen, M. (2019). *Reboot: My life, my time*. Reach Sport.

Pensgaard, A-M., Ivarsson, A., Nilstad, A., Solstad, B. E., & Steffen, K. (2018). Psychosocial stress factors, including the relationship with the coach, and their influence on acute and overuse injury risk in elite female football players. *BMJ Open Sport and Exercise Medicine*, *4*, e000317. DOI: 10.1136/bmjsem-2017-000317.

Philips, J. S., & Niyonsenga, J. D. (2013). Injuries among female Rwandan soccer players: Return to play decisions. *African Journal of Physical, Heath Education, Recreation and Dance*, *4*, 1135–1145.

Podlog, L., & Dionigi, R. (2010). Coach strategies for addressing psychosocial challenges during the return to sport from injury. *Journal of Sports Sciences*, *28*, 1197–1208.

Podlog, L., & Eklund, R. C. (2007). Professional coaches' perspectives on the return to sport following serious injury. *Journal of Applied Sport Psychology*, *19*, 207–225.

Podlog, L., Wadey, R., Stark, A., Lochbaum, M., Hannon, J., & Newton, M. (2013). An adolescent perspective on injury recovery and return to sport. *Psychology of Sport and Exercise, 14*, 437–446.

Roderick, M., Waddington, I., & Parker, G. (2000). Playing hurt: Managing injuries in English professional football. *International Review for the Sociology of Sport, 35*, 165–180.

Soligard, T., Nilstad, A., Steffen, K., Myklebust, G., Holme, I., Dvorak, J., Bahr, R., & Andersen, T. E. (2010). Compliance with a comprehensive warm-up programme to prevent injuries in youth football. *British Journal of Sports Medicine, 44*, 787–793.

Steffen, K., Meeuwisse, W. H., Romiti, M., Kang, J., McKay, C., Bizzini, M., & Emery, C. A. (2013). Evaluation of how different implementation strategies of an injury prevention programme (FIFA 11+) impact team adherence and injury risk in Canadian female youth football players: A cluster-randomised trial. *British Journal of Sports Medicine, 47*, 480–487.

Truong, L. K., Mosewich, A. D., Holt, C. J., Le, C. Y., Miciak, M., & Whittaker, J. L. (2020). Psychological, social and contextual factors across recovery stages following a sport-related knee injury: A scoping review. *British Journal of Sports Medicine*. Epub ahead of print. DOI: 10.1136/bjsports-2019-101206.

Van Wilgen, C. P., & Verhagen, E. A. (2012). A qualitative study on overuse injuries: The beliefs of athletes and coaches. *Journal of Science and Medicine in Sport, 15*, 116–121.

16

THE COFFEE BREAK TO CLOSE THE BOOK ... WHERE DO WE GO FROM HERE?

Dr Adam Gledhill and Dr Dale Forsdyke

When we were approached about editing this book, our first thought was 'but there are already a few psychology of sports injury books out there', so our first aim was to look at how we can do things a little differently. In doing this, we tried to look at this book from the perspective of the 5Rs of sports injury (Gledhill & Forsdyke, 2015): risk, responses, rehabilitation, return to sport and retirement, and hoped to be able to provide a type of injury life-cycle perspective in one book. We hope you found this interesting and informative, as well having facilitated thought and debate where you can challenge the arguments and opinions offered herein. After all, that is how we advance everything that we do (Gledhill, 2020a). In the spirit of this last point, the question now lingers: 'Where do we go from here?'

Time to take a coffee break (or beer, or water, or hot chocolate ... you see where we're going with this...) and we'll guide you through some reflections that have emerged through our experiences, not only of research and practice within the context of psychology of sports injury but, importantly, through the development of this book. Broadly, we've grouped these under three headings: (1) important subjects to consider, (2) population considerations and (3) methodological considerations, but there is some natural overlap.

IMPORTANT SUBJECTS TO CONSIDER

First and speaking broadly, there is a much greater breadth and depth of research available around post-injury factors than pre-injury factors. As such, an important research consideration is how we best enhance our understanding of pre-injury factors (i.e. injury risk factors or injury prevention). Specifically, we currently understand very little about the psychology of overuse injuries or how these might be best prevented or at least have their risk reduced (Gledhill et al., 2018; Ivarsson et al., 2017). We also understand very little about athletes' experiences of these pre-injury factors; however, intuitively, we can suggest with some confidence that overuse injuries will be caused by a complex interaction of personal, social, behavioural and cultural considerations (e.g. Appaneal &

Perna, 2014; Pensgaard et al., 2018; Richardson et al., 2008; Tranaeus et al., 2014). Further exploration of these considerations and their interactions would serve to enhance the area further.

Since 2016, the Bern Consensus Statement on Return to Sport (Ardern et al., 2016) has emerged as central to the return to sport landscape. Whilst the consensus statement asserts that there will be different psychosocial challenges associated with transitions through the different stages, there is little research that has examined this. Such research would refine our understanding of these transitions and, thus, better position us to provide appropriate support and facilitate those transitions. In a world where there are calls for interdisciplinary teamwork between sport science and medicine practitioners in order to best care for the athlete (e.g. Ekstrand et al., 2019; Gledhill et al., 2018; Johnson et al., 2020), positioning work within the Bern consensus statement is also likely to provide a consistent language of stages of return to sport that all team members understand.

Understanding more about sport socioculture and the team environment is also likely to add value to the body of research. Whilst we are aware that these are important in terms of cultural norms and their impact on injury risk and rehabilitation (Wiese-Bjornstal, 2010), what is less evident in the body of research is how we can best create facilitative environments that offer appropriate levels of psychological safety for the athletes experiencing them. Given that such environments may reduce injury risk through addressing some significant risk factors (e.g. stress, stress response; Ivarsson et al., 2017), understanding how they are best developed, in an interdisciplinary manner, would be a helpful addition.

Finally, understanding more about barriers and facilitators to the translation of research findings into practice will be an important step for the body of research. If we consider injury prevention, there is consistent evidence that psychological intervention can reduce the risk of injuries (see Gledhill et al., 2018; Gledhill & Ivarsson, 2020; Ivarsson et al., 2017), yet the adoption of these evidence-informed suggestions in to practice is still not common place (Gledhill et al., 2018; Gledhill & Ivarsson, 2020; Johnson et al., 2020). Understanding barriers and facilitators will place us in a better position to provide the highest quality of support for athletes, by better understanding how we can adopt these evidence-informed approaches.

IMPORTANT POPULATIONS TO CONSIDER

An important reflection on injury research is that we should caution against assuming that research findings from one study that took place with a given population, in a given context, or even within a given country or culture can automatically be translated into other areas (Carapinheira et al., 2018). This is important as, irrespective of which of the 5Rs of injury we refer to, we currently have a body of research with an under-representation of child and youth athletes, female athletes, parental perspectives, and research that understands dyadic (and beyond) relationships (Forsdyke et al., 2016; Gledhill et al., 2018; Johnson & Ivarsson, 2018). Moreover, a significant proportion of our understanding is based on athletes who have suffered Anterior Cruciate Ligament ruptures and/or surgical repair and is generally drawn from Europe and North America

(Forsdyke et al., 2016). Consequently, broadening our research populations to produce more contextually and culturally sensitive findings that can be used to inform practice will be an important step. These recommendations are especially important in child, adolescent and female athletes, given their significant vulnerability throughout different stages of the injury (e.g. increased injury risk, poorer rehabilitation outcomes; e.g. Forsdyke et al., 2016; Johnson & Ivarsson, 2018).

METHODOLOGICAL CONSIDERATIONS

As with all research, this body is not devoid of limitations. Naturally, your world view on what constitutes science and research will influence how relevant you perceive these methodological considerations to be (e.g. Gledhill, 2020b), but they are considerations nonetheless.

First, the research within this body of knowledge has been reported as having an overall moderate risk of reporting bias and some reported issues with methodological rigour (e.g. Forsdyke et al., 2016; Gledhill et al., 2018). Notwithstanding the aforementioned injury, gender and age biases we alluded to earlier, the area would also benefit from greater consideration of replication research in more emerging areas, greater consideration of sample size calculations and statistical power (Gledhill et al., 2018). In medical environments, decisions regarding health intervention adoption are informed by the veracity of the research trials that underpin investigations of efficacy and effectiveness. Perhaps increasing the confidence in our body of research, by reducing the risk of bias created by some of these methodological considerations, is one way that we might be able to increase the chances of translating research into practice. Further to this, the body of research is also, but for a few exceptions, largely dependent on retrospective, cross-sectional designs. This oft-single time point data collection suggests that the underlying psychological processes influencing injury rehabilitation happen almost instantaneously, as opposed to recognizing their changes and influence over time. Conducting more longitudinal (potentially mixed-methods) research, with multi-wave data collection that offers a lifespan perspective on the injury journey, is likely to advance the area further (Johnson et al., 2020).

TIME TO CLOSE THE BOOK

One of the unfortunate realities of sport is that athletes will get injured; that's just the way it is. Collectively, though, we (and by "we", we mean everybody surrounding the athlete with the athlete at the centre of our work) have a collective responsibility to reduce injury burden wherever we can and, where we can't, help athletes to navigate the choppy waters that are injury experiences. We know that there are ways in which we can help athletes take more control of their experiences, reappraise and redefine their experiences, reduce pain and plan for the worst in injury scenarios whilst highlighting the best in the same. Hopefully, this book has informed and developed your interest and understanding in how we can support our athletes to be happier, healthier and more productive, even in the most severe of injury circumstances. These are our collective responsibilities, after all.

References

Appaneal, R., & Perna, F. (2014). Biopsychosocial model of injury. In R. Eklund & G. Tenenbaum (Eds.), *Encyclopedia of sport and exercise psychology* (pp. 74–76). Sage Publications, Inc.

Ardern, C. L., Glasgow, P., Schneiders, A., Witvrouw, E., Clarsen, B., Cools, A., Gojanovic, B., Griffin, S., Khan K. M., Moksnes, H., Mutch, S. A., Phillips, N., Reurink, G., Sadler, R., Silbernagel, K. G., Thorborg, K., Wangensteen, A., Wilk, K. E., & Bizzini, M. (2016). 2016 Consensus statement on return to sport from the First World Congress in Sports Physical Therapy, Bern. *British Journal of Sports Medicine, 50*, 853–864.

Carapinheira, A., Mendes, P., Guedes Carvalho, P., Torregrossa, M., & Travassos, B. (2018). Career termination of Portuguese elite Football players: Comparison between the last three decades. *Sports, 6*, 155. https://doi.org/10.3390/sports6040155.

Ekstrand, J., Lundqvist, D., Davison, M., D'Hooghe, M., & Pensgaard, A-M. (2019). Communication quality between the medical team and the head coach/manager is associated with injury burden and player availability in elite football clubs. *British Journal of Sports Medicine, 53*, 304–308.

Forsdyke, D., Smith, A., Jones, M., & Gledhill, A. (2016). Psychosocial factors associated with outcomes of sports injury rehabilitation in competitive athletes: A mixed studies systematic review. *British Journal of Sports Medicine, 50*, 537–544.

Gledhill, A. (2020a). The final word with Dr Adam Gledhill, FBASES. *The Sport and Exercise Scientist, 64*, 31.

Gledhill, A. (2020b). Letter to the editor. *The Sport and Exercise Scientist, 65*, 5.

Gledhill, A., & Forsdyke, D. (2015, June). Rehabilitating the athlete, not just the injury. Invited International webinar for the British Association of Sport and Exercise Sciences and Human Kinetics. Available from: https://www.youtube.com/watch?v=p89x1_9s9fI.

Gledhill, A., Forsdyke, D., & Murray, E. (2018). Psychological interventions used to reduce sports injuries: A systematic review of effectiveness. *British Journal of Sports Medicine, 52*, 967–971.

Gledhill, A., & Ivarsson, A. (2020). Do you currently do everything to reduce sports injury risk? Making a case for psychological intervention. *The Sport and Exercise Scientist, 65*, 8–9.

Ivarsson, A., Johnson, U., Andersen, M. B., Tranaeus, U., Stenling, A., & Lindwall, M. (2017). Psychosocial factors and sports injuries: Meta-analyses for prediction and prevention. *Sports Medicine, 47*, 353–365.

Johnson, U., & Ivarsson, A. (2018). Managing injuries among young athletes. In C. J. Knight, C. G. Harwood, & D. Gould (Eds.), *Sport psychology for young athletes* (pp. 174–184). Routlege.

Johnson, U., Ivarsson, A., & Andersen, M. B. (2020). Afterword: Where are we and where may we be headed? In A. Ivarsson, & U. Johnson (Eds.), *Psychological bases of sports injuries* (4th ed.; pp. 311–316).

Pensgaard, A-M., Ivarsson, A., Nilstad, A., Solstad, B. E., & Steffen, K. (2018). Psychosocial stress factors, including the relationship with the coach, and their influence on acute and overuse injury risk in elite female football players. *BMJ Open Sport and Exercise Medicine, 4*.

Richardson, S. O., Andersen, M. B., & Morris, M. (2008). Overtraining athletes: Personal journeys in sport. *Human Kinetics*.

Tranaeus, U., Johnson, U., Engström, B., Skillgate, E., & Werner, S. (2014). Psychological antecedents of overuse injuries among Swedish elite floorball players. *Athletic Insight*, *6*(2), 155–172.

Wiese-Bjornstal, D. (2010). Psychology and socioculture affect injury risk, response, and recovery in high-intensity athletes: A consensus statement. *Scandinavian Journal of Science and Medicine in Sports*, *20*, 103–111.

INDEX

Page references in *italics* refer to figure and those in **bold** indicate table

activity-based rehabilitation (ABR) programme 198
acute injuries 7
Ahman, S. 182
amygdala activation, down-regulate 21
Andersen, M.B. 4–6, 20
Ang, K. 119
anterior cruciate ligament (ACL) injuries: adapted biopsychosocial model **165**; case study, 173–174; future return: prediction, 169–171; psychological response, and, 171–172; quality of life 173; locus of control 166; psychological aspect: impact of 163; reconstruction surgery after, psychological factors (*see* reconstruction surgery after ACL injuries); self-efficacy 165; theoretical model of return to sport after, 164–166
Anterior Cruciate Ligament Return to Sport after Injury (ACL-RSI) scale 168
anxiety 66; levels 22
Appaneal, R.N. 42
Ardern, C.L. 143, 168
Arvinen-Barrow, M. 42
athlete-centred therapeutic alliance 112
athletes, psychological programmes, use: barriers 23; evidence 23; implementation 23; other preventive techniques, and 23
athletic identity 6; following SCI 195–196; higher levels of RA 98; home cryotherapy completion and 100; home exercise completion and 100; loss of 77; lower optimism and 39; positive psychological adjustment and 197; psychological response 163; PTSD 66; self-motivation and 98; situational factors and 39
attempt at expedited rehabilitation (AER) 96

balance board training 16
Baltzell, A. 127
Bateman, A. 39
Beischer, S. 42
Bejar, M.P. 43, 49
biopsychological sport injury risk profile 4–5
Biopsychosocial Model of Athletic Injury and Health 1, 65, 203
Biopsychosocial Model of Sport Injury Rehabilitation 4, 140
Bittencourt, N.F.N. 8
Bramwell, S.T. 9
Brewer, B.W., 39, 98
Brinkman-Majewski, R.E. 49–50
Brown, C. 156
buffering effect 4
Busanich, R. 45
Butryn, T.M. 43

Carson, F. 40
Cassidy, C.M. 42
Castaldelli-Maia, J.M. 68
Cavallerio, F. 43
Chamari, K. 43
Chan, C.W.L. 195
Clement, D. 10, 49
clinic-based rehabilitation 98
coach: injury risk in sport, and: and -athlete interactions 203; case study 207; education and 204; injury rehabilitation and return, role in 204; injury rehabilitation environment and, 205–206; return-to-sport decision-making and 206; role in, 202–203; social support and injury rehabilitation 205; and -support team interactions, 203–204
coach–athlete relationships 8
Codonhato, R. 40
Cognitive Behavioural Techniques 69–70
Concussion in Sport Group (CISG) 181–182
confidence: ability to perform rehabilitation exercises 99; anxiety 142; in athletes returning to sport 166, 168–169; emotions and 168; injured body part 66; injury experience 91; injury-related 65, 144; knee 172–173; knowledge and prior experiences 82; loss of 76; motivation and 40, 141; overuse injuries 211; in performance 142; risk of bias 213; self 20, 98, **118**; training time 130

coping resources 5–7
Covassin, T. 183, 186
Cremades, J.G. 48
Crossman, J. 47
Cumming, J. 120

5-day exercise-induced pain protocol 45–46
Day, M.C. 40
depression and depressive symptoms 65–66
Devantier, C. 7
Doyle, M. 50
Driediger, M.V. 50
dropout reasons, from sport 8
Druckman, J.N. 43
Dugas, L.R. 44

effective/adaptive coping 5–6
Ekstrand, J. 10
Elbin, R.J. 42
Emotional Responses of Athletes to Injury Questionnaire (ERAIQ) 51
Evans, L., 77
'Exercise is Medicine' (EiM): issue with 196; movement 196; restitution 197

facilitators, to improve mental health: evaluation and diagnosis, 68–69; existing study limitations 70; goals 69; treatments/interventions, 69–70. *see also* mental health
fear of re-injury 65, 166–167; ACL 172–173; avoidant behaviour and 130; lower peak knee, hip and trunk flexion 172; psychological readiness 166, 174
Feller, J.A. 168, 171, 172
Fisher, A. 50
Forsdyke, D. 143
frequency, intensity, time (duration) and type (FITT) 34

Gayman, A.M. 47
Gledhill, A. 31, 91
goal setting 65
Goddard, K. 97
Goss, J. 17
Gouttebarge, V. 68

Hammer, C. 81, 82
Hewett, T.E. 172
Hilliard, R.C. 39
history-of-stressors 4
Hoisington, L. 50
home-based rehabilitation 98
Hsu, C.-J. 65
Hunt, E.R. 40

imagery, in injury rehabilitation 117; benefits 119; psychophysiological, neurobiological and neurocognitive underpinnings for 119; case study, 122–123; practice, in: PETTLEP approach, 119–120; skill 120; script, planning: set of guidelines, 121–122; theories and models **118**
individual differences factors: physical/biological 44; disordered eating 45; ergogenic aids, use of 44; genetics, 45–46; health and recovery status, 44–45; psychological 38; coping style 40; health locus of control 39; mental health 41; mood states 41; motivation 39; pain experience 40; personality 38; psychological skills 40–41; self-perceptions 38–39; sociodemographic: age 42; culture and ethnicity 42–43; gender 42; socioeconomic status 43; sport experience, 43–44
ineffective/maladaptive coping 5–6
Iñigo, M.M. 39
injury-prone athlete 9
Injury-Psychological Readiness to Return to Sport Scale (I-PRRS) 143
injury risk in sport: barriers and facilitators, research findings on 212; Bern Consensus Statement on Return to Sport 212; case study 25; coach: and -athlete interactions 203; education and 204; injury rehabilitation and return, role in 204; injury rehabilitation environment, 205–206; return-to-sport decision-making 206; role in, 202–203; social support and injury rehabilitation 205; and -support team interactions, 203–204; culturally sensitive findings 213; injury burden, responsibility to reduce 213; methodological considerations 213; pre-injury factors, research on 211; psychological intervention studies, reducing for: at-risk athletes 20; biofeedback training 20; characteristics of, 18–19; cluster randomization procedure 20; cognitive behavioural stress management 20; MAC approach, 20–21; randomized controlled trail (RCT) approach 17; relaxation

and breathing exercises 20; stress inoculation training programme 20; stress management 20; stress management training 17; systematic review and meta-analysis 17; psychological programmes, effect of: common factors, 22–23; methodological considerations and implications, 24–25; specific factors, 21–22; reducing, applied recommendations for 10; sport socioculture 212; team environment 212
Integrated Model of Psychological Response to the Sport Injury and Rehabilitation Process 33–34, *35*, 54
internal/personal variables 5
International Olympic Committee Consensus statement on mental health 70
Internet-based support interventions 70
irritability 6
Ivarsson, A. 10, 96, 97

Jayanthi, N.A. 43
Johnson, U. 5, 10, 20
Jowett, G.E. 38

Kabat-Zinn, J. 126
Kerr, G. 9, 17
Kinesiophobia 65, 166, 173
Kolar, E. 10
Kolt, G.S. 20
Kontos, A.P. 41, 42
Kroshus, E. 49
Kuhn, A.W. 187
Kvist, J. 166, 168, 172

Lam, K.C. 36
Landers, D.M. 9
Lasenby-Lessard, J. 43
Levy, A.R. 40, 98, 100
Lewin, K. 36
Lichtenstein, M.B. 42
life event stress 8
Life Experience Survey 9
locus of control 6

Maddison, R. 20
Madrigal, L. 39, 46
Markbreiter, J.G. 36
Martin, T.G. 186
Mayer, J. 50
McArdle, S. 37
McGannon, K.R. 47
McPherson, A.L. 173
mental health: case study, 71–72; facilitators, to improve: evaluation and diagnosis, 68–69; existing study limitations 70; goals 69; treatments/interventions, 69–70; symptoms and disorders, injured athletes in 64; anxiety 66; depression and depressive symptoms, 65–66; help-seeking behaviours, barriers to, 66–67; literacy 67; MHL 67; post-traumatic stress disorder 66; re-injury, fear of 66; sport culture 67; stigma 68; WHO definition 64
mental health literacy (MHL) 64, 67
Milliner, E.K. 65
Milne, M. 41
Minden, H. 9
mindfulness: approaches, sport psychology in 127; case study, 132–133; definition, 126–127; interventions, based, 130–132; interventions, comparison of **128**; literature for, sports injury rehabilitation 129; sports injury risk and rehabilitation: research 130
Mindfulness Acceptance Commitment (MAC) 20–21
Morgan, K.A.D. 39
Morrey, M.A. 164
Morrongiello, B.A. 43
Motivational Enhancement Techniques 69–70
muscle strength 22

Nadarajah, V. 195
Nagelli, C.V. 172
Nippert, A.H. 43, 48
Noh, Y-E. 20
Norlin, T. 48
Nyland, J. 39
Österberg, A. 168

Overbye, M.L. 44
overuse injuries: psychological risk factors for, model of, 5, *5*; factors combinations 6; outcome 6; proneness to 6; psychological risk factors in occurrence of, 7–8

passion for sport 6
Paterno, M.V. 172, 173
Performance Interview Guide (PiNG) 51
Perna, F.M. 7 personal factors: individual differences factors (*see* individual

differences factors); injury: factors 36; history 36; onset and healing status, 37–38; perceived cause 37; type and severity 37. *see also* psychological response to sport injuries
personal growth: case study 85; external/environmental factors 83; injury after, development, and 77; post-traumatic 78; research on, 78–80; terms, researchers employed 78; traumatic 78; intra-individual factors 81; organismic valuing theory 82; strategies for, 83–85; support for, 82–83
personality traits 8
Pluhar, E. 46
Podlog, L. 31, 49, 77, 82
Polman, R.C.J. 40, 99
post-traumatic stress disorder (PTSD) 66
Prapavessis, H. 20
psychoeducation 184
psychological flexibility and inflexibility: sports injury rehabilitation, in 129–130
psychological response to sport injuries: factors influencing 34; personal and situational factors 36; practitioner interview, *52–53*; sport injury and rehabilitation process, integrated model *35*
psychosocial risk factors in sports injury: case study, 11–12; coping resources 7; personality 6; stressors, history of, 6–7
public stigma 68
Puthucheary, Z. 45
Putukian, M. 65

readiness, psychological: associated with 142; case study, 146–147; decisions: elements 143; indicators 145; player-centred interdisciplinary perspective 146; valid and reliable measurement instruments, 143–146, **144**; modifiable and non-modifiable factors 143; multifaceted and multidimensional construct 142; situational factors 143. *see also* returning to sport
Reardon, C.L. 68
reconstruction surgery after ACL injuries: psychological factors: adverse consequence, 172–173; cut-off scores for predicting return **170**; fear of re-injury, 166–167; future return, prediction, 169–171; psychological readiness, 168–169; questionnaires and inventories **168**
Reel, J.J. 37, 45
rehabilitation adherence (RA): athletes and teams, burden 93; case study 102; compliance and, difference 94; enhancing 100; meaning, 93–94; measuring, methods of: athletic training 96; rehabilitation over adherence questionnaire 96; Sports Injury RA Scale (SIRAS), 95–96; psychosocial factors influencing 96; cognitive, 98–99; demographic 100; emotional, 98–99; personal, 97–98; social and contextual, 99–100; scale of rehabilitation non-adherence and impact, 94–95; self-determination theory, 100–101; sports injury 94
Rehabilitation Over Adherence Questionnaire (ROAQ) 96
re-injury anxiety 65–66, 117, 129, 167
relaxation activities 65
research, future directions 10–11
retirement, injury-related, from sport: case study, 157–158; experiences, improving 155; athlete involvement 157; financial planning and insurance 156; post-career, planning for 156; social support 156; staying physically active 157; psychosocial factors: reinjury emotions and cognitions, 153–154; support network, quality of 154; psychosocial impact of 154; life stressors 155
returning to sport: criteria testing 172; elements 140; evidences 140; performance outcomes 140; readiness to 140; holistic approach 141; physical and psychological, 141–142; quadrants of **141**
Rice, S. 41
Rogers, T.M. 9
Root, B.C. 48
Rothschild, J.E. 43
Roy-Davis, K. 81, 83
Rubio, V.J. 78
Ruddock-Hudson, M. 38
Russell, H.C. 37

Salim, J. 84
Sandel, N. 185
Schneider, S. 50
scholarship 48
SDT-based communication skills training (CONNECT) 101

self-determination theory 49–50
self-motivation 97–98
self-stigma 68
self-talk 65
Shannon, V.R. 49
situational factors: case study, 53–54; environmental: rehabilitation 50; sport ethic/philosophy, 50–51; social 48; coach influences 49; family dynamics 49; sports medicine team influences, 49–50; teammate influences, 48; sport 46; injury, timing of 47; level of competition 46–47; playing status, 47; scholarship status 48; type 46. *see also* psychological response to sport injuries
Smith, A.M. 37, 65 Social and Athletic Readjustment Rating Scale (SARRS): scores 9
social support 107; case study, 113; contextual factors 108; enhance, 111–112; injured athletes, help or hinder, 110–111; injured athletes, types of 109; interactions and messages 108; key providers, 109–110; pre-injury relationship, between support provider and athlete 108; sociocultural context 108
socioeconomic status (SES) 41–42, 43
Soligard, T. 44
spinal cord injury (SCI) and sport: case study, 197–198; causes of 193; degree of impairment 193; level of injury 194; neurological condition 193; patterns and occurrence rates 194; physical activity, after, 195–196; promotion, critical approach to, 196–197; review on 194; traumatic SCI, impact of 194; decreased self-esteem 195; depression and anxiety 195
sport injuries: emotional responses 3; implications: impacts 77; issues 76; prominent issues 76; rehabilitation phase, 76–77; sport-injury related growth, items reflecting, **79–80**; prevention programmes: FIFA 11+ program 16; risk factors 3
sport-related musculo-skeletal injury 66
Sports Injury RA Scale (SIRAS) 95–96
sport, sociocultural norm and rules 8
sports-related concussion (SRC): background to, 181–182; case study, 187–188; emotional responses to: frustration and anxiety 183; loss of identity 183; impact of: depression 182; long-term 182; neurodegenerative diseases 182; oft-quoted statistic 182; post-traumatic stress disorder, 182–183; management of, 186–187; media, effect of, 185–186; psychosocial interventions for, 184–185; social relationships and 184
state anxiety 6
Stein, C. 37
stigma 68
stress and athletic injury, model 4
injury relationship 6
susceptibility 6
suicide causes 66
Summers, J. 127
support-based interventions 70
Swanik, C.B. 6

Tagesson, S. 172
Tampa Scale of Kinesiophobia (TSK) 65, 172
Taylor, N.F. 168
trait anxiety 6
trauma-related symptoms 66
Trigsted, S.M. 172

Van Der Does, H. 45

Wadey, R. 38, 78, 84
Walker, N. 167
warm-up programmes 16
Wasserman, E.B. 184
Webster, K.E. 168, 171, 172
Weiss, W.M. 39, 50
Whatman, C. 50
Whitaker, L. 44
Whitehead, T.S. 168
Wiese-Bjornstal, D.M. 4, 8, 16, 36, 37, 39, 40, 41, 184
Wilkerson, J.M. 6
Williams, J.M. 4–6
Williams, S.E. 121
Willingness to Compete Hurt (WCH) 51

Yang, J. 9
youth sport, psychological risk factors and sports injury 8–9

For Product Safety Concerns and Information please contact our EU representative GPSR@taylorandfrancis.com
Taylor & Francis Verlag GmbH, Kaufingerstraße 24, 80331 München, Germany

www.ingramcontent.com/pod-product-compliance
Lightning Source LLC
LaVergne TN
LVHW021125300926
849160LV00010B/872